AF593559

Vascular Access for Hemodialysis—VII

Vascular Access for Hemodialysis—VII

MITCHELL L. HENRY, M.D.

W.L. Gore & Associates, Inc.
Precept Press

Library of Congress Cataloging-in-Publication Data
Vascular access for hemodialysis—VII / [edited by] Mitchell L. Henry.
p. ; cm.
Includes index.
ISBN 0-944496-67-9
1. Hemodialysis. 2. Arterial catheterization. 3. Arteriovenous shunts, Surgical.
[DNLM: 1. Renal Dialysis—methods. 2. Arteriovenous Shunt, Surgical. 3. Graft Occlusion, Vascular. 4. Kidney Failure, Chronic—therapy. 5. Vascular Surgical Procedures—methods. WJ 378 V33091 2001] I. Title: Vascular access for hemodialysis—7. II. Title: Vascular access for hemodialysis, seven. III. Henry, Mitchell L.
RC901.7.H45 V374 2001
617.4'61059--dc21

2001001487

05 04 03 02 01 5 4 3 2 1

Printed in the United States of America

CONTENTS

PREFACE

This is the seventh book reflecting the presentations and discussion of a wide variety of topics relating to vascular access for hemodialysis. Like the previous six, the motivations of the individuals who participated in Vascular Access for Hemodialysis-VII are diverse, but all share the common goal of optimizing the care of the dialysis patient. A great deal of information was presented in this meeting, which lasted a day and a half and was devoted to issues associated with dialysis access. The papers included in this book are intended to serve as a written account on the proceedings for future reference or refreshment of fact. The general discussions following the presentations are equally, if not more, beneficial. I believe these contributions by the many authors are a valuable source of information for the diverse topics relating to dialysis access, and I hope they will be used to improve the delivery of care to those with end-stage renal disease.

MITCHELL L. HENRY, M.D.

ACKNOWLEDGMENTS

Acknowledgements may occasionally be felt to be a perfunctory exercise. However, I would like to emphasize that my intent here is sincere. This meeting and the subsequent book took a great deal of effort by many individuals, and each person was important. Dr. Skip Campbell was a guest co-host of the meeting and his participation was invaluable. W.L. Gore invested substantial resources into this meeting, as well as past meetings, and their efforts are greatly appreciated. Don Lass, Ron Hron, Susan Boothe, and Marty Sylvain are some of those people who have aggressively supported this project from Gore. Laura Mouk, Cami Ackerman, and Sheila Zirkle of the Ohio State University, Columbus, devoted much energy in the organization of both the meeting and the book. Access Medical Group, Ltd. took care of the tiniest details and allowed the meeting and other arrangements to proceed smoothly. Sincere thanks go to all of those involved, and we look forward to May of 2002 for the production of *Vascular Access for Hemodialysis—VIII.*

ABOUT THE EDITOR

Mitchell L. Henry, M.D. is the clinical director of transplantation at Ohio State University Medical Center, Columbus, and professor in the Departments of Surgery and Veterinary Clinical Science. He has been a staff member of the university's Division of Transplantation since 1985. Dr. Henry's other professional appointments include associate attending surgeon at the James Cancer Hospital and Research Institute, Columbus; associate medical director and executive board member of Lifeline of Ohio Organ Procurement; and associate attending surgeon, Children's Hospital, Columbus.

Dr. Henry's medical degree is from the University of Nebraska, Omaha, where he graduated with high distinction in 1979. His internship and residency in surgery were at The Ohio State University Hospitals. He is a diplomate of the National Board of Examiners and the American Board of Surgery, a Fellow of the American College of Surgeons, and a founding member of the International Association for Pancreas and Islet Transplantation.

In addition to his role as one of the originators of a series of biannual conferences on vascular access for hemodialysis begun in 1988, Dr. Henry has served as co-editor of the books based on the meetings and is editor of this seventh of the series. He has published widely in medical specialty journals, authoring or co-authoring more than 150 articles, has contributed chapters to 20 books on vascular access and organ transplantation, and has presented papers at many conferences on this and related fields both here and abroad.

CONTRIBUTORS

Marwan S. Abouljoud, M.D., *Division of Transplantation, Henry Ford Hospital, Detroit, Michigan*

Diana J. Adams, R.H.I.A., *Medical City Dallas Hospital, Dallas, Texas*

Gregg A. Adams, M.D., *Santa Clara Medical Center, San Jose, California*

Michael Allon, M.D., *Department of Nephrology, The University of Alabama at Birmingham, Birmingham, Alabama*

Petros V. Anagnostopoulos, M.D., *Division of Transplantation, Henry Ford Hospital, Detroit, Michigan*

Aamer Ar'Rajab, M.D., Ph.D., *Department of Surgery, Division of Transplantation, Ohio State University Medical Center, Columbus, Ohio*

Gary W. Barone, M.D., *Department of Surgery, University of Arkansas for Medical Sciences, Little Rock, Arkansas*

Carolyn G. Birk, B.G.S., *Interventional Nephrology Section, Division of Nephrology and Hypertension, Department of Medicine, Louisiana State University Health Sciences Center, Shreveport, Louisiana*

David Buck, M.D., *Department of Interventional Radiology, Washington Hospital Center, Washington, D.C.*

Kent Bodily, M.D., *Department of Clinical Surgery, Oregon Health Sciences University, Portland, Oregon*

Pierre Bourquelot, M.D., *Department of Angio-Access Surgery, Centre Chirurgical Jouvenet, Paris, France*

Lisa C. Brown, R.N., *Department of Interventional Radiology, Washington Hospital Center, Washington, D.C.*

Francisco Cigarroa, M.D., *Department of Surgery, University of Texas Health Science Center at San Antonio, San Antonio, Texas*

Alexander W. Clowes, M.D., *Division of Veterans Affairs Puget Sound Health Care System, Department of Surgery, University of Washington, Seattle, Washington*

John K. Connolly, F.R.C.S.I., *Departments of Transplantation and Vascular Surgery, Belfast City Hospital, Northern Ireland*

Alan S. Coulson, M.D., Ph.D., *Department of Cardiovascular and Thoracic Surgery, Dameron Hospital Heart Institute, Stockton, California*

Ruben Dammers, M.Sc., *Department of Surgery, University Hospital Maastricht, Maastricht, the Netherlands*

Ingemar J. A. Davidson, M.D., Ph.D., F.A.C.S., *Division of Renal and Pancreas Transplantation, Medical City Dallas Hospital, Dallas, Texas*

Maurits de Brauw, M.D., Ph.D., *Department of Surgery, University Hospital Maastricht, Maastricht, the Netherlands*

Mark H. Deierhoi, M.D., *Department of Transplantation Surgery, The University of Alabama at Birmingham, Birmingham, Alabama*

Peter Dejanov, M.D., *Department of Nephrology, University of St. Kiril and Metodij, Skopje, Republic of Macedonia*

James W. Dennis, M.D., F.A.C.S., *Department of Surgery, Division of Vascular Surgery, University of Florida Health Sciences Center, Jacksonville, Florida*

Dale Distant, M.D., *Division of Transplantation, Department of Surgery, State University of New York Health Science Center at Brooklyn, Brooklyn, New York*

Paul Eggers, Ph.D., *Division of Kidney, Urology and Hematology, National Institute of Diabetes and Digestive and Kidney Diseases, Bethesda, Maryland*

Francisco S. Escobar III, M.D., *Division of Transplantation, Henry Ford Hospital, Detroit, Michigan*

Robert Esterl, Jr., M.D., *Department of Surgery, University of Texas Health Science Center at San Antonio, San Antonio, Texas*

Amanuel Fessahaye, M.D., *Department of Interventional Radiology, Washington Hospital Center, Washington, D.C.*

Michael H. Gallichio, M.D., *Department of Transplantation Surgery, The University of Alabama at Birmingham, Birmingham, Alabama*

Vesna Gerasimovska, M.D., *Department of Nephrology, University of St. Kiril and Metodij, Skopje, Republic of Macedonia*

Marc Glickman, M.D., *Department of Clinical Surgery, Oregon Health Sciences University, Portland, Oregon*

Rosario Gracia-Pajares, M.D., *Department of Vascular Access, Universitario Gregorio Marañón, Madrid, Spain*

Richard J. Gray, M.D., *Department of Interventional Radiology, Washington Hospital Center, Washington, D.C.*

Atul K. Gupta, M.D., *Department of Interventional Radiology, Washington Hospital Center, Washington, D.C.*

Glenn Halff, M.D., *Department of Surgery, University of Texas Health Science Center at San Antonio, San Antonio, Texas*

David R. Hasenstab, Ph.D., *Department of Veterans Affairs Puget Sound Health Care System, Seattle, Washington*

Jeffrey A. Hertz, M.D., *Department of Surgery, Division of Vascular Surgery, University of Florida Health Sciences Center, Jacksonville, Florida*

Toshiyuki Hiranaka, M.D., *Department of Surgery, Shirasagi Hospital, Osaka, Japan*

Joon H. Hong, M.D., *Division of Transplantation, Department of Surgery, State University of New York Health Science Center at Brooklyn, Brooklyn, New York*

Todd K. Howard, M.D., *Department of Surgery, Washington University in St. Louis School of Medicine, St. Louis, Missouri*

Kathleen A. Jablonski, Ph.D., *Department of Interventional Radiology, Washington Hospital Center, Washington, D.C.*

Beverley L. Ketel, M.D., *Department of Surgery, University of Arkansas for Medical Sciences, Little Rock, Arkansas*

Thomas R. Kirkman, B.A., *Division of Veterans Affairs Puget Sound Health Care System, Seattle, Washington*

Ted R. Kohler, M.D., *Division of Veterans Affairs Puget Sound Health Care System, Department of Surgery, University of Washington, Seattle, Washington*

Ulf Kruger, M.D., *Department of Vascular Surgery, Queen-Elizabeth-Hospital, Berlin, Germany*

Miltos K. Lazarides, M.D., *Division of Vascular Surgery, Democritus University of Thrace Medical School; Alexandroupolis University Hospital, Alexandropoulis, Greece*

Abraham Levitin, M.D., *Department of Interventional Radiology, Washington Hospital Center, Washington, D.C.*

Meredith L. Lightfoot, M.D., *Department of Surgery, University of Arkansas for Medical Sciences, Little Rock, Arkansas*

Jill Lindberg, M.D., *Department of Clinical Surgery, Oregon Health Sciences University, Portland, Oregon*

Jeffrey A. Lowell, M.D., *Department of Surgery, Washington University in St. Louis School of Medicine, St. Louis, Missouri*

Keelee J. MacPhee, M.D., *Department of Surgery, Division of Vascular Surgery, University of Florida Health Sciences Center, Jacksonville, Florida*

Chrisostomos Maltezos, M.D., *Division of Vascular Surgery, Democritus University of Thrace Medical School; Alexandroupolis University Hospital, Alexandropoulis, Greece*

Richard L. McCann, M.D., *Department of Surgery, Duke University Medical Center, Durham, North Carolina*

Cruz Menárguez, M.D., *Department of Vascular Access, Universitario Gregorio Marañón, Madrid, Spain*

William D. Middleton, M.D., *Department of Radiology, Washington University in St. Louis School of Medicine, St. Louis, Missouri*

Roger Milam, M.S., *Office of Strategic Planning, Health Care Financing Administration, Baltimore, Maryland*

David E. Morris, M.D., *Division of Transplantation, Henry Ford Hospital, Detroit, Michigan*

Carolyn E. Munschauer, B.A., *Medical City Dallas Hospital, Dallas, Texas*

David D. Oakes, M.D., F.A.C.S., *Department of Surgery, Stanford University School of Medicine, Stanford, California; Santa Clara Medical Center, San Jose, California*

Mark Odland, M.D., *Department of Clinical Surgery, Oregon Health Sciences University, Portland, Oregon*

Angel Oncevski, M.D., *Department of Nephrology, University of St. Kiril and Metodij, Skopje, Republic of Macedonia*

William D. Paulson, M.D., *Interventional Nephrology Section, Division of Nephrology and Hypertension, Department of Medicine, Louisiana State University Health Sciences Center, Shreveport, Louisiana*

Arun D. Pherwani, M.S., D.N.B., F.R.C.S., *Departments of Transplantation and Vascular Surgery, Belfast City Hospital, Belfast, Northern Ireland*

Michael Petzold, M.D., *Department of Vascular Surgery, Queen-Elizabeth-Hospital, Berlin, Germany*

Karen Petzold, M.D., *Department of Vascular Surgery, Queen-Elizabeth-Hospital, Berlin, Germany*

Iraklis I. Pipinos, M.D., *Division of Transplantation, Henry Ford Hospital, Detroit, Michigan*

Jorge Polo, M.D., *Department of Vascular Access, Universitario Gregorio Marañón, Madrid, Spain*

José R. Polo, M.D., *Department of Vascular Access, Universitario Gregorio Marañón, Madrid, Spain*

Timothy Lane Pruett, M.D., *Department of Surgery, University of Virginia Health System, Charlottesville, Virginia*

John Raheb, D.O., *Department of Surgery, University of Texas Health Science Center at San Antonio, San Antonio, Texas*

Sunanda J. Ram, Ph.D., *Interventional Nephrology Section, Division of Nephrology and Hypertension, Department of Medicine, Louisiana State University Health Sciences Center, Shreveport, Louisiana*

Venkataraman Ramachandran, M.D., *Department of Surgery, Washington University in St. Louis School of Medicine, St. Louis, Missouri*

Julie A. Reid, M.R.C.S., *Departments of Transplantation and Vascular Surgery, Belfast City Hospital, Belfast, Northern Ireland*

Michelle Robbin, M.D., *Department of Radiology, The University of Alabama at Birmingham, Birmingham, Alabama*

John R. Ross, M.D., *Department of Surgery, Bamberg Hospital, Bamberg, South Carolina*

Hans Scholz, M.D., *Department of Vascular Surgery, Queen-Elizabeth-Hospital, Berlin, Germany*

Earl S. Schuman, M.D., *Department of Clinical Surgery, Oregon Health Sciences University, Portland, Oregon*

Mary Jo Shaver, M.D., *Department of Medicine, University of Arkansas for Medical Sciences, Little Rock, Arkansas*

Surendra Shenoy, M.D., Ph.D., *Section of Transplantation, Division of Surgery, Washington University in St. Louis School of Medicine, St. Louis, Missouri*

John P. Sherck, M.D., F.A.C.S., *Santa Clara Medical Center, San Jose, California*

Bruce Sommer, M.D., *Division of Transplantation, Department of Surgery, State University of New York Health Science Center at Brooklyn, Brooklyn, New York*

Yvonne H. Sparling, M.S., *Department of Interventional Radiology, Washington Hospital Center, Washington, D.C.*

Demetrios N. Staramos, M.D., *Division of Vascular Surgery, Democritus University of Thrace Medical School; Alexandroupolis University Hospital, Alexandropoulis, Greece*

Nabil Sumrani, M.D., *Division of Transplantation, Department of Surgery, State University of New York Health Science Center at Brooklyn, Brooklyn, New York*

Jan H. M. Tordoir, M.D., Ph.D., *Department of Surgery, University Hospital Maastricht, Maastricht, the Netherlands*

Luc Turmel-Rodrigues, M.D., *Department of Vascular Radiology, Clinique Saint-Gatien, Tours, France*

Vasilios D. Tzilalis, M.D., *Division of Vascular Surgery, Democritus University of Thrace Medical School; Alexandroupolis University Hospital, Alexandropoulis, Greece*

Nirmal K. Veeramachaneni, M.D., *Department of Surgery, Washington University in St. Louis School of Medicine, St. Louis, Missouri*

Henry C. Veldenz, M.D., F.A.C.S., *Department of Surgery, Division of Vascular Surgery, University of Florida Health Sciences Center, Jacksonville, Florida*

Thomas Vesely, M.D., *Department of Radiology, Washington University in St. Louis School of Medicine, St. Louis, Missouri*

William Washburn, M.D., *Department of Surgery, University of Texas Health Science Center at San Antonio, San Antonio, Texas*

Kerri A. Welch, R.N., C.N.N., *Vascular Access Coordinator, RenalCare Associates, S.C., Peoria, Illinois*

David W. Windus, M.D., *Department of Internal Medicine, Washington University in St. Louis School of Medicine, St. Louis, Missouri*

Jack Work, M.D., *Interventional Nephrology Section, Division of Nephrology and Hypertension, Department of Medicine, Louisiana State University Health Sciences Center, Shreveport, Louisiana*

Carlton J. Young, M.D., *Department of Transplantation Surgery, The University of Alabama at Birmingham, Birmingham, Alabama*

Jurgen Zanow, M.D., *Department of Vascular Surgery, Queen-Elizabeth-Hospital, Berlin, Germany*

SECTION I

1

INTIMAL HYPERPLASIA

Ted R. Kohler, M.D., Thomas R. Kirkman, B.A., David Hasenstab, Ph.D., and Alexander W. Clowes, M.D.

The vast majority (80%) of polytetrafluoroethylene (PTFE) access failure is caused by stenosis at the venous end of the graft.[1] The lumen is encroached upon by a lesion composed of smooth muscle cells and their matrix (collagen and proteoglycans). Similar lesions form at the distal end of grafts placed in arterial circulation, but they are much less common and slower to develop.[2]

Several differences between arteriovenous grafts (AVGs) and artery-to-artery grafts can help to explain this disparity. The most obvious difference is the extremely high fistula flow in AVGs and the resulting wall vibration, which is palpable as a thrill. This may directly injure the wall. Also, high flow may increase platelet accumulation on the injured vessel.[3,4] The resulting thrombus contributes to intimal hyperplasia due to the release of growth factors from activated platelets and generation of thrombin and other clotting factors that are mitogenic.[5,6] Thin-walled recipient vessels, distal vessel bathing with activated platelets (and their products) during dialysis, abnormal plasma factors present in uremia, and graft puncture are additional problems associated with arterial graft use. The end result of intimal hyperplasia following injury is similar in both access grafts and arteries. Detailed animal models of the cellular and molecular events leading to wall thickening can help us to better understand dialysis access failure in humans.

Animal models of intimal hyperplasia. Intimal hyperplasia is a response to injury by smooth muscles cells, which migrate to the site of injury (usually crossing the internal elastic lamina into the intima), proliferate, and deposit matrix. Thrombi that accumulate at the site of injury also contribute to lesion formation by providing a fibrin scaffolding that is invaded and organized by inflammatory cells and smooth muscle cells, resulting in lesions similar to those of the primary injury. The smooth muscle response to injury has been studied extensively in a rat model.[7] In this model, 3 passes of a balloon catheter through the common carotid artery cause denudation and wall injury with loss of about 20% of medial smooth muscle cells. The injured surface is almost immediately coated with a thin layer of activated platelets, which release platelet-derived growth factors (PDGF) and other cytokines. Thrombosis is limited, with very little fibrin formation and almost no thrombus after 24 hours, due to the passiveness of the surface caused by adsorbed plasma proteins. Early thrombosis is related to a rapid but transient induction of tissue factor. Tissue factor reaches maximum levels 2 hours after injury, declines significantly by 24 hours, and is back to baseline after 3 days.[8]

Within 1 to 2 days, about 40% of smooth muscle cells leave their quiescent state and enter the cell cycle, modulating from the contractile phenotype (rich in actin) to the synthetic phenotype (with prominent rough endoplasmic reticulum and Golgi apparatus). These cells are then able to break down attachments to the matrix, migrate, and produce abundant amounts of elastin and collagen. The primary stimulus for proliferation is probably the release of basic fibroblast growth factor (bFGF) from injured smooth muscle cells. Antibodies that block the action of bFGF can reduce proliferation, while the addition of bFGF to smooth muscle cells enhances proliferation.[9] Heparin given in the first 24 hours after injury reduces intimal hyperplasia by blocking smooth muscle cell migration and proliferation.[10] Cells must detach from the surrounding matrix in order to divide and migrate, and heparin may act by inhibiting the production of metalloproteinases necessary for cell detachment.[11] Migration into the intima is stimulated by PDGF;[12] blocking PDGF activity reduces the amount of neointima that forms without affecting proliferation.[13]

Observations in human access failure. Studies of stenotic lesions from human dialysis fistulae have documented increased smooth muscle cell proliferation.[14] Rekhter et al. have described the histology of stenotic lesions at the venous anastomosis of 7 human PTFE access grafts.[15] Lesions consisted primarily of smooth muscle cells (α-actin positive) but macrophages and lymphocytes were also present, particularly in association with microvessels. High rates of cell proliferation (positive for cell nuclear antigen proliferation) were found in cells in the microvessels (smooth muscle and endothelial cells). Macrophages in this region also displayed a high rate of proliferation. Cell proliferation and angiogenesis may result from the paracrine and autocrine effects of mitogens made by these cells. Hemosiderin was found in the media and adventitia of most specimens, suggesting that thrombosis may be a feature of human lesion formation, as it is in our sheep model (table 1–1).

Possible role of thrombosis in dialysis access graft failure. Some data suggest that antiplatelet therapy can reduce intimal hyperplasia following arterial injury or bypass. Platelet GP IIa/IIIb antagonists have shown lasting benefit by reducing the need for repeat intervention following coronary angioplasty.[16] However, there are no data that demonstrate this therapy actually reduces restenosis. Another

Table 1-1. Tissue Factor and Fibrin in Sheep Dialysis Access Grafts (n=4, P<0.05).

Location	Tissue Factor Activity (±SD)	Tissue Factor Protein	Fibrinin
Normal artery	22.0 (±18.0)	–	–
Graft near artery	113.5 (±10.9)	++	+
Graft near vein	194.5 (±15.2)	+++	+
Normal vein	32.0 (±1.5)	–	–

Tissue factor activity is reported as optical density units, which correspond to the quantity of chromogenic Factor Xa generated during the assay. Results of immunohistochemistry analysis for tissue factor protein and fibrin are qualitative. The number of pluses correspond with the intensity of immunostaining.

antiplatelet agent, ticlopidine, has been shown to improve the long-term (2 year) patency of lower extremity saphenous vein bypass grafts.[17] Previous work revealed that aspirin could improve the short-term patency of coronary bypass grafts, but it did not appear to affect later development of intimal hyperplasia and had no effect on lower extremity bypass grafts. Little work has been done to assess the effect of antiplatelet therapy in dialysis access grafts, even though there was interest initially when AV shunts were first used for dialysis in the 1970s. Sulfinpyrazone was shown to improve patency of these external, silastic devices.[18] While commonly prescribed for patients with dialysis access grafts, clinical evidence for the benefit of low-dose aspirin is lacking. Another approach to reducing thrombosis is to make the PTFE surface less thrombogenic. Hanson et al. treated canine AV PTFE grafts with phosphorylcholine and found a reduction in platelet update, intimal hyperplasia, and smooth muscle cell proliferation.[19] This same group demonstrated that local infusion of heparin reduces intimal hyperplasia in experimental PTFE grafts placed in the arterial circulation.[20] As noted above, heparin's effect may result from inhibition of smooth muscle cell migration rather than from its antithrombotic properties.

Effect of flow on graft failure. Flow patterns at the venous anastomosis are likely to include turbulence, abnormally high shear, and flow separation regions (with vortices and low, oscillating shear). Similar regions of flow separation are associated with atherosclerotic plaque development at the carotid bifurcation.[21] In access grafts, some regions at the venous end may be exposed to exceptionally wide variations in shear throughout the cardiac cycle. Instability of the endothelium, thrombus formation, and production of mitogens by surface endothelial or smooth muscle cells may all be influenced by these patterns.[22] Experimentally, high flow rates are associated with increased platelet thrombus on injured vessels.[3,4] Tissue factor expression is increased in normal veins when they are subjected to arterial flow conditions ex vivo.[23]

Previous work suggests that the proliferation of smooth muscle cells in the neointima of PTFE grafts is under the control of many different growth inhibitors and promoters, several of which have flow-responsive expression that may be different for high, low, and turbulent flows.[24] Shear upregulates transcription of the PDGF B chain gene.[25] Messenger ribonucleic acid for the PDGF A chain has been found in the subendothelial region of neointima in porous PTFE grafts.[26] Smooth muscle cell proliferation is greatest both in experimental grafts and in human lesions of graft and AV fistula stenosis.[14] Flow regulates smooth muscle cell proliferation and neointimal growth in PTFE grafts in primates. Proliferation and rapid growth of the neointima is induced when flow is abruptly reduced, from high fistula flow to normal arterial levels.[27] This growth may result, in part, from an increase in PDGF gene expression and protein,[28] and release of growth inhibition may also play a role. Intima regresses when flow is increased, and expression of nitric oxide, a growth inhibitor, is enhanced.

One of the primary differences between arterial grafts, which tend not to develop severe stenosis, and AV grafts, which develop severe stenosis, is that the distal anastomosis connects to a thin-walled vein rather than an artery. Vein walls are much thinner than arteries and may not be well suited for handling the hemodynamic stress associated with the distal anastomosis of access grafts. Vessel thickness is proportional to pressure and diameter. This relationship maintains wall tension in a narrow, physiologic range. While veins and arteries carry similar flows, arteries have significantly higher intraluminal pressure and, therefore, have thicker walls. Although intraluminal pressure may be decreased to near normal venous levels at this location, high flow causes turbulence and vibration (this can be heard as a bruit on the graft and can be detected by color Doppler duplex scanning). Vibratory energy may cause injury to the vessel wall that contributes to continued smooth muscle cell proliferation.

Fillinger's work on a canine model for dialysis access grafts showed that vessel vibration causes injury that stimulates wall thickening. In this model, the vein wall thickens opposite the venous anastomosis. The degree of thickening correlates with the extent of the bruit (acoustic vibration) around the vessel, as seen on color Doppler scanning. Reducing blood flow by narrowing the arterial inlet, either by banding or use of tapered grafts, results in less vibration and less wall thickening.[29,30] Tapered grafts are now used clinically, but their benefit has not been proven. Other graft configurations, such as creation of a distal hood, have been devised in an attempt to reduce turbulence, vibration, and wall injury at the venous anastomosis. Surface modification (to decrease thrombogenicity), alteration of PTFE structure (to improve healing via nodal architecture and increased internal distance), alteration of graft compliance, use of different materials, impregnation of the graft with agents to improve capillary ingrowth and endothelial coverage, and seeding of grafts with endothelium are all types of graft modifications currently under consideration. Improved graft endothelialization seen with high-porosity PTFE, for example, could result in a more stable graft surface, less thrombosis, and less intimal hyperplasia.

Abnormal fistula flow alone does not produce stenosis. AV fistulae consisting of anastomoses between native arteries and veins, such as the radiocephalic fistula, function better in the long term than do PTFE bridge fistulae. When native fistulae do thrombose, it is usually due to narrowing along the segment of vein that has been repeatedly punctured for dialysis. Stehbens has demonstrated that native artery-to-vein fistulae in sheep function very well for years. His group found ultrastructural changes at the electron microscope level in these fistulae with very little wall thickening.[31,32] This suggests that the interaction of the prosthetic material with the native vessel is an important component of access graft failure. This may be caused by blood interactions with the prosthetic surface, compliance mismatch, or instability of the developing neointima as it grows onto the prosthetic surface.

Effect of uremia on access failure. Because only end-stage clinical lesions are available for pathologic study, fundamental questions regarding development of hyperplasia and the role of renal failure have been unanswered. Graft stenosis may be accelerated by renal failure (uremia). This is suggested by the finding that serum from uremic patients contains factors that stimulate proliferation of smooth muscle cells in vitro[33] and patients who develop stenoses in autogenous access fistulae have lipid abnormalities and increased levels of certain cytokines and plasminogen activator inhibitors.[34]

Materials and Methods

The discovery of hyperplasia inhibition by high flow led us to wonder why venous stenosis is a problem in AV access grafts. We developed a sheep model of dialysis access failure in order to answer this question.[35] Standard PTFE grafts (with normal porosity), the same as those used clinically, were placed from the carotid artery to the jugular vein in the neck. Sheep were chosen because of the well-established sheep model of chronic uremia, which can be used to assess the effects of renal failure on access stenosis, and the coagulation system, which is similar to that of humans.[36-38]

In an effort to determine why thrombus is present in the sheep access grafts, we assayed the graft and adjacent vessel surfaces for tissue factor activity at various points of time. Elevated tissue factor expression may result in increased fibrin deposition (that may provide a provisional matrix for smooth muscle cell migration) and may chronically disturb flow or release platelet factors. We examined sheep grafts for tissue factor expression to see if increased tissue factor expression could be found at the venous anastomosis.

The graft with adjoining artery and vein was removed between 2 and 3 weeks following engraftment. The graft and vessels were flushed and longitudinally opened, then placed in a modified Boyden chamber. We isolated 7 mm^2 regions along the length of the vessel for a tissue factor assay. Factor VIIa and Factor X were added to the chamber, then added to a chromogenic substrate for Factor Xa. Tissue factor activity is reported as OD405 of Factor Xa substrate. Fluorescent-labeled tissue factor ligand was used to localize tissue factor in paraffin embedded sections. Fibrin accumulation was identified by use of immunohistochemistry.

Results

Venous anastomoses developed thick neointima within the PTFE graft by 4 weeks. Lesions at the venous end were significantly thicker than those at the arterial end by 8 weeks and had greater cross-sectional area at both 4 and 8 weeks (figure 1-1), and this pattern persisted in one animal studied at 12 weeks. Seventy-five percent of grafts thrombosed within 3 months. Lesions were composed of smooth muscle cells, matrix, and thrombus of various ages (figure 1-2). Cellular proliferation was prominent in some developing regions of intimal hyperplasia, such as neointima adjacent to thrombus and granulation tissue surrounding the graft (figure

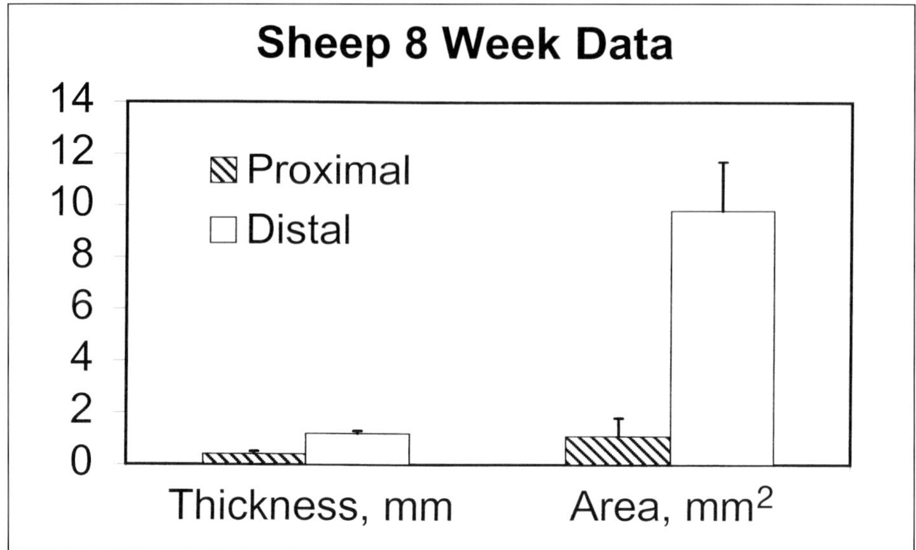

Figure 1-1. Areas and thickness of lesions of intimal hyperplasia at the proximal (arterial) and distal (venous) anastomosis at 4 and 8 weeks in the sheep model.

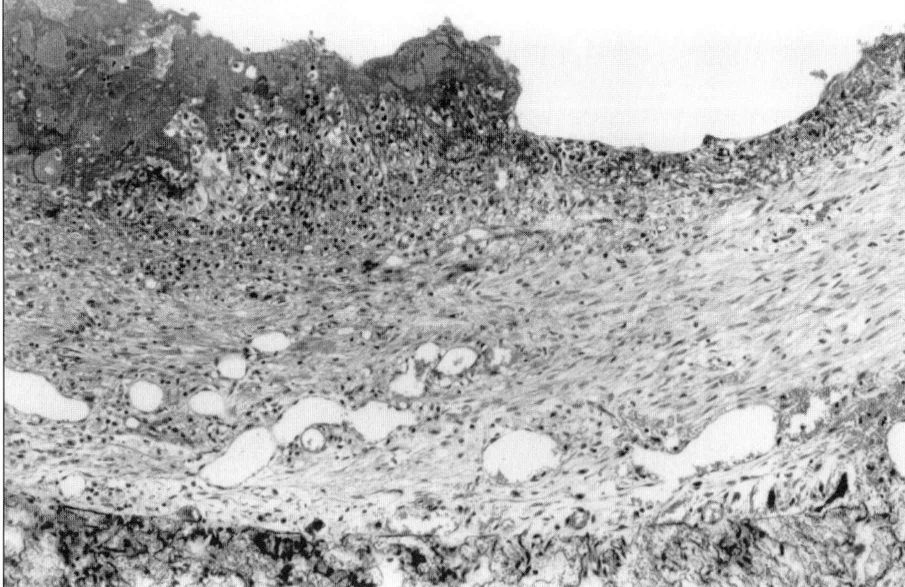

Figure 1-2. Neointimal lesion at the venous end of a 1-month graft demonstrating acute thrombus at the surface, abundant neovascularization is seen at the bottom just above the PTFE graft (hematoxylin-eosin, original magnification X64).

1-3). Organizing thrombus contributed significantly to luminal narrowing. The continued presence of thrombus and high rates of cellular proliferation suggest that ongoing injury is an important cause of lesion formation. Rapid development of lesions morphologically similar to clinical specimens makes this model ideally suited for the study of the cellular mechanisms of dialysis failure.

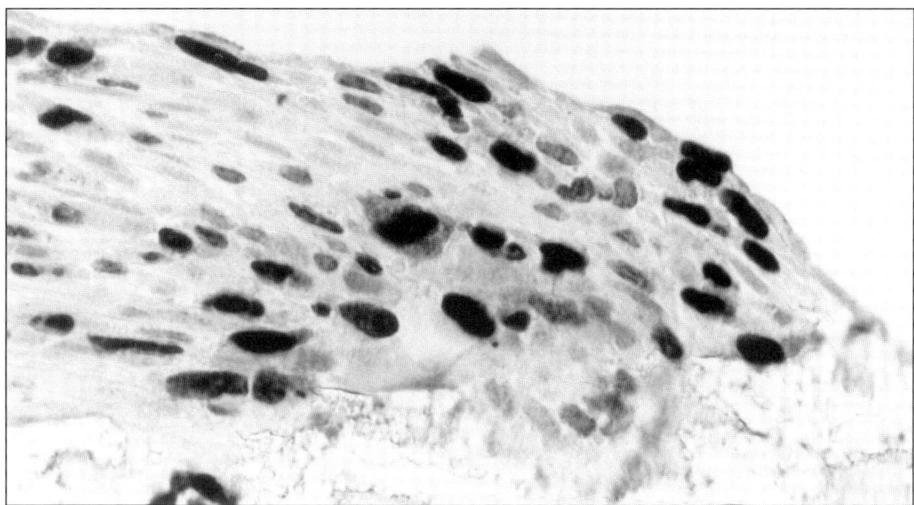

Figure 1-3. Section of neointima near an arterial anastomosis demonstrating frequent cellular proliferation (positive immunoreactivity in the cell nucleus with the antibody Ki-67, original magnification X250).

Tissue factor activity and protein were increased at the venous anastomosis compared with the arterial anastomosis or adjoining vein and artery 3 weeks following graft placement. Increased tissue factor expression colocalized with fibrin deposition (figure 1-4). Two weeks following engraftment, there was a similar increase in tissue factor activity at the venous end of the graft compared with the arterial end (n=3, $P<0.05$, figure 1-5).

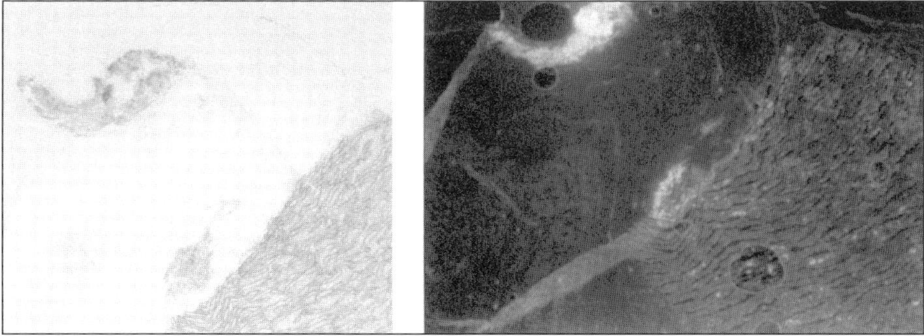

Figure 1-4. Immunohistochemistry showing fibrin (left) and tissue factor (right) localization from adjacent cuts through a section taken from a venous anastomosis. Areas of fibrin accumulation co-localize with tissue factor expression. PTFE is at the lower right (original magnification X20).

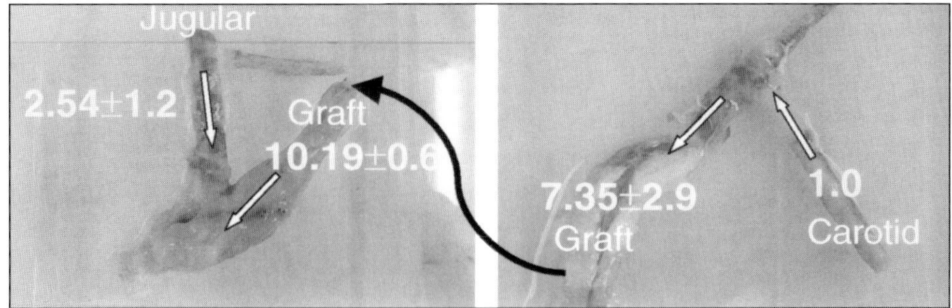

Figure 1-5. Tissue factor activity at 2 weeks following graft placement. Tissue factor activity is expressed as fold increase (±SD above the uninjured carotid artery. Activity levels are displayed for the carotid artery and jugular vein adjacent to the graft and for the proximal and distal ends of the graft. Open arrows indicate direction of blood flow and closed arrow indicates original position of graft prior to dissection.

Discussion

The sheep model of dialysis access failure has been useful in gaining information regarding the development of intimal hyperplasia and the possible methods for controlling it. The advantage of this model is that lesions develop quickly and have cellular characteristics that are very similar to clinical pathology. A prominent component of surface thrombus and a lack of involvement of the adjacent vein are important differences between this model and human stenosis. We have found that intimal hyperplasia at the venous anastomosis in these sheep grafts is associated with increased tissue factor expression and fibrin accumulation. Thrombus at the venous anastomosis may contribute to intimal hyperplasia by stimulating smooth muscle cell migration and inflammatory cell accumulation. Thrombus also serves as a framework for ingrowth of mesenchymal cells, which organize the thrombus into the cellular lesion that characterizes access stenosis. Experiments using antithrombotic agents to locally inhibit tissue factor activity are underway to determine the importance of thrombosis in the development of intimal hyperplasia. Our model can also be used to assess other ways to improve access function through brachytherapy, antiproliferative drugs, mechanical means of reducing flow-induced injury, and modification of the prosthetic material and its surface lining.

References

1. Morbidity and mortality of dialysis. NIH Consens Statement 1993; 11:1-33.
2. Cantelmo NL, Quist WC, Lo Gerfo FW. Quantitative analysis of anastomotic intimal hyperplasia in paired dacron and PTFE grafts. J Cardiovasc Surg (Torino) 1989; 30:910-15.
3. Ouriel K, Donayre C, Shortell CK, et al. The hemodynamics of thrombus formation in arteries. J Vasc Surg 1991; 14:757-62.

4. Mailhac A, Badimon JJ, Fallon JT, et al. Effect of an eccentric severe stenosis on fibrin(ogen) deposition on severely damaged vessel wall in arterial thrombosis. Relative contribution of fibrin(ogen) and platelets. Circulation 1994; 90:988-96.
5. Harker LA, Hanson SR, Runge MS. Thrombin hypothesis of thrombus generation and vascular lesion formation. Am J Cardiol 1995; 75:12B-7B.
6. Ross R, Glomset JA. The pathogenesis of atherosclerosis. N Engl J Med 1976; 295:369-77.
7. Clowes AW, Reid MA, Clowes MM. Mechanisms of stenosis after arterial injury. Lab Invest 1983; 49:208-15.
8. Marmur JD, Rossikhina M, Guha A, et al. Tissue factor is rapidly induced in arterial smooth muscle after balloon injury. J Clin Invest 1993; 91:2253-59.
9. Lindner V, Reidy MA. Proliferation of smooth muscle cells after vascular injury is inhibited by an antibody against basic fibroblast growth factor. Proc Natl Acad Sci USA 1991; 88:3739-43.
10. Clowes AW, Clowes MM. Kinetics of cellular proliferation after arterial injury. Inhibition of smooth muscle growth by heparin. Lab Invest 1985; 52:611-16.
11. Kenagy RD, Nikkari ST, Welgus HG, Clowes AW. Heparin inhibits the induction of three matrix metalloproteinases (stromelysin, 92-KD gelatinase, and collagenase) in primate arterial smooth muscle cells. J Clin Invest 1994; 93:1987-93.
12. Jawien A, Bowen-Pope DF, Lindne V, Schwartz SM, Clowes AW. Platelet-derived growth factor promotes smooth muscle migration and intimal thickening in a rat model of balloon angioplasty. J Clin Invest 1992; 89:507-11.
13. Ferns G, Raines EW, Sprugel KH, Motani AS, Reidy M, Ross R. Inhibition of neointimal smooth muscle accumulation after angioplasty by an antibody to PDGF. Science 1991; 253:1129-32.
14. Hofstra L, Tordoir JH, Kitslaar PJ, Hoek AP, Daemen MJ. Enhanced cellular proliferation in intact stenotic lesions derived from human arteriovenous fistulas and peripheral bypass grafts. Circulation 1996; 94:1283-90.
15. Rekhter MD, Nicholls SC, Ferguson M, Gordon D. Cell proliferation in human arteriovenous fistulas used for hemodialysis. Arterioscler Thromb 1993; 13:609-17.
16. Coller BS, Anderson K, Weisman HF. New antiplatelet agents: Platelet GPIIb/IIIa antagonists. Thromb Haemost 1995; 74:302-08.
17. Schomig A, Neumann FJ, Kastrat A, et al. Randomized comparison of antiplatelet and anticoagulant therapy after the placement of coronary-artery stents. N Engl J Med 1996; 334:1084-89.
18. Kaegi A, Pineo GF, Shimizu A, Trivedi H, Hirsh J, Gent M. Arteriovenous-shunt thrombosis prevention by sulfinpyrazone. N Engl J Med 1974; 290:304-06.
19. Gupta AK, Bandyk DF, Johnson BL. In situ repair of mycotic abdominal aortic aneurysms with rifampin-bonded gelatin-impregnated dacron grafts: A preliminary case report. J Vasc Surg 1996; 24:472-76.
20. Chen C, Lumsden AB, Hanson SR. Local infusion of heparin reduces anastomotic neointimal hyperplasia in aortoiliac expanded polytetrafluoroethylene bypass grafts in baboons. J Vasc Surg 2000; 313:54-63.
21. Zarins CK, Giddens DP, Bharadvaj BK, Sottiurai VS, Mabon RF, Glagov S. Carotid bifurcation atherosclerosis: Quantitative correlation of plaque localization with flow velocity profiles and wall shear stress. Circ Res 1983; 53:502-14.

22. Mattsson E, Kohler T, Vergel S, Liao JK, Clowes AW. Gene expression of nitric oxide synthase increases and intimal hyperplasia regresses with increased blood flow in baboons. J Vasc Res 1996; 33 (Supp 1).
23. Muluk SC, Vorp DA, Severyn DA, Gleixner S, Johnson PC, Webster MW. Enhancement of tissue factor expression by vein segments exposed to coronary arterial hemodynamics. J Vasc Surg 1998; 27:521-27.
24. Topper JN, Cai J, Falb D, Gimbrone MA Jr. Identification of vascular endothelial genes differentially responsive to fluid mechanical stimuli: Cyclooxygenase-2, manganese superoxide dismutase, and endothelial cell nitric oxide synthase are selectively up-regulated by steady laminar shear stress. Proc Natl Acad Sci USA 1996; 93:10417-22.
25. Resnick N, Collins T, Atkinson W, Bonthron DT, Dewey CF Jr, Gimbrone MA Jr. Platelet-derived growth factor B chain promoter contains a cis-acting fluid shear-stress-responsive element. Proc Natl Acad Sci USA 1993; 90:4591-95.
26. Golden MA, Au Y, Kirkman TR, et al. Platelet derived growth factor activity and MRNA expression in healing vascular grafts in baboons. J Clin Invest 1991; 87:406-14.
27. Geary RL, Kohler TR, Vergel S, Kirkman TR, Clowes AW. Time course of flow-induced smooth muscle cell proliferation and intimal thickening in endothelialized baboon vascular grafts. Circ Res 1994; 74:14-23.
28. Kraiss LW, Geary RL, Mattsson EJ, et al. Acute reductions in blood flow and shear stress induce platelet-derived growth factor-A expression in baboon prosthetic grafts. Circ Res 1996; 79:45-53.
29. Fillinger MF, Reinitz ER, Schwartz RA, Resetarits DE, Paskanik AM, Bredenberg CE. Beneficial effects of banding on venous intimal-medial hyperplasia in arteriovenous loop grafts. Am J Surg 1989; 158:87-94.
30. Fillinger MF, Reinitz ER, Schwartz RA, et al. Graft geometry and venous intimal-medial hyperplasia in arteriovenous loop grafts. J Vasc Surg 1990; 11:556-66.
31. Stehbens WE. Blood vessel changes in chronic experimental arteriovenous fistulas. Surg Gynecol Obstet 1968; 127:327-38.
32. Stehbens WE. The ultrastructure of anastomosed vein of experimental arteriovenous fistulae in sheep. Am J Path 1974; 76:377-400.
33. Bagdade JD. Chronic renal failure and atherogenesis-serum factors stimulate the proliferation of human arterial smooth muscle cells. Atherosclerosis 1979; 34:243-48.
34. De Marchi S, Falleti E, Giacomello R, et al. Risk factors for vascular disease and arteriovenous fistula dysfunction in hemodialysis patients. J Am Soc Nephrol 1996; 7:1169-77.
35. Kohler TR, Kirkman TR. Dialysis access failure: A sheep model of rapid stenosis. J Vasc Surg 1999; 30:744-51.
36. Eschbach JW, Adamson JW, Dennis MB. Physiologic studies in normal and uremic sheep: I. The experimental model. Kidney Int 1980; 18:725-31.
37. Mladenovic J, Eschbach JW, Garcia JF, Adamson JW. The anaemia of chronic renal failure in sheep: Studies in vitro. Br J Haematol 1984; 58:491-500.
38. Tillman P, Carson SN, Talke, L. Platelet function and coagulation parameters in sheep during experimental vascular surgery. Lab Anim Sci 1981; 31:263-67.

2

DIAGNOSING THE FAILING VASCULAR ACCESS

Aamer Ar'Rajab M.D., Ph.D., and Mitchell L Henry, M.D.

Arteriovenous graft patency rates have been reported at 60% and 20% for 1 year and 3 years, respectively. Fifteen percent of hospitalizations for patients with end-stage renal disease are caused by vascular access complications, and thrombosis is the main complication for all types of vascular access. Many dialysis patients run out of sites for access, and therefore, measures to improve the longevity of vascular access are needed. Thrombosis and access failure can be prevented through preoperative evaluation when selecting the site and type of access and through surveillance of the access to detect and remove any developing lesions.

Diagnosis Techniques

Access monitoring. The goals of access monitoring are: (1) to ensure ongoing optimal delivery of adequate dialysis; (2) to extend the graft life and to minimize thrombosis; and (3) to predict access failure and consequently to correct a lesion prior to access thrombosis or loss. While rising venous pressure and poor flow characteristics may signal impending graft thrombosis, many such episodes occur without warning. Accurate prediction of imminent graft failure allows elective revision in a great number of patients.

In 153 hemodialysis accesses (56 fistulae and 97 polytetrafluoroethylene [PTFE] grafts), elective access revision prior to thrombosis improved the longevity of the access in both primary fistulae (999 days versus 358 days) and PTFE grafts (1023 days versus 689 days).[1] In addition, early revision prior to thrombosis significantly decreased the number of clotting episodes for primary fistulae (0.5 clots per patient years versus 4.8 clots per patient years) and PTFE grafts (1.1 clots per patient years versus 3.6 clots per patient years).[1] The methods used for access monitoring included:

1) Physical exam
2) Venous pressure monitoring
3) Doppler ultrasound
4) Recirculation studies
5) Intra-access flow

Physical exam. A physical exam is routinely performed at the time of cannulation. It is easy and the patient can be taught to perform a self exam. It uses simple clinical parameters such as needle insertion, a thrill changing to a pulse (venous stenosis), a "full" graft changing to an empty graft (arterial abnormalities), and swelling that results in an aneurysm with collateral formation. The physical exam, however, is a subjective assessment and its value is limited because many grafts thrombose without any clinical warnings.

Venous pressure monitoring. Venous pressure monitoring is based on the premise that as stenosis develops in the venous outflow, the resistance to flow will increase. Increased resistance results in increased pressure in the access proximal to the stenosis. Venous pressure measured from the dialysis machine is a useful screening test for vascular access dysfunction, although it is a crude reflection of intragraft hemodynamics.

Dynamic venous pressure monitoring utilizes pressure measured at a standard pump speed. It represents the total sum of the actual intra-access pressure, the hydrostatic pressure between the needle and the measuring site, and the pressure gradients through the external venous return tubing and the venous needle. This technique requires consistent dialyzer flow and standardization for different dialysis machines. Schwab et al.[2] measured venous pressures during dialysis at blood flows of 200 to 255 cc/min. They found that 73 patients had a venous pressure greater than 150 mm Hg. Fifty (86%) of 58 patients who agreed to angiography had a venous stenosis rate greater than 50%.

Static pressure measures intra-access venous pressure at a blood flow of 0. Besarab et al.[3] used this technique in 133 patients using an "in-line" 3-way stopcock adjacent to the venous return needle. Patients with a venous pressure or systolic blood pressure greater than 0.4 were referred for angiography. On 80 occasions, accesses with significant stenosis had overall sensitivity and specificity rates of 91% and 91%, respectively.

Increased pressure in the access proximal to a stenosis is a result of increased resistance to flow. Van Stone et al.[4] evaluated access outlet stenosis by measuring the relative resistance of the outflow segment. Graft resistance is determined by comparing the arterial and venous dialysis line pressures with the graft open to these pressures when the graft is occluded by digital compression between the needles. When the graft is occluded, the arterial line pressure is equal to the systemic arterial pressure and the venous line pressure is equal to peripheral venous pressure. Because there is no flow through the graft, these pressures are not affected by any stenosis. The difference between the occluded and nonoccluded line pressure equals the pressure decrease caused by graft blood flow across the graft segment and venous system distal to the venous needle. The resistance of the outflow segment relative to total graft resistance is equal to the difference between systemic arterial pressure and peripheral venous pressure. The relative outflow resistance is thus calculated by dividing the difference between non-occluded and occluded arterial line pressure and occluded venous line pressure. Van Stone et al. found that a relative resistance of 0.4 has a sensitivity of 90% and a specificity of 53% for detecting hemodialysis access outlet obstruction.[4]

Duplex ultrasonography. Only Doppler ultrasound has proven to be effective in evaluating both anatomic vascular features and blood flow parameters. Its value in the follow-up of the vascular bypass graft is well established. This technique has also been adopted for patients with vascular accesses.

Strauch et al.[5] used color Doppler flow imaging to study the predictive value for future episodes of thrombosis. They evaluated the degree of stenosis as well as the access volume flow in vascular access graft patients. They found that 57% of patients with a stenosis of greater than 50% had clotting episodes within 6 months. In contrast, only 11% of patients with stenosis less than 50% had clotting episodes. Patients with a low access flow had more clotting episodes than those with a high flow.

Shackleton et al.[6] evaluated flow characteristics using Duplex scanning in 18 patients with a forearm PTFE vascular graft. They found that mean Doppler flow in grafts that subsequently thrombosed was significantly lower than in those that did not thrombose (544 ± 218 mL/min versus 843 ± 391 mL/min, $P<0.001$). The interval from exam to thrombosis ranged from 13 to 58 days.

Sands et al.[7] used ultrasonography to evaluate access flow rates in 253 patients (177 PTFE grafts and 76 arteriovenous fistulae). They found that patients with a flow rate less than 800 cc/min had a 92.9% incidence of thrombosis within 6 months, compared with a 25% thrombosis rate in patients with higher flow rates. Low-flow grafts with an elective revision of an area with greater than 50% stenosis had a thrombosis rate of 5.6% over 6 months, compared with 42% in patients with no revisions.

Bay et al.[8] found that quantifying blood flow in the access graft using color Doppler ultrasound could predict graft failure. The relative risk of graft failure increased by 40% when the blood flow in the graft decreased to less than 500 cc/min, and the relative risk doubled when the blood flow was less than 300 cc/min. However, duplex ultrasound flow measurement in native fistulae did not accurately predict fistula survival.

Bakran[9] used Doppler duplex ultrasound before, during, and after operation in 60 patients who underwent placement of primary AV fistulae. Preoperative ultrasound evaluation was better than clinical assessment at predicting both successful and unsuccessful outcomes. Intraoperative Doppler duplex ultrasound flow measurements were widely variable, possibly due to vascular spasm.

Problems with routine use of Doppler ultrasound in vascular access screening have been: (1) the variability of flow measurements from 1 hand to the other; (2) the high capital costs of the equipment coupled with technician and physician costs; and (3) the lack of reimbursement for screening.

Measurement of dialysis access recirculation. Recirculation is defined as the immediate return of venous (dialyzed) blood to the dialyzer, which effectively truncates the patient's blood flow. When blood is pumped out of the access into the dialyzer, a low-resistance circuit is created that is designed to increase the total access blood flow. As a result, the venous drainage of the access is increased during dialysis. If the venous outflow is restricted, the likelihood of recirculation will be increased. Recirculation also will be facilitated by an increase in negative pressure at the arterial needle. Therefore, the measurement of dialysis access recirculation has important diagnostic implications. The presence of recirculation is confirmed by demonstrating the concentration of a dialyzable solute in dialyzer afferent (arterial line) blood is lower than that in systemic blood.

Recirculation can be measured directly using classical solute dilution techniques or indicator dilution methods provided by a variety of newly developed devices. The blood flow entering the dialyzer (Qa) is composed of a mixture of true systemic blood (Qs) and recirculated blood (Qr). Qa is measured as the sum of Qs and Qr. The rate of solute (such as blood-urea-nitrogen [BUN]) delivery to the dialyzer can be expressed by the equation: $Ca \chi Qa = Cs \chi Qs + Cv \chi Qr$, where Ca is dialyzer arterial solute concentration, Cs is the systemic concentration, and Cv is the dialyzer venous concentration. The fraction of arterial flow that consists of recirculated blood is calculated by the equation

$$Fr = \frac{Qr}{Qa} = \frac{Cs - Ca}{Cs - Cv}$$

Thus recirculation can be calculated from BUN concentrations measured in 3 blood samples drawn simultaneously. The arterial and venous samples are obtained from blood samples drawn simultaneously from the arterial and venous ports in the bloodline.

Recirculation may also be detected indirectly from the results of urea modeling. Urea is the most widely used solute for the measurement of recirculation because it is easily measured and extracted in large quantities by the dialyzer. The difference between modeled and expected urea clearance is a measure of recirculation, provided that no other error (eg, blood flow) contributes to the difference. Recently it has been suggested that dialysis access recirculation measurement has the potential to substantially overestimate actual recirculation. Sherman suggested that most of the potential error in this measurement could be reduced by using an arterial, rather than a venous, specimen for the systemic sample.[10]

Access flow measurement. Low or falling access blood flow rates are predictive of access dysfunction, and the dilution method has been used to measure access blood flow. In 1995, Krivitski introduced the reversed line approach for measuring access flow during hemodialysis.[11] This technology was based on reversing the delivery of the dialyzer outflow and placing it upstream from the arterial line with respect to the vascular access flow. In this arrangement, the indicator introduced through the venous line into the vascular access mixes with the incoming access flow. After mixing, a portion of the mixed blood reenters the dialyzer via the arterial inlet, which is downstream from the mixing site due to the line reversal.

Blood flow measurement is based on the Stewart-Hamilton principle. The most commonly used formula for flow measurement is Qa = Qb (1/R-1), where Qb is blood flow in the venous line, R is access recirculation measured with reversed lines, and Qa is access blood flow. Several methods are available for measuring access blood flow based on this approach, including: ultrasound dilution, thermal dilution, and conductivity dilution. Lindsay et al.[12] compared access flow rates measured with several indicator dilution methodsm, including: ultrasound dilution, optical dilution, and conductivity dilution. They found that ultrasound dilution and conductivity dilution yielded essentially identical flow rate data. Measurement with optical dilution correlated with both other techniques but consistently measured higher access flow.

May et al.[13] studied flow rates in 172 PTFE grafts for 12 weeks using the ultrasound dilution technique. They observed 34 episodes of thrombosis and found the accesses that thrombosed had a significantly lower flow rate than those that remained open (875 cc/min versus 1193 cc/min). Similarly, Depner et al.[14] followed PTFE grafts prospectively after obtaining baseline flow volume measurements. They found a 77% failure rate in grafts with a baseline access flow less than 600 mL/min over 6 months.

Conclusions

Early detection of dialysis access dysfunction and elective timely intervention may result in a prolongation of access function. Several methods are available for diagnosis of failing accesses. Doppler ultrasound has the advantage of evaluating both anatomic and flow parameters. This method, however, is associated with potential problems, including a lack of availability, the need for trained personnel, the variability of data among machines, and a high cost. Though static venous pressure avoids many of these issues, it is able to represent intra-access pressure only. Access flow measurements have important diagnostic implications, but the technology is still evolving. A sensitive and noninvasive method is needed for routine evaluation of the accesses and determination of further interventions.

References

1. Sands JJ, Miranda CL. Prolongation of hemodialysis access survival with elective revision. Clin Nephrol 1995; 44:329-33.
2. Schwab SJ, Raymond JR, Saeed M. Prevention of hemodialysis fistula thrombosis: Early detection of venous stenoses. Kidney Int 1998; 36:707-11.
3. Besarab A, Moritz M, Sullivan K. Venous access pressures and the detection of intra-access stenosis. Artif Organs 1992; 38:519-23.
4. Van Stone JC, Jones M, Van Stone J. Detection of hemodialysis access outlet stenosis by measuring outlet resistance. Am J Kidney Dis 1994; 23:562-68.
5. Strauch BS, O'Connell RS, Geoly KL, Grundlehner M, Yakub N, Tietjen DP. Forecasting thrombosis of vascular access with doppler color flow imaging. Am J Kidney Dis 1992; 19:554-57.

6. Shackleton CR, Taylor DC, Buckley AR, Rowley A, Cooperberg PL, Fry PD. Predicting failure in polytetrafluoroethylene vascular access grafts for hemodialysis: A pilot study. Can J Surg 1987; 30:442-44.
7. Sands J, Young S, Miranda C. The effect of doppler flow screening studies and elective revisions on dialysis access failure. Artif Organs 1992; 38:524-31.
8. Bay WH, Henry ML, Lazarus JM, Lew NL, Ling J, Lowrie EG. Predicting hemodialysis access failure with color flow doppler ultrasound. Am J Nephrol 1998; 18:296-304.
9. Bakram A. The arteriovenous fistula: Can we do it better? In: Henry ML, ed. Vascular access for hemodialysis-VI. Chicago: W.L. Gore & Associates and Precept Press, 1999:431-43.
10. Sherman RA. The measurement of dialysis access recirculation. Am J Kid Dis 1995; 22:616-21.
11. Krivitski NM. Vascular access flow measurement by dilution during hemodialysis: Overview of first four years' experience. In: Henry ML, ed. Vascular access for hemodialysis-VI. Chicago: W.L. Gore & Associates and Precept Press, 1999:79-89.
12. Lindsay RM, Blake PG, Malek P. Hemodialysis access blood flow rates can be measured by a differential conductivity technique and are predictive of access clotting. Am J Kidney Dis 1997; 30:475-82.
13. May RE, Himmelfarb J, Yenicesu M. Predictive measures of vascular access thrombosis: A prospective study. Kidney Int 1997; 52:1656-62.
14. Depner TA, Rizwan S, Cheer AY, Wagner JM, Eder LA. High venous urea concentration in the opposite arm. A consequence of hemodialysis-induced compartment dysequilibrium. Artif Organs 1991; 37:141-43.

3

STATE OF THE ART RADIOLOGIC INTERVENTION

Thomas M. Vesely, M.D.

Polytetrafluoroethylene (PTFE) grafts continue to be the most prevalent type of vascular access for hemodialysis in the United States.[1,2] The durability of PTFE grafts is limited; recent studies have reported 1 year primary patency rates of only 43% to 54%.[3-5] Graft failure occurs through the progressive development of intimal hyperplastic stenoses, a relentless and predictable process. Lesions can be difficult to treat and tend to recur quickly and aggressively. Our current methods for percutaneous treatment of intimal hyperplastic stenoses, unfortunately, typically provide only a short interval of additional graft patency.

Angioplasty continues to be the primary percutaneous technique for the treatment of intimal hyperplastic stenoses. Atherectomy devices have been used to cut away and remove intimal lesions, and vascular stents have been inserted to oppose elastic recoil and optimize luminal diameter. Unfortunately, the use of these newer technologies has not proven to be more effective than conventional angioplasty.[6-8]

Our continuing efforts to improve vascular access for hemodialysis has turned our attention to new possibilities that include the use of alternative types of vascular access and improved methods for graft surveillance. These topics cross specialty lines. The development and clinical implementation of future improvements will require collaboration and cooperation among the various physicians who comprise the vascular access team.[9,10]

Alternative Vascular Access

Throughout the 1990s, there was a widespread and well-documented shift away from arteriovenous fistulae toward the use of PTFE grafts as the initial vascular access for hemodialysis patients.[1] This shift occurred despite clinical evidence that had demonstrated the decreased longevity and increased complication rates of grafts when compared with native fistulae. Recently, the acceptance and implementation of the Dialysis Outcomes Quality Initiative (DOQI) Clinical Practice Guidelines, which strongly advocate the use of arteriovenous fistulae, have begun to reverse this trend.[11] The prevalence of arteriovenous fistulae is increasing. Many surgeons and interventionalists are learning new skills for the diagnosis and treatment of problems related to native fistulae.

Recent reports regarding the use of percutaneous interventions in arteriovenous fistulae are encouraging. The primary patency rates for angioplasty of stenoses in dysfunctional but patent fistulae are 60% at 1 year and 40% at 2 years.[12,13] This is substantially better than the 60% 6-month and 40% 1-year primary patency rates achieved by angioplasty of dysfunctional PTFE grafts.[6,14] Percutaneous treatment of thrombosed arteriovenous fistulae can be laborious, often taking 2 hours or more for the procedure, but the results seem to be worth the effort. Reported primary patency rates for the treatment of thrombosed fistulae are 50% to 70% at 6 months and 30% to 60% at 1 year.[15,16] Again, these results are much better than the expected primary patency rate of 40% at 3 months for treatment of thrombosed PTFE grafts.[11] As the prevalence of arteriovenous fistulae continue to increase, the use of percutaneous interventions will continue to provide a viable alternative to open surgical procedures.

The use of implantable hemodialysis ports may potentially serve as alternative primary vascular accesses for some patients.[17,18] Two different types of hemodialysis ports, the LifeSite® (Vasca Inc, Tewksbury, MA) and the Dialock® (Biolink Corp, Middleboro, MA) are undergoing clinical trials in the United States. The use of a completely subcutaneous vascular access device may decrease the infectious complications associated with conventional tunneled hemodialysis catheters. In addition, the development of new catheter locking solutions, which have both anticoagulant and antimicrobial effects, may also contribute to the long-term viability of hemodialysis ports.[18,19]

Finally, the growing interest in nocturnal hemodialysis may have an effect on the future of vascular access.[20] A typical duration for nocturnal hemodialysis treatment is 8 to 10 hours per night. Unlike conventional hemodialysis, which requires vascular access blood flow rates of 400 to 500 mL/min, nocturnal hemodialysis may only need blood flow rates of 200 to 300 mL/min. These lower performance standards may provoke the development of a new type of vascular access that is more durable and less susceptible to complications than those utilized today.

Graft Surveillance

As previously mentioned, recent technological advances in endovascular therapy have failed to improve the outcome of percutaneous interventions in hemodialysis grafts. Inventive surgical approaches, including the use of new graft materials and novel constructions of anastomoses, have also failed to substantially increase the longevity of vascular access grafts. Currently, the most effective method to improve long-term graft patency is the implementation of a graft surveillance program.

Routine, periodic monitoring of hemodialysis grafts can detect the development of intimal hyperplastic stenoses. Early treatment of hemodynamically significant stenoses, using angioplasty, can prevent thrombosis. Avoiding thrombosis leads to increased long-term graft survival and decreased procedural costs. Sullivan and colleagues reported a substantial reduction in the incidence in graft thrombosis, from 0.58 thromboses per patient per year to 0.19 thromboses per patient per year, following the implementation of a graft surveillance program.[21,22] In addition, they also reported that the mean graft age increased by approximately 1 year using graft surveillance and early treatment of stenoses.

Data from the interventional radiology literature also supports the concept that early treatment will prolong patency. Angioplasty of a significant stenosis in a dysfunctional, but patent, hemodialysis graft should achieve a 6-month primary patency rate of 50% to 65%.[14] In comparison, a combined percutaneous thrombectomy and angioplasty procedure will yield a 6-month patency rate of only 25% to 35%.[6] The reasons for this difference have not yet been elucidated. Despite the benefits of early treatment, angioplasty causes vascular injury and may incite intimal hyperplasia. DOQI guidelines suggest that interventions should be avoided until the stenosis becomes hemodynamically significant (>50%) and is associated with a clinical or physiologic abnormality.

The guidelines also suggest that a variety of different methods can be used for graft surveillance. Sequential measurements of graft function are more predictive of developing stenoses than a single, isolated measurement. Several reports have now demonstrated that sequential measurements of intragraft blood flow are the most useful predictor of impending thrombosis.[23-25] Although there are several methods to measure intragraft blood flow, the ultrasound dilution technique (Transonic Systems Inc, Ithaca, NY) has become the most widely used. Using the Transonic system, intragraft blood flow can be easily and noninvasively measured while the patient is connected to the hemodialysis machine. A blood flow of less than 600 mL/min and an incremental decrease of 25% are predictive of impending graft thrombosis. These patients are referred to radiology for a diagnostic fistulogram and treatment of significant stenoses.

Interestingly, the routine measurement of intragraft blood flows has provided new insights into the hemodynamics of vascular access. Intragraft blood flow is significantly higher than many physicians would have imagined. An unpublished analysis of monthly blood flows obtained from 100 patients with PTFE grafts at the author's institution revealed a mean intragraft blood flow of 1000 mL/min, with a range of 120 mL/min to 3300 mL/min. A well-functioning graft often has a blood flow of nearly 1500 mL/min. A significant portion of the patient's cardiac output is shunted through a vascular access.[26] In addition, prior to placement of a PTFE graft, the typical blood flow in the brachial artery is 75 to 150 mL/min. Following insertion of a graft, the brachial artery blood flow increases more than 10-fold in response to the vascular shunt.

Measurement of intragraft blood flow has also provided a new method to assess the effectiveness of percutaneous or surgical interventions. A successful repair of a stenosis should return the intragraft blood flow to normal levels. But we now know that there is no normal or optimal blood flow that should be achieved. The baseline or normal intragraft blood flow is patient dependent and highly variable. A recent study compared postangioplasty blood flows to the blood flow measured in the graft and demonstrated that a successful intervention can return the blood flow to baseline.[27]

Assessment of intragraft blood flow has also provided evidence for a higher than expected incidence of arterial problems. A recent study reported that despite successful angioplasty, intragraft blood flow failed to improve in 39% of treated patients.[28] Further evaluation of these patients often reveals significant arterial pathology, primarily atherosclerotic stenoses located in the proximal inflow arteries. Although at first surprising, this high incidence of arterial stenoses could have been predicted by the growing number of elderly and diabetic hemodialysis patients. As previously mentioned, the hemodynamics of the inflow arteries are substantially altered by the placement of the vascular shunt. Arterial lesions, which had been of little clinical significance, can become a substantial impediment to optimal blood flow following placement of a vascular access. Previously, our attention had been primarily focused on identification and treatment of stenoses at the venous or arterial anastomoses, in the native veins, and within the graft. It is likely that additional studies will further substantiate the necessity of evaluating the inflow arteries during diagnostic fistulography.

Conclusion

Technological advances, both radiological and surgical, have failed to extend the longevity of vascular access for hemodialysis. Significant improvements can be achieved by implementing graft surveillance programs and increasing the prevalence of arteriovenous fistulae. The development of new types of vascular access may provide additional benefits.

References

1 Hirth RA, Turenne MN, Woods JD, et al. Predictors of type of vascular access in hemodialysis patients. JAMA 1996; 276:1303-08.

2 Stehman-Breen CO, Sherrard DJ, Gillen D, Caps M. Determinants of type and timing of initial permanent vascular access. Kidney Int 2000; 57:639-45.

3. Cinat ME, Hopkins J, Wilson SE. A prospective evaluation of PTFE graft patency and surveillance techniques in hemodialysis access. Ann Vasc Surg 1999; 13:191-98.

4. Hodges TC, Fillinger MF, Zwolak RM, Walsh DB, Bech F, Cronenwett JL. Longitudinal comparison of dialysis access methods: Risk factors for failure. J Vasc Surg 1997; 26:1009-19.

5. Ascher E, Gade P, Hingorani A, et al. Changes in the practice of angioaccess surgery: Impact of dialysis outcomes and quality initiative recommendations. J Vasc Surg 2000; 31:84-92.

6. Gray RJ. Percutaneous intervention for permanent hemodialysis access: A review. J Vasc Interv Radiol 1997; 8:313-27.

7. Schwab SJ. Vascular access for hemodialysis. Kidney Int 1999; 55:2078-90.
8. Hoffer EK, Sultan S, Herskowitz MM, Daniels ID, Sclafani SJ. Prospective randomized trial of a metallic intravascular stent in hemodialysis graft maintenance. J Vasc Interv Radiol 1997; 8:965-73.
9. Allon M, Bailey R, Ballard R, et al. A multidisciplinary approach to hemodialysis access: Prospective evaluation. Kidney Int 1998; 53:473-79.
10. Gelbfish GA. Surgery versus percutaneous treatment of thrombosed dialysis access grafts: Is there a best method? J Vasc Interv Radiol 1998; 9:875-77.
11. NKF-DOQI clinical practice guidelines for vascular access. National Kidney Foundation-Dialysis Outcomes Quality Initiative. Am J Kidney Dis 1997; 30(suppl 3) S150-91.
12. Lay JP, Ashleigh RJ, Tranconi L, Ackrill P, Al-Khaffaf H. Results of angioplasty of Brescia-Cimino hemodialysis fistulae: Medium-term follow-up. Clin Radiol 1998; 53:608-11.
13. Turmel-Rodrigues L, Pengloan J, Blanchier D, et al. Insufficient dialysis shunts: Improved long-term patency rates with close hemodynamic monitoring, repeated percutaneous balloon angioplasty, and stent placement. Radiology 1993; 187:273-78.
14. Vesely TM. Percutaneous transluminal angioplasty in the treatment of failing hemodialysis grafts and fistulae. Semin Dialysis 1998; 11:351-59.
15. Turmel-Rodrigues L, Pengloan J, Rodrigue H, et al. Treatment of failed native arteriovenous fistulae for hemodialysis by interventional radiology. Kidney Int 2000; 57:1124-40.
16. Haage P, Vorwerk D, Wildberger JE, Piroth W, Schurmann K, Gunther RW. Percutaneous treatment of thrombosed primary arteriovenous hemodialysis access fistulae. Kidney Int 2000; 57:1169-75.
17. Levin NW, Yang PM, Hatch DA, et al. Initial results of a new access for hemodialysis. Kidney Int 1998; 54:1739-45.
18. Sodemann K, Feldmer B, Polaschegg HD, Thon P, Lubrich-Birjner I, Baumert J. Clinical results of the German Dialock access study: A new subcutaneous port system and a novel antimicrobial lock solution [abstract]. J Am Soc Nephrol 1999; 10:218A.
19. Wentworth DW, Kim FJ, Lentino JR, Hatch DA, Gandhi VC. Citrate may be the anticoagulant of choice to prevent clotting of antibiotic locks used in vascular access devices [abstract]. J Am Soc Nephrol 1999; 10:222A.
20. Pierratos A, Ouwendyk M, Francoeur R, et al. Nocturnal hemodialysis: Three-year experience. J Am Soc Nephrol 1998; 9:859-68.
21. Sullivan KL, Besarab A. Hemodynamic screening and early percutaneous intervention reduce hemodialysis access thrombosis and increase graft longevity. J Vasc Interv Radiol 1997; 8:163-70.
22. Besarab A, Sullivan KL, Ross RP, Moritz MJ. Utility of intra-access pressure monitoring in detecting and correcting venous outlet stenosis prior to thrombosis. Kidney Int 1995; 47:1364-73.
23. May RE, Himmelfarb J, Yenicesu M, et al. Predictive measures of vascular access thrombosis: A prospective study. Kidney Int 1997; 52:1656-62.
24. Bosman PJ, Boereboom FT, Eikelboom BC, Koomans HA, Blankenstijn PJ. Graft flow as a predictor of thrombosis in hemodialysis grafts. Kidney Int 1998; 54:1726-30.

25. Neyra NR, Ikizler T, May RE, et al. Change in access blood flow over time predicts vascular access thrombosis. Kidney Int 1998; 54:1714-19.
26. Ori Y, Katz M, Korzets A, Chagnac A, Weinstein T, Gafter U. Hemodynamic effects of arteriovenous access for hemodialysis [abstract]. J Am Soc Nehrol 1999; 10:214A.
27. Murray BM, Ali B, Rojczak S, Mepani B. Utility of access blood flow measurements in evaluating the efficacy of radiological angioplasty of arteriovenous shunts [abstract]. J Am Soc Nephrol 1999; 10:213A.
28. Levine MI, Wallach JD. Inflow stenoses of AV hemodialysis accesses can be found more frequently in patients monitored with regular intra-access flow measurements [abstract]. J Am Soc Nephrol 1999; 10:209A.

4

STATE OF THE ART SURGICAL TREATMENT FOR FAILING GRAFTS

José R. Polo, M.D., Cruz Menárguez, M.D., Jorge Polo, M.D., and Rosario Gracia-Pajares, M.D.

Stenosis and thrombosis of dialysis grafts are the most frequent complications affecting the graft's life and increasing the hospitalization of dialysis patients.[1] The purpose of this presentation is to analyze the surgical methods available for the treatment of stenosis and thrombosis of dialysis grafts.

Stenosis in dialysis grafts. The aim of surgical treatment for stenosis in dialysis grafts is to prevent thrombosis, a flow dependent pathology,[2] by increasing the access flow and improving dialysis efficiency by decreasing the dialysis venous pressure and the recirculation rate.[3] Prevention of thrombosis by elective treatment of stenosis has been well documented.[4,5] Surgical and radiological methods cannot be considered competitive but complementary.

A multidisciplinary approach, with close collaboration and agreement between surgeons and radiologists, is necessary to offer the best possible treatment to patients with dialysis access stenosis. Comparative studies regarding the efficiency of surgery or interventional radiology in the treatment of stenosis are controversial.[6,7] Either radiology or surgery should be considered depending on such variables as the location, length and tightness of the stenosis, resources of the hospital, and experience in managing vascular access by the radiologists and surgeons in each center. Our unit's approach is to treat all peripheral stenoses (distal to proximal axillary vein) by surgical methods, by bypassing to a proximal dilated vein. Proximal stenoses, or stenoses difficult to reach under local anesthesia, are treated with interventional radiology.

There are 4 possible locations of dialysis grafts stenosis: (1) graft-vein stenosis, in which myo-intimal hyperplasia affects the last centimeters of grafts and the portion of the vein close to the anastomosis; (2) mid-graft stenosis, located at the puncture sites; (3) arterial-graft stenosis (quite infrequent), affecting either the graft close to the anastomosis or the artery close to the graft, mainly observed in small arteries such as the radial artery; and (4) central vein stenosis, usually associated with previous central catheters.

Graft-vein stenosis. Stenosis affecting the graft-vein junction is the most frequent finding in graft dysfunction (figure 4-1). One surgical solution can be a polytetrafluoroethylene (PTFE) bypass to a proximal dilated vein, the procedure favored by the authors. The first papers dealing with graft revision advised this technique.[8,9] In 1984, the first large series with more than 300 procedures was published in the French literature.[10] The old anastomosis can be excluded, thus avoiding the dissection in scarred tissue. Both anastomoses, graft-to-graft and graft-to-vein, are performed in an end-to-end fashion (figure 4-2). A mean survival of 72% of bypasses at 2 years was presented in a publication in which this technique was individually analyzed.[10] We have treated 97 cases of graft-vein stenosis by this method, also called extended graft or jump graft. Cumulative primary patency after this procedure was 70% and 45%, at 1 and 4 years respectively, after the bypass construction. Secondary patency was of 87% and 71%, at 1 and 4 years. The rate of surgical procedures used to obtain this secondary patency (eg, surgical thrombectomy or graft curettage) was 0.32 per graft-year (1 procedure every 3 years).[11]

Patch angioplasty is another method. This involves longitudinal incision of the stenosed segment and placement of either a venous or graft patch to enlarge the lumen (figure 4-3).[12] This method may be used for the treatment of short and not too narrow stenosis. To our knowledge, there is no published experience regarding the

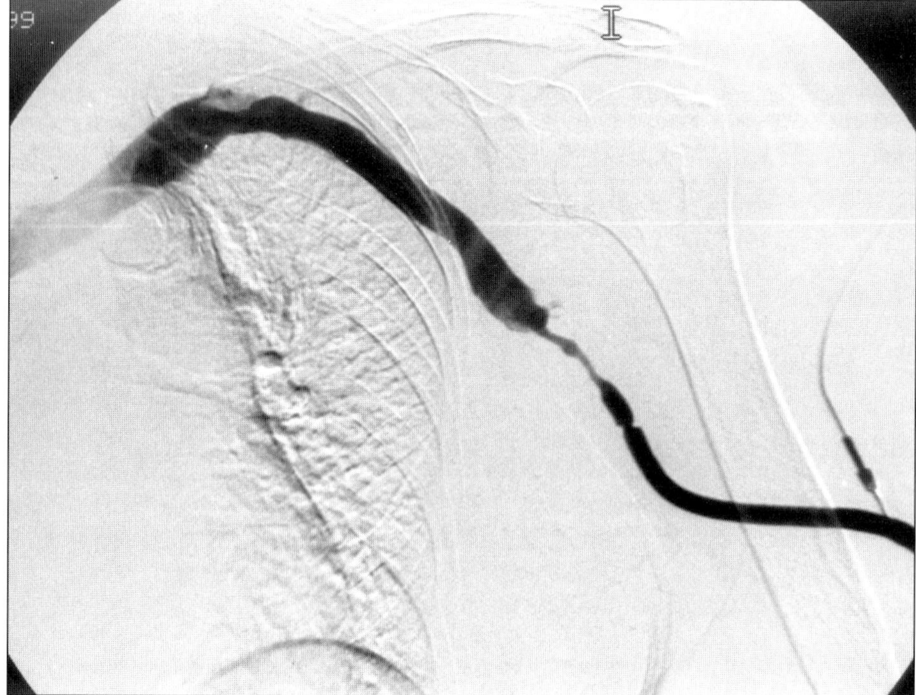

Figure 4-1. Graft-vein stenosis affecting a brachioaxillary graft.

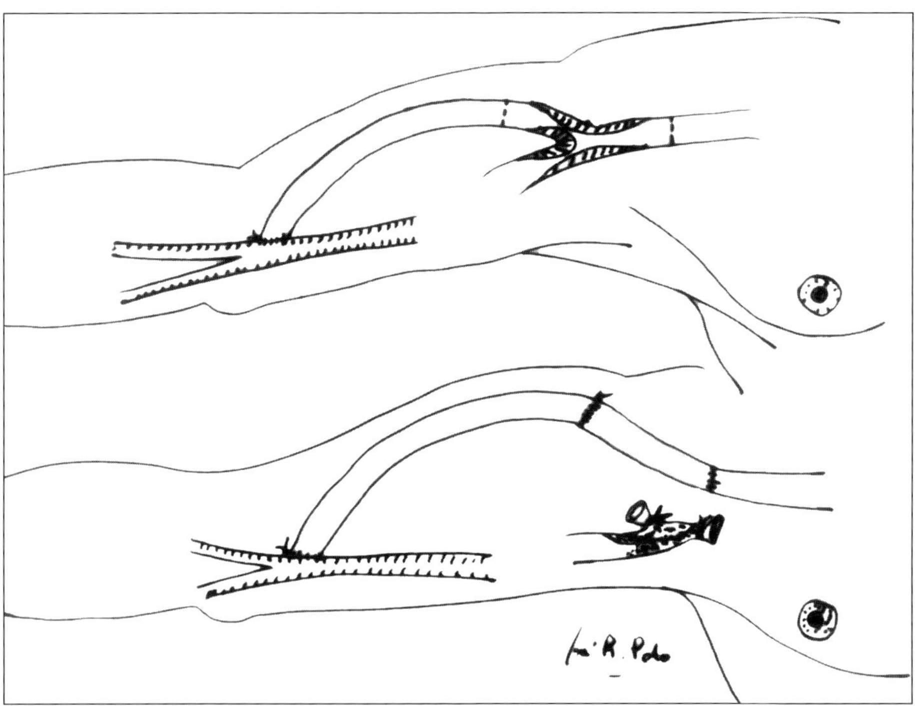

Figure 4-2. Bypass to a proximal vein. The old anastomosis is excluded, avoiding dissection in a scarred tissue.

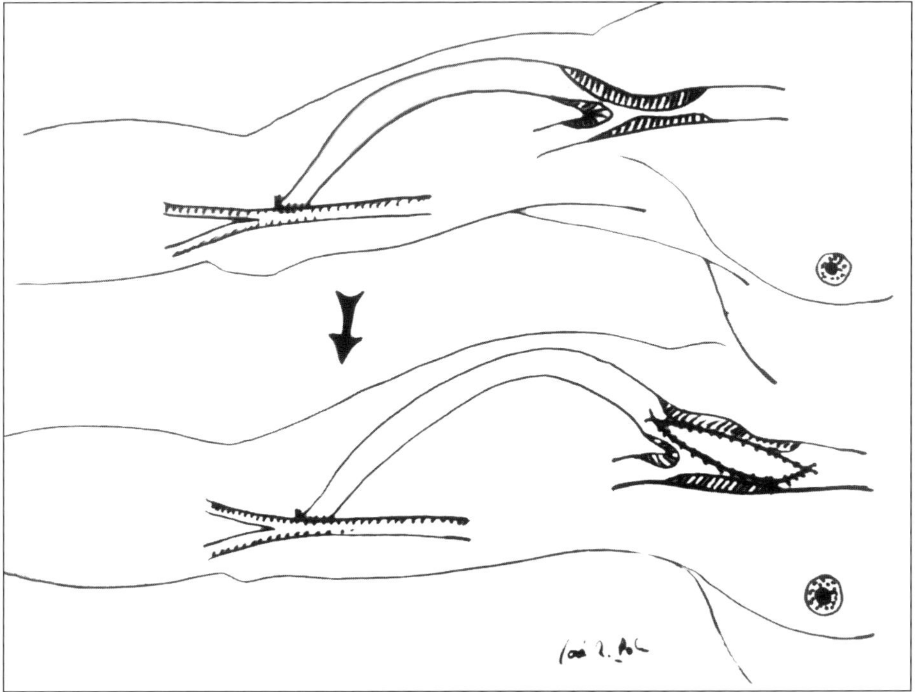

Figure 4-3. Patch angioplasty for treatment of short, but not too narrow stenosis.

long-term performance of this technique, because patch angioplasty, bypass graft, and dilation with probes are usually studied together in most publications. In a recent study, patch angioplasty was analyzed in 22 patients for a period of 2 years. Primary patency was 17% at 6 months.[13]

As in cases with radiological treatment, the secondary patency rate is improved by continuous monitoring of the graft and early treatment of restenosis.[14]

Mid-graft stenosis. This kind of stenosis is observed at the puncture sites. Stenosis is not only induced by intimal hyperplasia, but also by organized thrombus and calcification of the neointimal layer (figure 4-4). Whenever the stenosis is distal to the venous puncture, an increase in dialysis venous pressure is not observed. The only way to detect early mid-graft stenosis is by frequent evaluation of access flow. The use of graft flow measurement will allow more and more mid-graft stenosis detection.

Graft curettage (using a uterine curette) can be performed to treat this condition. Vascular rings and Volkmann curettes are other useful tools for this procedure, which

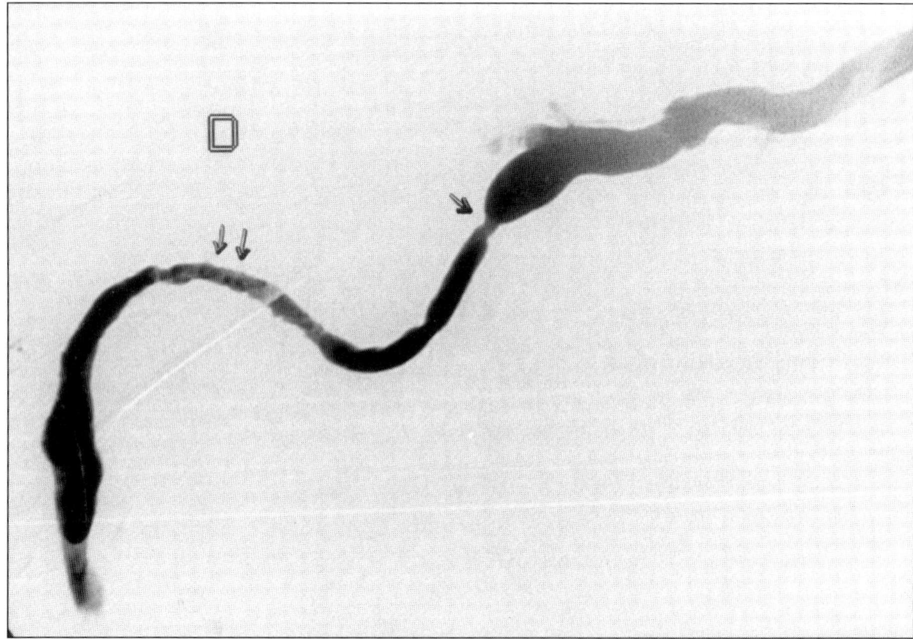

Figure 4-4. Mid-graft stenosis affecting the distal middle of a brachioaxillary graft (double arrow). Mild graft-vein stenosis is also observed (single arrow).

is performed with a graft approach close to the arterial anastomosis. The hyperplastic debris are then removed using a Fogarty catheter. Occasionally, a second approach, close to the venous anastomosis, becomes necessary in order to control the back flow or to complete the graft curettage (figure 4-5).[15] Restenosis is frequently observed after this procedure. After repeated curettage, a new graft, parallel to the previous one, must be considered. In these cases, a short segment of the old graft must be left in place to permit single needle dialysis during the 2-week period required for graft maturation (figure 4-6).

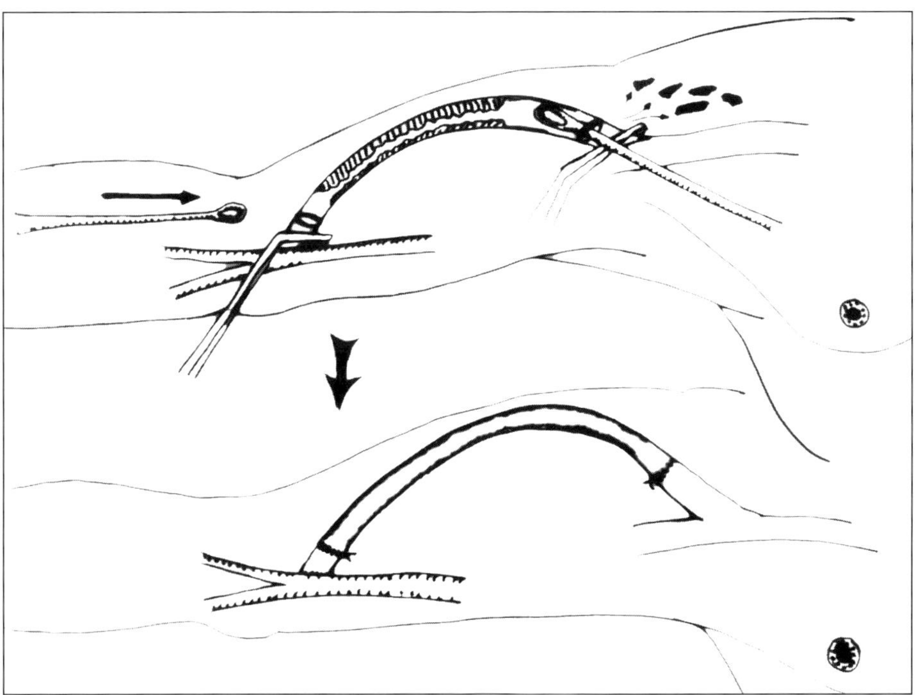

Figure 4-5. Graft curettage for treatment of mid-graft stenosis.

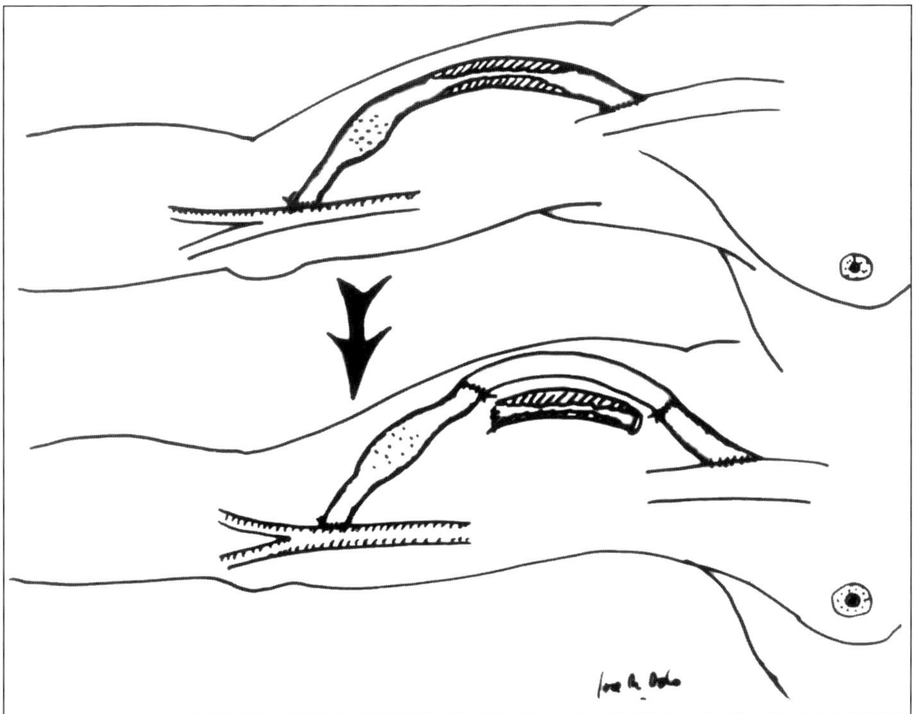

Figure 4-6. Partial graft substitution for treating localized mid-graft stenosis.

Arterial-graft stenosis. This kind of stenosis is rarely observed. In our experience, it was observed in 5 out of 238 cases in which a fistulography was performed. These cases were successfully treated by performing a bypass from the proximal artery to the nonstenotic portion of the graft close to the arterial anastomosis (figure 4-7).

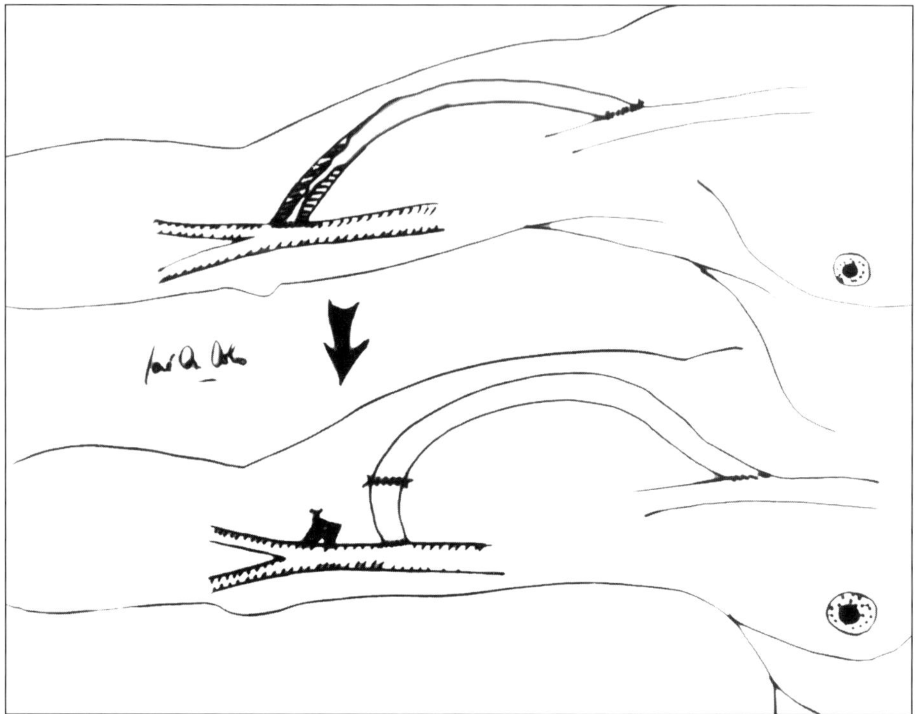

Figure 4-7. Bypass to proximal artery for treating arterial-graft stenosis.

Central vein stenosis. Central vein stenoses tend to be diagnosed a considerable amount of time after they develop, because collateral circulation precludes most cases from either increasing dialysis venous pressure or decreasing access flow. Only when critical stenosis forms will distal edema or high venous pressure allow detection of this condition. Although complex intrathoracic procedures have been performed to solve this problem,[16,17] most patients with this condition can be treated with interventional radiology.[18,19] Brachiojugular or axillary-axillary grafts can be used in cases of isolated subclavian vein occlusion (figure 4-8).[20,21] In a long-term analysis of 41 brachiojugular grafts, primary and secondary patencies at 2 years were 39% and 71%, respectively.[22,23]

Surgical treatment of thrombosed grafts. Most graft thromboses are associated with some degree of stenosis. Therefore, the purpose of graft thrombectomy is not only the removal of the clot in order to clear the access, but also detection and treatment of every associated stenosis to avoid new episodes of graft clotting in the future. Direct visualization of Fogarty balloon withdrawal is a reasonable and practical method of venous stenosis detection. Other methods include: arterial probes (for mid-graft stenosis detection), angioscopy, and perioperative angiography. We

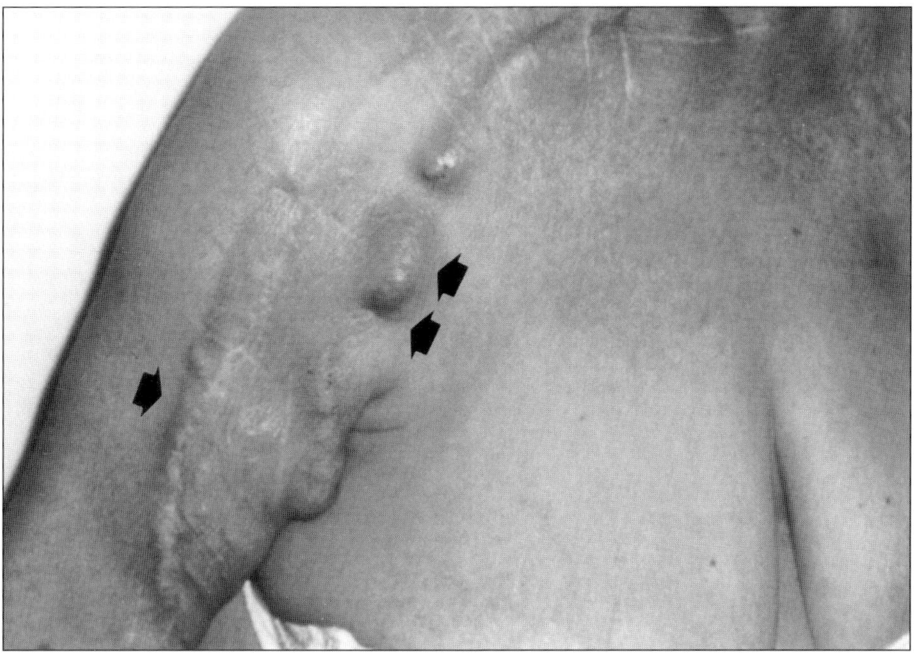

Figure 4-8. Patient with bilateral subclavian vein occlusion due to dialysis catheters used for several months. Brachiojugular graft (external jugular vein) (single arrow) was used for 3 years. Another brachiojugular graft (internal jugular vein) is currently used for more than 7 years. Left arm remains free for further jugular accesses.

believe that all episodes of graft thrombosis should be managed without delay in order to avoid a temporary dialysis catheter. Our group performed all procedures with local anesthesia in an ambulatory surgical facility.[23] If the procedure was successful, the patient was dialyzed immediately and sent home after dialysis, avoiding both an unnecessary hospital stay and a temporary catheter.

Surgical thrombectomy includes a series of steps that should be followed sequentially:

1. The graft is approached at the graft-vein anastomosis. The graft and the first few centimeters of the proximal vein are visualized and a horizontal incision is performed in the graft 3 to 4 cm away from the graft vein junction. A Fogarty catheter is passed into the vein and a proximal thrombectomy is performed. Eventually, a venous stenosis can be detected during this maneuver by observing the narrowing of the balloon as it passes through the stenosed segment. Further stenosis that affects only the last part of the graft can be detected by using arterial probes of different sizes (graft stenosis never behaves like a recoil stenosis). Whenever a graft-vein stenosis is detected, a graft bypass to a proximal dilated vein is performed. Patch angioplasty can be performed in very short stenoses, but not narrow stenoses. Intraoperative balloon dilation can be also used.[24]
2. The second step is removal of the clot in the midpart of the graft and determination of the graft lumen size. These maneuvers should be performed without

removal of the arterial plug (the white thrombus placed at the arterial-graft anastomosis). After the clot is withdrawn from the graft by a Fogarty catheter, arterial probes are used to detect midgraft stenosis, and an eventual removal of hyperplastic fibrotic tissue and organized thrombus (mainly observed at the puncture sites) is performed, using uterine curettes, Volkmann curettes, or vascular rings. Intimal debris is then removed with a Fogarty catheter. Whenever the approach to the middle part of the graft is difficult from the graft-vein junction, a second incision is performed near the arterial-graft anastomosis to clean the prosthesis along both sides of the graft. Due to the simplicity of this maneuver, systematic graft curettage should be advised in all cases of surgical graft thrombectomy. Whenever the graft cannot be cleaned by curettage (most times this is due to severe calcification of the prosthesis), a parallel graft substitution can be performed. Some segment of the old graft should be preserved in order to allow single needle dialysis until the new graft matures (2 weeks in our experience).

3. Once the graft and the graft-vein junction are found to have a proper lumen (at least 70% of the graft size), intravenous heparin is administered (the same heparin dose that is used to begin dialysis), the arterial plug is removed, and the graft is sutured (we use a fine Gore-Tex suture CV-7, TT-13). Failure to completely remove the arterial plug can lead to an incomplete thrombectomy.

Regardless of procedure used (simple thrombectomy or thrombectomy associated with graft curettage or bypass), an elective fistulography should be performed as soon as possible after the post-thrombectomy dialysis in order to find undetected stenosis during surgery. These stenoses can be treated with surgical or radiological methods according to the hospital resources or center preferences.

Personal experience. A complete follow-up of 716 grafts placed between 1982 and 1997 was performed at the end of 1997.[25] The overall follow-up time was 2226 months. Six hundred and sixty-four episodes of thrombosis were observed, yielding a thrombosis rate of 0.35 episodes per graft-year. Table 4-1 depicts the surgical procedures used for treatment of 474 episodes of thrombosis. One hundred and ninety grafts were abandoned because of repeated episodes or severe hypotension. Rates

Table 4-1. Procedures used for treatment of 664 episodes of graft thrombosis.

Procedure	Number	%
Simple thrombectomy	236	35.5
Thrombectomy + patch angioplasty	91	13.7
Thrombectomy + graft extension	84	12.6
Thrombectomy + partial graft substitution	36	5.4
Thrombectomy + graft curettage	27	4
Graft abandoned. Access in other limb, CAPD, other causes	190	28.6

for early success are depicted in table 4-2. Cumulative primary patencies after these procedures are shown in figure 4-9. Thrombectomy plus bypass to a proximal vein (extended graft) showed the best results (95% early success and 1 year primary patency rate of 59%). Making log-rank comparisons, the primary curve of this procedure displayed a significantly better result than those of other procedures

Table 4-2. **Success rates (at least 1 week of dialysis use) after several surgical procedures for treating graft thrombosis.**

Procedure	%
Simple thrombectomy	83
Thrombectomy + graft curettage	89
Thrombectomy + patch angioplasty	91
Thrombectomy + partial graft substitution	92
Thrombectomy + graft extension (bypass to a proximal dilated vein)	95
Overall (474 procedures)	89

(P<0.001).[26] Significant stenoses were detected in 238 cases (50%). Some stenoses were missed during simple thrombectomy in our series, being later detected by fistulography.

Analysis of the literature. Procedures associated with thrombectomy (eg, angioplasty or graft extension) were heterogeneous in the published literature and generally mingled together for analysis. The overall early success rate for all procedures (at least 1 week of use for dialysis) was 89% in our series. Early success ranged from 83% in simple thrombectomy to 95% in thrombectomy associated with graft extension.[26] These results were similar to those published in the literature for surgical thrombectomy, which ranged from 80% to 94%.[27-31] One year cumulative primary patency varied in our series from 38% in simple thrombectomy to 59% in thrombectomy associated with graft extension.[26] One year primary patency after

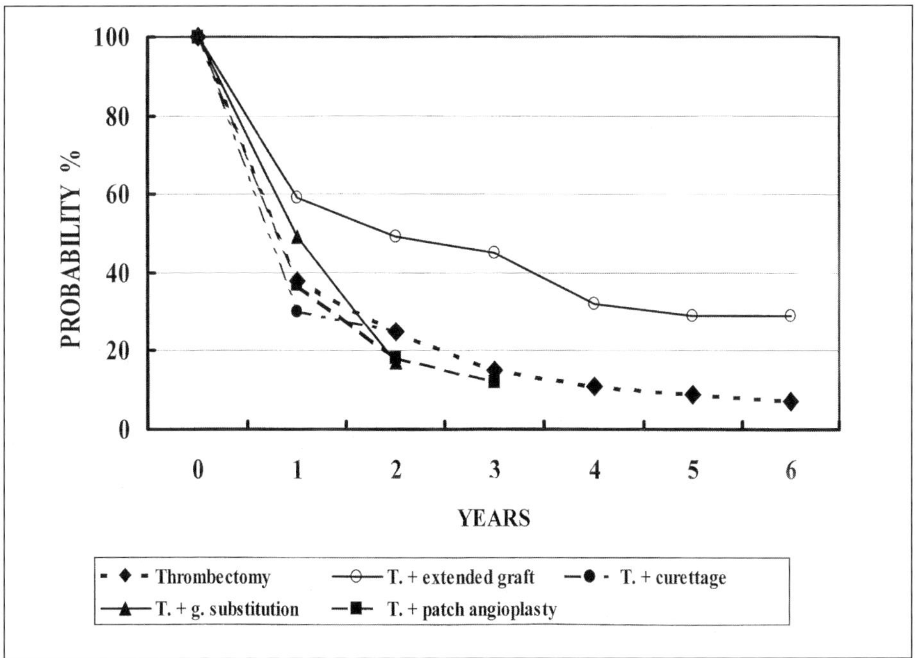

Figure 4-9. Cumulative primary patencies of different surgical procedures for treating graft thrombosis. (T = thrombectomy; g = graft). Standard error at 1 year: P<0.05.

surgical thrombectomy (associated or not with adjuvant procedures) ranged between 25% and 58% in those studies in which 1 year results were analyzed.[27,31-32] In our series, the best results were observed when thrombectomy was associated with bypass to a proximal vein for vein stenosis graft treatment. Similar experiences were published in other reports.[33-34]

Some kind of associated stenoses have been found in most grafts during thrombectomy.[35] Thus, detection and treatment of all types of stenoses should be encouraged after thrombectomy, through either radiological or surgical means. Patients with failing grafts (stenosis or thrombosis), however, should be considered at high risk for dysfunction and must be closely monitored through repeated measurement of both access flow (dilution techniques or echodoppler)[2,36,37] and venous dialysis pressure,[38] in order to treat recurrences as soon as possible. The definition of criteria for high-risk access permits concentration of angioaccess monitoring efforts for this patient population. Perhaps more frequent measurements of access flow and venous pressure should be performed in this high-risk access population.

Conclusions

1. Early detection and treatment of stenosis affecting dialysis grafts prolongs the patency of the access.
2. The best surgical treatment for graft-vein stenosis is bypass to a healthy proximal vein.
3. Graft curettage or partial graft substitution yields the same results for midgraft stenosis treatment. Restenosis after these procedures is quite frequent.
4. Graft thrombosis should be approached as soon as possible in order to avoid temporary catheters.
5. Whenever possible, graft thrombectomy should be followed by evaluation and treatment of every stenosis affecting the graft in the same surgical stage.
6. Graft fistulography should be performed after surgical thrombectomy in the radiological suit and as soon as possible in order to detect a missed stenosis.
7. Every graft treated for stenosis or thrombosis should be considered high risk for recurrence. They should be followed closely by frequent measurements of both access flow and dialysis venous pressure, in order to detect and treat restenosis as early as possible.

References

1. Feldman HI, Held PJ, Hutchinson JT, Stoiber RM. Hemodialysis vascular access morbidity in the United States. Kidney Int 1993; 43:1091-96.
2. Bay WH, Henry ML, Lazarus JM, Lew NL, Ling J, Lowrie EG. Predicting hemodialysis access failure with color flow doppler ultrasound. Am J Nephrol 1998; 18:296-304.

3. Martin LG, MacDonald MJ, Kikeri D, Cotsonis GA, Harker LA, Lumsden AB. Prophylactic angioplasty reduces thrombosis in virgin ePTFE arteriovenous dialysis grafts with greater than 50% stenosis: Subset analysis of a prospectively randomized study. J Vasc Interv Radiol 1999; 10:389-96.
4. Sands JJ, Miranda CL. Prolongation of hemodialysis access survival with elective revision. Clinical Nephrology 1995; 44:329-33.
5. Schwab SJ, Raymond JR, Saeed M, Newman GE, Denis PA, Bollinger RR. Prevention of hemodialysis fistula thrombosis. Early detection of venous stenosis. Kidney Int 1989; 36:707-11.
6. Brooks JL, Sigley D, May KJ, Mack RM. Transluminal angioplasty versus surgical repair for stenosis of hemodialysis grafts. Am J Surg 1987; 153:530-31.
7. Dapunt O, Feurstein M, Rendl KH, Prenner K. Transluminal angioplasty versus conventional operation in the treatment of hemodialysis fistula stenosis: Results from a 5-year study. Br J Surg 1987; 74:1004-05.
8. Etheredge EE, Haid SD, Maester MN, Sicard GA, Anderson CB. Salvage operations for malfunctioning polytetraflouroethylene hemodialysis access grafts. Surgery 1983; 94:464-70.
9. Munda R, First MR, Alexander JW, Linneman CC, Fidler JP, Kittur D. Polytetrafluoroethylene graft survival in hemodialysis. JAMA 1983; 249:219-22.
10. Valverde JP, Maillet R, Nussaume O. Stènoses des greffons d'hèmodialyse. Treatment par courte greffe. Press Med 1984; 13:1957-58.
11. Polo JR, Echenagusia A, Menarguez C, Polo J, Sanabia J, Jimenez P. Bypass to a proximal vein to treat peripheral venous stenosis in PTFE grafts for hemodialysis. In: Henry ML, Ferguson RM eds. Vascular access for hemodialysis-V. Tucson: W.L. Gore & Associates and Precept Press, 1997; 127-36.
12. Henry ML. Options for restoration of thrombosed vascular access: surgery. In: Conlon PJ, Schwab SJ, Nicholson ML. Hemodialysis vascular access: Practice and problems. Oxford: Oxford University Press, 2000:229-39.
13. Bitar G, Yang S, Badosa F. Balloon versus patch angioplasty as an adjuvant treatment to surgical thrombectomy of hemodialysis grafts. Am J Surg 1997; 174:140-42.
14. Turmel-Rodrigues L, Pengolan J, Blanchier D, et al. Insufficient dialysis shunts: Improved long-term patency rates with close hemodynamic monitoring, repeated percutaneous balloon angioplasty, and stent placement. Radiology 1993; 187:273-78.
15. Puckett JW, Lindsay SF. Midgraft curettage as a routine adjunt to salvage operation for thrombosed polytetrafluoroethylene hemodialysis access grafts. Am J Surg 1988; 156:139-43.
16. Williams IR, Flinn WR, Yao JST. Spiral vein graft bypass of subclavian obstruction complicating arm dialysis access. In: Sommer BG, Henry ML eds. Vascular access for hemodialysis-II. Chicago: W.L. Gore & Associates and Precept Press, 1991; 237-45.
17. Duncan MJ, Baldwing, Caralis JP, Cooley DA. Subclavian vein-to-right atrial bypass for symptomatic venous hypertension. Ann Thorac Surg 1991; 52:1342-43.
18. Schwab SJ, Quarles LD, Middleton JP, Cohan RH, Saeed M, Dennis VW. Hemodialysis-associeted subclavian vein stenosis. Kidney Int 1988; 33:1156-59.

19. Mickley V, Görich J, Rillinger N, Stork M, Abendroth D. Stenting of central vein stenosis in hemodialysis patients: Long-term results. Kidney Int 1994; 51:277-80.
20. Polo JR, Sanabia J, Garcia-Sabrido JL, Luño J, Menarguez C, Echenagusia A. Brachial-jugular polytetraflouroethylene fistulas for hemodialysis. Am J Kidney Dis 1990; 16:465-68.
21. McCann RL. Axillary grafts for difficult hemodialysis access. J Vasc Surg 1996; 24:457-62.
22. Polo JR, Sanabia J, Calleja J. Brachial-jugular expanded PTFE grafts for dialysis. In: Henry ML, Ferguson RM eds. Vascular access for hemodialysis-IV. Chicago: W.L. Gore & Associates and Precept Press, 1995; 203-09.
23. Polo JR, Sanabia J, Serantes A, Morales R. Ambulatory surgery for vascular access for hemodialysis. Nephron 1993; 64:323-24.
24. Woodle ES, Knoerzer MP, Newell KA, Hackworth C, Rosenbloom J, Leef J. Stenotic lessions associated with A-V grafts for hemodialysis: Experience with intraoperative ballon angioplasty and postoperative endovascular stent placement. In: Henry ML, Ferguson RM eds. Vascular access for hemodialysis-IV, Chicago: W.L. Gore & Associates Inc and Precept Press, 1995; 169-74.
25. Polo JR, Menarguez MC, Sanabia J, Flores A, Rueda JA, Polo J. Long-term results of 716 grafts for dialysis: Analysis of different graft sizes and configurations. Br J Surg 1999; 85(Suppl 2):4.
26. Polo JR, Polo J, Vega D, Pacheco D, Garcia-Pajares R. Surgical treatment of stenoses and thromboses in dialysis grafts. Dialyse-Journal 1999; 18:242-45.
27. Schuman E, Quinn S, Standage B, Gross G. Thrombolisis versus thrombectomy for occluded hemodialysis grafts. Am J Surg 1994; 167:473-76.
28. Beathard GA Thrombolysis versus surgery for the treatment of thrombosed dialysis access grafts. J Am Soc Nephrol 1995; 6:1619-24.
29. Vesely TM, Idso MC, Audrin J, Windus DW, Lowel JA. Thromboslysis versus surgical thrombectomy for the treatment of dialysis graft thrombosis: Pilot study comparing costs. J Vasc Interv Radiol 1996; 7:507-12.
30. Uflaker R, Rajapopalan PR, Vujic I, Stutley JE. Treatment of thrombosed dialysis access agrafts: Randomized trial of surgical thrombectomy versus mechanical thrombectomy with the Amplatz device. J Vasc Interv Radiol 1996; 7:185-92.
31. Marston WA, Criado E, Jaques PF, Maturo MA, Burnham SJ, Keagy BA. Prospective randomized comparison of surgical versus endovascular management of thrombosed dialysis access grafts. J Vasc Surg 1997; 26:373-80.
32. Dougherty MJ, Calligaro KD, Schinder N, Raviola CA, Ntoso A. Endovascular versus surgical treatment for thrombosed hemodialysis grafts: A prospective, randomized study. J Vasc Surg 1999; 30:1016-23.
33. Palder SB, Kirkman RL, Whitmore AD, Hakim RM, Lazarus JM, Tinley NL. Vascular access for hemodialysis. Patency rates and results of revision. Ann Surg 1985; 202:235-39.
34. Halpin DP, Stack MM, Knoll K, Gaskin TA. Arteriovenous graft salvage in hemodialysis patients. In: Henry ML, Ferguson RM eds. Vascular access for hemodialysis-IV. Chicago, W.L. Gore & Associates and Precept Press; 1995,153-57.

35. Beathard GA, Welch BR, Maidment HJ. Mechanical thrombolysis for the treatment of thrombosed hemodialysis access grafts. Radiology 1996; 200:711-16.
36. Krivitski NM, MacGibbon D, Gleed RD, Dobson A. Accuracy of dilution techniques for access flow meassurement during hemodialysis. Am J Kidney Dis 1998; 31:502-08.
37. Neyra NR, Ikizler TA, May RE, et al. Change in access blood flow over time predicts vascular access thrombosis. Kidney Int 1998; 54:1714-19.
38. Agarwal R, Davis JL. Monitoring interposition graft venous pressure at high blood-flow rates improves sensitivity in predicting graft failure. Am J Kidney Dis 1999; 34:212-17.

DISCUSSION

Panelists:

Thomas Vesely, M.D.
Mitchell L. Henry, M.D.
José R. Polo, M.D.
Alan Lumsden, M.D.
Ted R. Kohler, M.D.
Jeffrey Sands, M.D.
Steven Schwab, M.D.
Brian Hague, M.D.

Discussant: I would like to address a paper that describes the frequent flyers, or patients that are having frequent clotting episodes and separated those patients out from the patients that were having infrequent episodes. Basically when he separated those out from his total group he found that the long-term patency of grafts treated with thrombectomy was comparable to those that just had angioplasty. I wonder if the panel may comment on that?

Dr. Vesely: I reviewed that paper. It is actually a very bad paper. The data analysis did not substantiate a lot of his statements. I would actually disagree with a lot of his things. His concept was great and I think he has anecdotal experience. It is really not supported by appropriate data analysis so really all of his statements he made at that presentation, and he has given that talk several times now, it is strictly anecdotal and needs to be taken in that light. That is all I want to say about that.

Dr. Henry: Well I'll throw in that he really wanted to be here and present that exact data but he had a family conflict. So he was not able to be here.

Discussant: We have all seen a lot of patients, I'm sure, that we have seen huge variations in the amount of the intimal hyperplasia that develops. The graft that Dr. Polo just showed with the patient that has had it for 15 years, I bet those grafts that have been there for ten to 15 years, those particular patients don't really develop the same degree of intimal hyperplasia as the ones that have the failure in 3 months or 2 months. You take those out and they may be filled with that intimal hyperplasia. I wonder if there is any comment as far as why there may be such huge variation among patients like that? I would also like to hear some comments on the nephrology literature using regarding the use of dipyridamole in trying to prevent this.

Discussant: That is a really interesting question. There are very different propensities for this smooth muscle cell proliferative process from species to species, and even within a species. For example, we have noticed in studying carotid intimal hyperplasia following balloon injury, you can see different degrees of response to injury from animals from different vendors. As we all know, there are patients who have a very marked propensity towards this problem, just as patients have a difference in the way they heal scars. Some make keloid, which is a very hyperplastic response, and some scar little at all. John Wolfe looked at this in patients undergoing vein bypass for lower extremity arterial disease. He took segments of unused vein and removed the smooth muscle cells, placed them in culture and gave them a mitogenic stimulus to see how well those smooth muscle cells responded to the stimulus. He found that patients, who had a very robust proliferative response in vitro, also tended to be in the group that had re-stenosis later. There is probably a genetic variance in the propensity for smooth muscle cells to proliferate in response to stimulus or injury. With regard to anti-platelet agents, aspirin was shown way back in the 70s when Scribner shunts came out with sialastic external dialysis access techniques. Aspirin was shown in a *New England Journal of Medicine* article to improve patency in those devices. Most of the patients are on aspirin now, but I am not aware of any good studies showing that anti-platelet agents improve dialysis access. They have been shown following coronary procedures to improve immediate rate of thrombosis, but not to inhibit intimal hyperplasia later on. I am not familiar with dipyridamole or any studies. I wonder if anybody in the panel knows perhaps more than I do?

Dr. Henry: Dipyridamole as a single agent really showed no advantage in long-term outcomes as compared to no treatment at all. There is a question from the floor about whether you use a 6 or 8 mm jump graft, and secondly, how do you do the curettage?

Dr. Polo: For a healthy proximal vein, I use the same size as the graft. Fifty percent of the grafts that I place are upper arm grafts that are 6 to 8 mm. I use the same size of graft for performing the bypass. For the second question, I use 2 small incisions, one on the arterial side, and the other in the vein size to allow the graft to be free from blood flow. I use the uterine curettes. I think it is a very good instrument. I have never broken a graft. I then remove the debris by balloon catheter.

Dr. Henry: We also use routine curettage, and I really think it is valuable, not only in the graft, but gently in the outflow veins. We use a circular pituitary curette rather than a uterine curette.

Dr. Lumsden: I have 2 questions. The first one is for Dr. Kohler. I think you have a fascinating model. One of the things we have done at Emory is look at proliferation in the venous anastomosis in human AV grafts at the time that we revise them. It differs dramatically from the balloon angioplasty model, because even 4 or 5 years later, these grafts are still going. When you are looking at smooth muscle cell proliferation, you have overall proliferation compared with a balloon angioplasty model. That has huge implications in terms of therapy. I was interested in your comments about initial smooth muscle cell suppression. Clearly, that may apply in a balloon angioplasty type model, but I am interested in your thoughts on how we are going to tackle the venous anastomotic intimal hyperplasia. It is just a different, much more aggressive model than we are going to get elsewhere. I would be surprised if 1-time therapy rather than on-going therapy is going to have any influence.

Dr. Kohler: That is an obvious, very important point, that there is ongoing injury in this dialysis access model, where as a lot of experimental models are a 1-time injury. So, any method that we are going to use to suppress that ongoing injury has to be ongoing as well. There are various methods that are being devised to try to deliver ongoing therapy. You are probably aware of Steve Hanson's infusion device that can deliver agents into the boundary layer along the inner surface of the graft over a period of time. There are various methods to be tried locally which have slow release. You may envision injecting things over time or using brachy-radiation therapy over time. One thing with the increased porosity of grafts-we are experimenting with actually seeding those devices with transduced smooth muscle cells, so you have a way of biologically delivering either an anti-proliferative or anti-thrombotic agent over time.

Dr. Vesely: Did you go to the SCBR meeting? It was about a month ago, and the day before the meeting started, there was an entire day on gene therapy, brachytherapy, sort of new technologies in endovascular treatment. I was actually extremely disappointed with how this stuff is working for vascular access. Brachy-therapy, burning it just doesn't work. The one thing that sticks out in mind has to do with exactly what you were talking about. At the time of the surgical creation of the anastomosis, they take an antiproliferative and they wrap the anastomosis in it. That was decreasing smooth muscle migration into it. Honestly, from all of the techniques that were being advertised that day, that seemed to be the best.

Dr. Lumsden: And now for the second, more controversial question. A recurring theme has been graft monitoring and prophylactic intervention. That has been proposed as a national policy. That is very expensive. Where is the level 1 data to support all of the contentions, whether it is balloon angioplasty or surgical revision, that it is the cost effective way of prolonging graft patency?

Dr. Kohler: Well, we know, you are very knowledgeable. You are aware of the data as much as we are.

Dr. Lumsden: That is why I am setting you up to answer these questions.

Dr. Kohler: As you know, that is the feeling, because there are a lot of little pieces, when they are all put together, that is leading us to believe that is the truth. Is there a study that proves it? No. It is hard for me personally to discount a lot of the work that has been done. Because the reality is, in my own program, when the dialysis people do very heavy duty graft surveillance, and we do a lot of angioplasties, our patency rates increase. When we cannot fund the graft surveillance anymore, and it drops off, all I do are thrombectomies. It is anecdotal, I agree, but...

Dr. Lumsden: I agree with you. It seems logical. But, to propose that we study every dialysis patient across the nation without having that data also seems equally absurd to me, quite frankly. The study we published clearly has its flaws, but in 32 patients that we treated, we charged over half a million dollars to achieve almost no improvement in patency. You are advocating something that is unbelievably expensive based upon very little data. That is my concern. It may be the right thing to do, but I don't know if we have the data to support doing that across the country at the moment.

Dr. Henry: Well, you also know that there are other single-center studies and single individual studies that show exactly the opposite, that there are actually improvements in care of long-term patency rate and decreased costs. The real question you are asking is do we have a multi-center national study that is going to show that, and it is clearly not currently available. Now, the NIH just recently had out some RFPs, which I have not had privy to, and hopefully within those there are people that have made some attempts to quantify those issues. You are right, it has not been done.

Dr. Kohler: There is no better forum than this to put that kind of project together.

Dr. Sands: Alan and I have known each other for a long time. I think it is a national disgrace that we spend billions of dollars on care and do not devote the kind of money to research to make any kind of rational decisions and so we have all of these little studies and we can debate about what is best. I am a monitoring guy, as you know, but it is embarrassing to stand up here and not have that data.

Dr. Sands: I wonder if you would comment on the variability in access flow measurement week to week, month to month, and in the same patients, and its implications on false positive readings or negative angiography, and what that implies for patients.

Dr. Henry: You probably know that data better than I do, because you follow it very closely as well. Clearly, there are physiologic changes in cross-sectional areas that are going to improve or decrease flow. Cardiac output, for example, on a particular day is going to change the flow in your graft. That is why studies over sequential time periods are really important to measure, and you do not do it once or twice, but you try to follow it very carefully over time. Again, single-center studies have shown that it is quite advantageous, and that between a majority of the time, you can find a significant stenosis of patients that have decreasing flows with whatever measurement you want to look at, particularly either duplex or intra-access flow monitoring.

Dr. Sands: That is exactly my concern. Let's say, at best, you have an 80% sensitivity and 80% specificity. That means that if your program goes to angiogram, 20 times out of 100, you are doing a study that is unnecessary. If you have significant residual GFR, and you start giving these people dye, we may be doing these people a disservice. Aside from the amount of money you are going to spend doing negative angiograms. I wonder if other people are seeing that kind of issue.

Discussant: Sort of a side thought on that. Something we have learned that I think is extremely interesting with the blood flow stuff. It kind of points to what you are talking about. What we do is do blood flow measurements ahead of time, get them upstairs, do an angiogram, and 80% of the time we find or treat a problem. That leads us to study native inflow arteries. For every fistulogram that we do now, I run a catheter up to the arch and actually shoot all the arteries coming down. Where most people have been lead to believe that about 5% or less than 5% of problems are arterial inflow problems, we are at nearly 25%. It is a whole new paradigm. I have elderly black diabetics, and so I find FMD not irregularly. I am finding all of these inflow arterial problems that I have been ignoring for the last 10 years. Your concern about dye is not insignificant, but as a caveat to that there is ionic and non-ionic dye. The patent just went off of non-ionic dye, so we use that almost exclusively now since there is so little cost difference compared to regular dye. Maybe you could try to convince your radiologists to use non-ionic dye, which is more renal friendly, and much cheaper than it used to be.

Dr. Henry: I tend to agree with you about the arterial inflow abnormalities, although you have to be careful that just an anatomic abnormality by angiography may not actually identify that it is a significant physiologic abnormality. But my bias is that you are right, we need to look a little bit more carefully at that.

Discussant: At the San Diego VA, we have been very impressed with physical exam and angioplasty can actually preserve the lifetime of both fistulas and grafts extremely well, and that physical exam provides a good exam of monitoring. In my view, a procedure of 30 to 45 minutes from the angiographer once every 3 to 9 months, ought to be viewed as expected maintenance of a graft. I think we need to make an appeal for 4 levels of definitions: primary patency, assisted primary patency, secondary patency-meaning a second operating room procedure, and group 4 is the truly failed vascular access that needs to be abandoned until this type of 4 different analyses takes place. I think we will not have either a clinical or cost-effective analysis of these interventions. My plea is that definitions and follow-up need to be slightly more complicated-we need 4 channels, not 2. Primary and secondary patency is no longer good enough.

Dr. Vesely: I agree with you. There is also another question that someone from the audience has added: Why do we not standardize nomenclature and definitions in dialysis access quality review? In actuality, that has been done. Our society, The Society of Cardiovascular and Interventional Radiology, has done that, and has now published standards of publication for vascular access cases. They were published 2 or 3 months ago in the *Journal of Vascular and Interventional Radiology*. For anyone who is interested in this sort of thing, or are writing on this subject, I strongly suggest that you get a copy of these standards. They are really quite good. It is what the vascular surgeons asked us radiologists to do 5 years ago. We standardized the data.

Dr. Henry: The SVS also has a paper on that.

Discussant: It was recommended that we do monthly graft surveillance. How do we get reimbursed for that?

Dr. Henry: You don't.

Dr. Kohler: You are right. HCFA is working on it. The Transonics are free. Actually doing it is free. Once you purchase it, there are no more costs except labor. We almost have a full-time person doing it. It looks like HCFA will probably reimburse for it, hopefully by the end of this year.

Dr. Henry: It is a little bit like electrocautery devices, as long as you use the pens that are attached to it, they will give you the machine.

Discussant: A comment about graft blood flow monitoring. It is true that a graft with a low blood flow is much more likely to thrombose. It is also true that a graft with a large decrease in blood flow is much more likely to thrombose. But, generally, we find that half the grafts that thrombose do not have a low blood flow, and half do not have any significant decrease in blood flow. We think that we have a long way to go before we can predict graft thrombosis with acceptable accuracy. I think there are some implications about national implementation of graft monitoring programs. I wonder if you would comment on that.

Dr. Vesely: There are 5 pretty decent papers written on the use of blood flow for following these. Although they acknowledge the fact that patients who have high blood flows do thrombose, the majority of the time, those would not match yours. Most of these are fairly predictive of impending graft thrombosis, although it is not exact. It is still the best method. You probably should be using something.

Dr. Schwab: I think the concept of prospective monitoring is something that the DOQI dealt with in 1997 and 2000. The DOQI guidelines were charged with evaluating the preponderance and the weight of the evidence. You are right; there was no randomized, prospective, single, multi-centered trial. But when you look at practice guidelines in cardiology, pulmonary, critical care and indeed, surgery, there are precious few randomized, multi-centered, prospective clinical trials that define the way we practice. In the practice guidelines dealing with monitoring, in the 2000 edition, 26 prospective trials, all single-centered trials, were evaluated. Twenty-four of the 26 showed a substantial and significant benefit from prospective monitoring. Two studies showed no significant benefit from prospective monitoring. It was the unanimous opinion of the committee that 24 out of 26 endorsed the concept that prospective monitoring improves access patency. The way you monitor is more difficult, but the weight of the evidence is moving, as you suggested, toward flows, and the 2000 guidelines will basically say that if you look at the studies that are out there now, the majority of the single-centered studies published in the literature suggest that flows are most sensitive in fistulas and grafts in terms of evaluating patency.

The other comment that swayed the committee was the fact that the data on prospective monitoring comes from the United States, Europe, and Asia. So, the preponderance of the evidence comes from 3 different continents and suggests that prospective monitoring, when combined with prospective intervention, improves patency of both fistulas and grafts. The committee came down heavily in the practice guidelines that prospective monitoring, based on the preponderance of the evidence, is the way we should go.

Discussant: Tom, I just wanted to confirm what you were saying about the arterial inflow. I think that the arterial inflow is the ignored part of the access. We reported in the last ASN that in our experience, that there was a 40% incidence of arterial inflow problems. We included the native feeding artery, the arterial anastomosis, and the segment of the graft in front of the arterial needle. We found that because the pre- and post-intervention access flow measurements would improve after we would angioplasty the outflow, it would prompt us to go back and look at the inflow. We would see maybe a little pinch, and feel that was significant, so we would angioplasty that and flow would go up significantly. A quick comment about Dr. Polo's good talk. I thought I heard you implying that intra-graft and inflow lesions need to be treated with surgery. We find those lesions are very amenable to percutaneous intervention.

Discussant: Another question for Dr. Polo. I noticed that you did not make any comment about steal syndromes. You talked about 6- to 8-mm grafts, and we know that Dr. Lumsden is going to talk to us about step grafts. Either your population is a lot different than ours, or we are not doing something right because those size grafts would lead to steal syndrome problems. Do you have any comment regarding that?

Dr. Polo: I have performed about 300 cases of 6 to 8 upper arm brachioaxillary grafts. In the first 150 cases, about 5% had steal syndrome. I had to use banding to a more narrow part of the graft at 5 mms more or less. Then, because of that experience, I avoided putting this kind of graft in patients over 65 years old and diabetics, because it is worse in these 2 populations. In young people, this type of 6- to 8-mm graft is perfect. Probably with 8-mm grafts, you can avoid one of the most important part of stenosis which is significant mid-graft stenosis. On the other hand, an 8-mm graft is easier to puncture by the nurses and with fewer complications. Currently, I avoid using this type of graft in 65 years old and diabetics.

Dr. Henry: Dr. Vesely, there are several questions up here that ask at what point do you give up on angioplasty and lesion multiple times over a long period of time?

Dr. Vesely: That is a tough question, and my thoughts on this are in the minority compared to several of my other colleagues in the room. I tend to give up fairly early. Luc Turmel-Rodrigues, as well as Dr. Beathard in his landmark paper in 1992 showed that repeated angioplasty has equivalent patency. In other words, your second and third angioplasty of the venous anastomosis should have about the same patency. In my data, we published a paper that actually showed that there is decreasing patency with each subsequent angioplasty of the same lesion. Our results showed that after that second angioplasty, the results of the third and fourth are really pretty lousy. So, we will angioplasty 2 or 3 times. I could show you picture after picture, case after case, that show once you angioplasty, the next time it comes back it is more aggressive. It comes back nastier and longer. But, again, my thoughts are in the minority. There is a lot of data out there that would substantiate that angioplasty after angioplasty is ok. There is really some discourse in the literature with that. Where I automatically send them to my surgeons is when the graft is patent but yet the primary venous outflow is occluded. Now, you may think that does not make sense, but it is not that unusual for the venous outflow vein to be occluded with the graft being kept via collaterals. If a network of collaterals is keeping the graft open, I am done. I cannot do anything with that. If the pressure is 300, that is going to my surgeons, and also very long stenoses. In Dr. Beathard's paper, he was treating and reported on short, medium and long stenoses. He showed that he was getting equivalent results with longer stenoses. I might do it once or twice, but my surgeons are innovative. They are doing as many interesting on vascular access as I am, so I actually trust them. They are doing good, innovative, surgical work on these types of lesions.

Dr. Henry: You are making me nervous, with radiologists trusting surgeons.

Dr. Vesely: We should all work together, and we do. That is why I trust them. When I think I have given up, I give them to the surgeons.

Dr. Hague: We have developed a very complicated patient-driven algorithm in our hospital to manage these grafts. I thought I would share it with you. When the nephrologist finds out at 7 o'clock in the morning that a patient has clotted, he calls his secretary. The secretary then calls the radiology department and says, "When can you get to this graft?" She writes that number down and then calls my secretary and says, "When can Dr. Hague get to this graft?" Then she picks the smallest number, that is about how it seems. Alan has opened a wonderful topic that needs a lot of discussion, but I think there are 2 real issues here that we could solve that would not cost millions of dollars. The reason I say that is because by the time I see most of these people for access, they already have already been in the hospital, they already have a perma-cath in place, and frequently, they have already had one episode of staph sepsis before I am ever called to see them. As a surgeon, I would like to see diabetics in my office with a creatione of 4 or 5. Then we are going to get fistulas in these people. The other point I want to make is that when DOQI came out, I kind of thought that I was not very important. But, my behavior has changed as a surgeon because while I thought I was doing as many fistulas as I possibly could, but I do not think I really was. In our institution, we are doing more upper arm fistulas. These are 2 cheap things that will not cost this country another 12 billion dollars. When this started, years ago, it was about 70 million. Now it is about 12 billion. So, I think that early referral from nephrologists and surgeons being honest with themselves about fistulas will save a lot of money.

SECTION II

5

PATENCY AND SURVIVAL OF PRIMARY ARTERIOVENOUS FISTULAE

Arun D. Pherwani, M.S., D.N.B., F.R.C.S., F.R.C.S.I., Julie A. Reid, M.R.C.S., and John K. Connolly, F.R.C.S.I.

The Dialysis Outcomes Quality Initiative (DOQI) guidelines recommended that at least 40% of prevalent dialysis accesses should be provided through native arteriovenous fistulae (AVF).[1] The literature suggests that wrist or elbow AV fistulae are the preferred type of access due to excellent patency, lower complication rates, and lower morbidity.[1-3] The guidelines, however, fail to make any recommendations regarding targets for patency rates in AVF. Specifically, it recommended that primary patency rates should not be used as an indicator of quality to encourage fistula construction in higher risk patients.

The Regional Nephrology and Hemodialysis Unit at the Belfast City Hospital in Northern Ireland has a hemodialysis population of approximately 400 patients. Our policy is to create primary AV fistulae in all patients referred for vascular access procedures. This is a study evaluating the primary patency and overall survival of these AV fistulae.

Patients and Methods

Data were collected from 276 patients with 313 primary AV fistulae created from January 1997 to June 1999. The minimum follow-up period was 6 months with a mean follow-up of 18 months. Fistulae occlusion from all causes (eg, a failing fistula, inadequacy for dialysis requiring revision, or death of the patient) were used as endpoints of follow-up, and determinations of fistula survival. Primary patency was defined as the time until first thrombosis or inadequacy for dialysis.

Pre-operative assessment was through evaluation of clinical history and examination. Allen's test was performed to assess the status of the palmar arch. A standard distal to proximal approach was followed with regards to placing of the fistula. However, the elbow fistula was used preferentially in patients with sub-optimal vessels at the wrist as detected by clinical examination. All fistulae were created under local anesthesia as day cases. Standard vascular surgical techniques were used to create side-to-end radiocephalic fistulae at the wrist or side-to-end brachial artery, to either the median cubital, cephalic, or basilic vein at the elbow. All patients received intra-operative intravenous heparin (2000 IU) to prevent peri-operative thrombosis. Patency of the draining vein was confirmed by passage of a 6 French feeding tube with instillation of heparinised saline. Patients were followed up and data retrospectively entered into a database.

Data on the patient's age, sex, diabetes status, and site of fistula were subjected to univariate analysis. Actuarial survival was calculated using the Kaplan-Meier survival analysis, and differences between groups compared by log-rank tests. Statistical significance was obtained using the chi-square test. SurvanXL (copyright S.G. Shering, 1995-1997) was used to plot survival curves that assessed the influence of variables such as age, gender, site of fistula, and diagnosis of diabetes to primary patency.

Results

A total of 313 fistulae were created in 276 patients. Of these, 202 were in men and 111 were in women. The mean age was 58 ± 0.95 years (range 18 to 95 years of age). Fifty percent of men (n=101), and 58% of women (n=64) were over 60 years of age. Of the 313 fistulae, 123 were wrist fistulae and 190 were sited at the elbow. The causes of renal failure are shown in table 5-1. Ninety-seven patients (31%) had an AV fistula created prior to the onset of hemodialysis.

There were a total of 78 failures (25%) throughout the follow-up period. Of these, 36 were early failures, occurring within 30 days, of which 24 (66%) were determined to have little prospect of success at operation. Patients with poor arterial inflow or stenosed or occluded venous outflow were counted as primary patency failures. The

Table 5-1. Etiology of Renal Failure

Cause of Renal Failure	Percent of Study Patients
Glomerulonephritis	20
Diabetes mellitus	18
Chronic pyelonephritis	12
Renovascular hypertension	8
Polycystic renal disease	5
Other	5
Unknown/uncertain aetiology	32

30-day failure rate was 8% (n=16) for elbow fistulae and 18% (n=20) for wrist fistulae. Overall, 41 (22%) of 190 elbow fistulae and 37 (30%) of 123 wrist fistulae failed.

During the follow-up period, 70 (22%) patients died, 53 of whom were aged 60 years or older. Of the 70 deaths, 61 patients died with a functioning fistula. The overall primary patency rates obtained were 77% at 1 year, 72% at 2 years and 69% at 3 years.

Age. Primary patency in patients aged less than 60 years or less was 73%, 69%, and 69% at 1, 2, and 3 years, compared with 81%, 74% and 69%, respectively, in patients 60 years of age or above (P=0.20). Of the 148 fistulae created in patients under 60 years of age, the majority (53%) were created at the wrist, but in patients 60 years of age or above, 70% (n=101) of the 165 fistulae were created at the elbow. In patients less than 60 years of age there were 17 deaths (11%). There were 53 (32%) deaths in patients 60 years of age or more.

Gender. Women in the study had significantly worse outcomes than men. Primary patency rates at 1, 2, and 3 years were 82%, 78%, and 78% for men compared with 68%, 60%, and 54%, respectively, for women (P=0.0036). Of the 202 fistulae in male patients, 56% (n=114) were created at the elbow, and 44% (n=88) at the wrist. In contrast, of the 111 fistulae created in female patients, 68% (n=76) were created at the elbow, and only 32% (n=35) were created at the wrist. Over the study period, the death rates for men and women were comparable (23% in men versus 20% in women). The influence of age and gender on fistula survival is shown in figure 5-1. Elderly women in particular were associated with the poorest outcomes.

Site. There was no significant difference in the primary patency rates of elbow and wrist fistulae, 81%, 75%, and 71% for elbow fistulae, compared with 71%, 67%, and 67% at 1, 2 and 3 years, respectively (P=0.089). Of the 190 elbow fistulae created, the majority, 121 (64%) were in patients over 60 years of age, whereas the majority (n=79, 64%) of the 123 wrist fistulae were in patients under 60 years of age. In all, 28% (n=54) of patients with elbow fistulae died compared with 13%

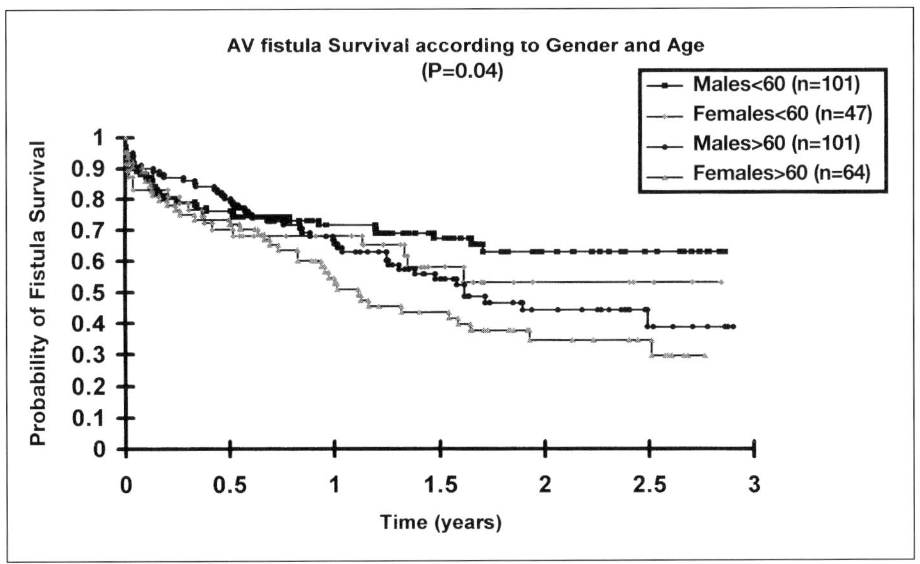

Figure 5-1. Life table analysis of AV fistula survival based on age and gender.

(n=16) of patients with wrist fistulae. Site of fistulae placement had no apparent influence on fistula survival, as seen in figure 5-2.

Diabetes. Eighteen percent (n=56) of patients were affected by diabetes mellitus. In this group, there were 17 failures and 17 deaths. The primary patency rates obtained for diabetics were 70% at 1 year, 62% at 2 years, and 61% at 3 years compared with 79%, 74%, and 69% in nondiabetics, respectively (P=0.18). Elbow fistulae accounted for 63% (n=35) of fistulae in this group, while only 37% (n=21) were created at the wrist. The death rate among diabetics was 30% (17 of 56), compared

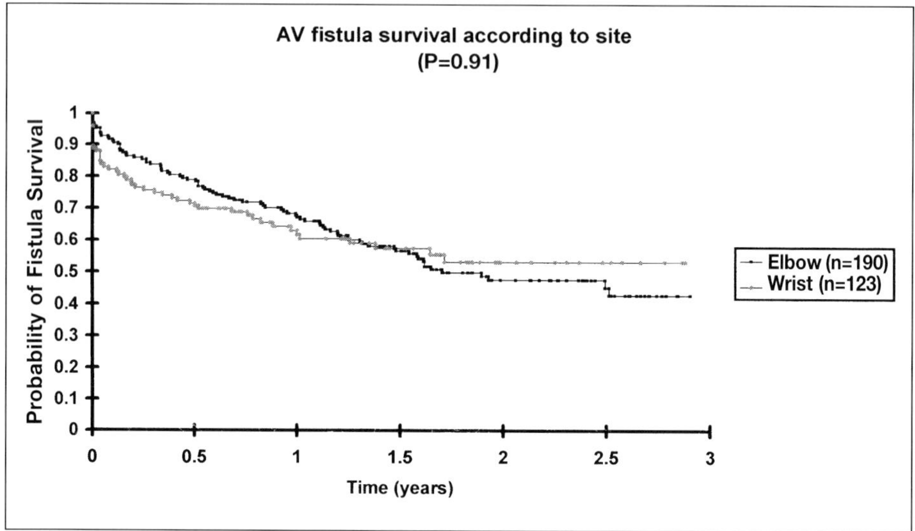

Figure 5-2. Life table analysis of the effect of site on overall AV fistulae survival.

with 21% (53 of 257) among nondiabetics. Patients with diabetes also had a fistula survival rate significantly worse than nondiabetics (P=0.05), as seen in figure 5-3.

Discussion

Access creation is not just a technical exercise. Accesses should be trouble-free and suit the individual patient, because survival of the patient is dependent on the quality of dialysis. Factors that affect the quality of dialysis (eg, prolonged use of central venous catheters, failed surgical procedures, recirculation and poor flow related to venous stenoses, and quality of life with repeated admissions for thrombectomy, declotting, or treatment of sepsis) are directly related to the type of access created. Provision of satisfactory dialysis from suitable access has indirect effects on control of hypertension, erythropoietin (EPO) resistant anemia, and development of bone disease.

Native AV fistulae are associated with excellent patency, lower complication rates, and lower morbidity, providing high flows for high-flux dialysis. This has

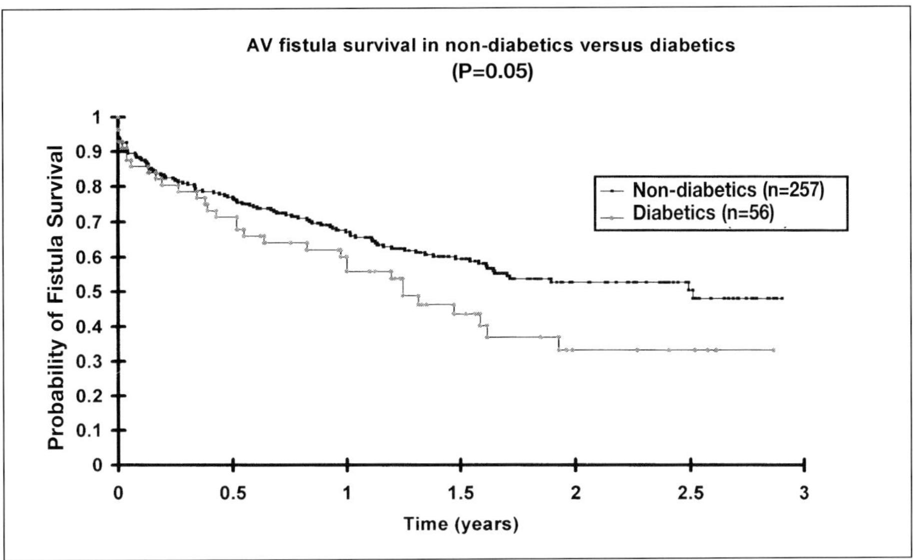

Figure 5-3. Life table analysis of the effect of diabetes on overall AV fistulae survival.

been well understood and the DOQI guidelines recommend that at least 40% of dialysis accesses should be provided by native AV fistulae.[1] However, the guidelines fail to make any recommendations regarding targets for patency rates in AV fistulae. Specifically, they recommend that primary patency rates should not be used as an indicator of quality, in order to encourage fistulae construction in high-risk patients.

Conventional methods of reporting outcomes with fistulae take into account factors such as primary patency, assisted primary patency, secondary patency, and cumulative patency. These terms, however, do not provide a true indication of survival rates, as these figures fail to address the main problem associated with high-risk patients (ie, the high mortality in this patient population). Rather than reporting primary patency alone, therefore, we have estimated fistula survival. This takes into account both failures recognized at the time of operation and those due to death of the patient. The significance of this concept is that resources should be directed toward maximizing the AV fistulae proportion in patients deemed to have the greatest prospect of long-term survival.

The results we obtained in this study support this claim. During the study period, almost a quarter of the study patients died. Operative failures accounted for two thirds of early failures and in each case the cause was determined, either due to poor arterial inflow or stenosed or occluded venous outflow. These factors could have been excluded, or patients offered a more appropriate procedure, if selection was not based purely on clinical examination. Improved pre-operative methods of assessing the vasculature and better patient selection could identify those patients in whom long-term life expectancy is poor or those who are likely to fail immediately. This is illustrated in figure 5-4, which shows primary patency excluding deaths and operative failures. Slight improvement of our overall primary patency rates to 80% at 1 year, 74% at 2 years, and 71% at 3 years are achievable goals. Alternative forms of vascular access, such as central venous catheters, could be

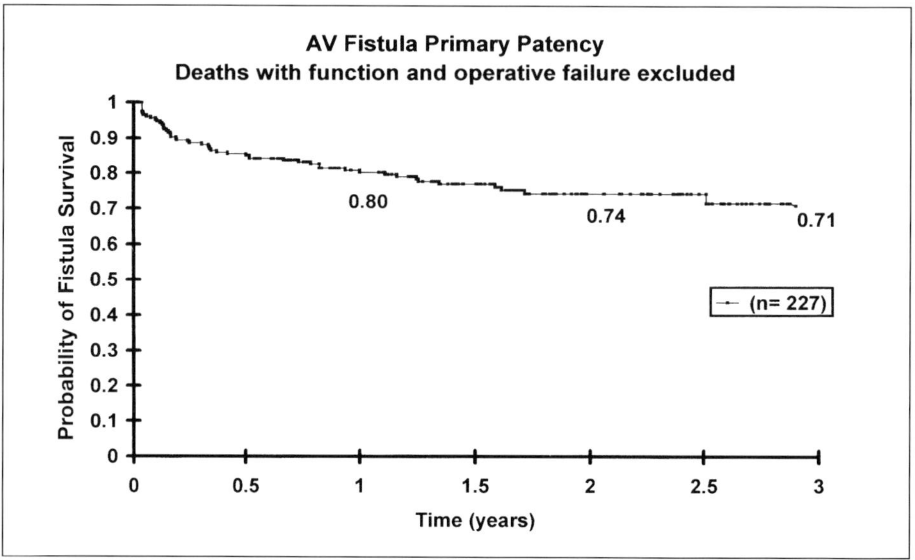

Figure 5-4. Life table analysis showing achievable patency rates of AV fistulae, excluding death with a functional fistula and those that failed at the time of the operation.

preferentially used, freeing resources to create more AV fistulae in patients approaching dialysis with end-stage renal failure. Not only would this improve primary patency rates as shown, but perhaps more importantly, this would improve survival rates with fistulae and would also increase the proportion of patients commencing dialysis with a functioning fistula (31%).

These results compared well with reported patency rates for wrist and elbow fistulae. Initial failure rates of 8% to 30% with 1 year primary patency rates from 48% to 76%, and 2 year primary patency rates from 24% to 67% have been reported for wrist fistulae.[4-7] The 30-day failure rate in our series was 18% for wrist fistulae, with primary patency rates of 71%, 67%, and 67% at 1, 2, and 3 years respectively. Early failure rates of 5% to 12%, and primary patency rates of 75% to 93% at 1 year, 63% to 80% at 2 years, and 53% to 80% at 3 years have been reported for elbow fistulae.[7-9] The 30 day failure rate in our series was 8% for elbow fistulae. Primary patency rates were 81%, 75%, and 71% at 1, 2, and 3 years respectively.

The primary patency rates obtained for older patients were better than those seen in younger patients. Without a doubt, this is because significantly more elbow fistulae were created than wrist fistulae in the older patients. Several series have demonstrated poorer outcomes in older patients with the wrist fistula as the site of access.[5,6] This was not meant to be a comparison of the site of access with age. Instead, it demonstrated that it is possible to achieve good primary patency rates in older patients, with the elbow fistula used as the preferred site.[10] Not surprisingly, fistulae survival rates were worse in older patients because of their higher death rate.

Female patients, particularly elderly women, did poorly compared with men, both in terms of primary patency and survival of fistulae, a feature reported in other series.[4,5,10] This is despite greater use of the elbow fistula in women as suggested by Miller and colleagues.[10]

Our findings in diabetics are in contrast to reported findings.[4-6] We were able to obtain comparable primary patency rates in diabetics and nondiabetics. However, there was a definite trend of worse fistulae survival in diabetics, approaching statistical significance. There are 3 reasons for this. First, there are relatively smaller numbers of patients with diabetes as a cause of end-stage renal disease in the United Kingdom. Second, the higher proportion of fistulae created in diabetics were elbow fistulae,[10] and third, the higher death rates in diabetics compared with nondiabetics.

We have demonstrated that it is possible to achieve good primary patency rates with AV fistulae in an unselected patient group. These findings support the use of the elbow AV fistula in the older patient population, female patients, patients with diabetes, and in patients with previous damage to the veins at the wrist.[7-10] The concept of reporting fistulae survival is unique but is important, given the poor long-term survival of patients with end-stage renal disease.

References

1. NKF-DOQI clinical practice guidelines for hemodialysis adequacy. National Kidney Foundation. Am J Kidney Dis 1997; (3 Suppl 2):S15-66.
2. Burkhart HM, Cikrit DF. Arteriovenous fistulae for hemodialysis. Semin Vasc Surg 1997; 10:162-65.
3. Connolly JK. Vascular access surgery. In: Essential surgical practice-II 2000. Cuscheri A, Steele R, Moosa AR, eds. Woburn, Mass: Butterworth-Heinemann (In press).
4. Golledge J, Smith CJ, Emery J, Farrington K, Thompson HH. Outcome of primary radiocephalic fistula for hemodialysis. Br J Surg 1999; 86:211-16.
5. Leapman SB, Boyle M, Pescovitz MD, Milgrom ML, Jindal RM, Filo RS. The arteriovenous fistula for hemodialysis access: Gold standard or archaic relic? Am J Surg 1996; 62:652-57.
6. Prischl FC, Kirchgatterer A, Brandstatter E, et al. Parameters of prognostic relevance to the patency of vascular access in hemodialysis patients. J Am Soc Nephrol 1995; 6:1613-18.
7. Bender MH, Bruyninckx CM, Gerlag PG. The brachiocephalic elbow fistula: A useful alternative angioaccess for primary hemodialysis. J Vasc Surg 1995; 20:808-13.
8. Gessaroli M, Faggioli GL, Freyrie A, Gargiulo M. Regarding "the brachiocephalic elbow fistula: A useful alternative angioaccess for primary hemodialysis". J Vasc Surg 1995; 22:195-96.
9. Elcheroth J, de Pauw L, Kinnaert P. Elbow arteriovenous fistulas for chronic hemodialysis. Br J Surg 1994; 81:982-84.
10. Miller PE, Tolwani A, Luscy CP, et al. Predictors of adequacy of arteriovenous fistulas in hemodialysis patients. Kidney Int 1999; 56:275-80.

6

VENO-VENOUS BYPASS OF CENTRAL VEIN OCCLUSIONS FOR SALVAGING HEMODIALYSIS GRAFTS AND FISTULAE: LONG-TERM RESULTS

David E. Morris, M.D., Petros V. Anagnostopoulos, M.D., Iraklis I. Pipinos, M.D., Francisco S. Escobar III, M.D., and Marwan S. Abouljoud, M.D.

Most patients on hemodialysis will at some time require the placement of a central venous catheter for hemodialysis access. Central vein stenosis or occlusion is a common complication and has been reported to occur in 11% to 46% of the patients who undergo catheterizations.[1-3] Although some stenoses or occlusions remain asymptomatic, the subsequent placement of an ipsilateral arteriovenous fistula (AVF) or arteriovenous graft (AVG) may unmask in an extremity previously unrecognized central vein lesions, creating venous hypertension in that extremity.

Venous hypertension may manifest clinically as edema of the hand, forearm, or arm with throbbing of the affected extremity, formation of collateral vasculature over the upper arm and chest wall, and prolonged bleeding from the hemodialysis access site. Furthermore, patients may experience repeated episodes of AVF or AVG thrombosis. Until relatively recently, the most common treatment for these manifestations has been ligation of the AVF or AVG.[4,5] There is, however, a segment of the hemodialysis population that dies each year due to lack of vascular access and any additional patency that might be preserved at a given access site is therefore desirable.

Although central vein lesions proximal to an existing AVF or AVG have been addressed surgically[4-6], endovascular approaches have become more attractive as an initial approach. Percutaneous transluminal angioplasty (PTA) of central vein stenoses have good initial results but the recurrence rate of the lesions is high. Shoenfeld reported a 62% restenosis rate at 17 months[7], and others have reported an approximately 66% restenosis rate at 1 year after PTA.[8,9]

Percutaneous intravascular stenting of central lesions has improved long-term patencies over PTA alone. Shoenfeld has reported 68% and 93% primary and secondary patencies, respectively, at 17 months after PTA with stenting of central vein lesions.[7] Using the absence of clinical symptoms with a functioning AVF or AVG in the ipsilateral upper extremity as an endpoint, Bhattia reported a 71% 1 year success rate after PTA with stenting.[10]

Multiple approaches to the operative reconstruction of central vein stenoses or occlusions have been described.[4-6,10,11] Post-operative patency and subsequent interventions required to maintain the patency of such reconstructions, however, are not well described. This study will review our patencies and subsequent interventions with extrathoracic veno-venous bypass grafts (VVBGs) to salvage AVFs and AVGs with central vein lesions.

Patients and Methods

Between March 1994 and April 1999, 8 hemodialysis patients (2 women, 6 men) of average age 55.2 years (range 32 to 71 years) developed signs of upper extremity venous hypertension in the extremity containing a functioning AVF or AVG (table 6-1). Four patients underwent venography with endovascular therapy (PTA with or without stenting), but later developed recurrent lesions that were not amenable to further endovascular treatment. In 4 patients, initial venography revealed an occlusive lesion that could not be crossed with angiocatheters (table 6-2). These 8 patients underwent operative reconstruction to bypass their central vein occlusions.

Surgical technique. VVBGs extended from the cephalic or axillary vein (distal anastomosis) to the ipsilateral internal jugular, contralateral internal jugular, or the

Table 6-1. Demographic data for patients undergoing VVBG.

Patient	Age (y)	Sex	ESRD DX	HD Access Site
1	32	F	GN	right wrist fistula
2	52	M	HTN	left elbow fistula
3	46	M	HTN	right forearm graft
4	36	M	DM	left elbow fistula
5	67	M	HTN	right forearm fistula
6	71	M	DM	right elbow fistula
7	70	M	HTN	left elbow fistula
8	67	F	HTN	right forearm graft
	Avg 55	F 25%	GN=1	Fistulae=6
			HTN=5	Grafts=2
			DM=2	

Table 6-2. Endovascular interventions for venous hypertension prior to placement of a VVBG.

Patient Number	Number of Prior HD Accesses	Time from Access Placement to V-V Bypass (months)	Prior Endovascular Therapy
1	3	14	PTA & Stent
2	1	2	PTA Only
3	2	3	PTA & Stent
4	0	37	None (Occluded veins)
5	0	55	None (Occluded veins)
6	0	15	None (Occluded veins)
7	0	22	None (Occluded veins)
8	1	53	PTA Only
	Avg 0.9	Avg 25.1	Endo Rx 50%
			Occluded Veins 50%

contralateral axillary vein (table 6-3). These extrathoracic VVBG were performed under general anesthesia followed by a 1 to 3 day in-patient stay. Patients were not routinely treated with anticoagulation or antiplatelet agents.

Axillo-ipsilateral internal jugular veno-venous bypass. An incision was made in the midaxilla and the axillary vein was islolated with vessel loops. The internal jugular vein was approached through a second incision between the sternal and clavicular heads of the sternocleidomastoid muscle. A third incision was made just inferior to the clavicle at its midpoint and the dissection was carried through the pectoralis major along its fibers. Using blunt dissection, a subpectoral tunnel was created between the axillary and infraclavicular incisions. A ringed polytetrafluoroethylene (PTFE) graft was then tunneled from the axillary vein, subpectorally, to the infraclavicular space (figure 6-1). The graft was further

Table 6-3. Sites of VVBGs.

Patient Number	Inflow Vein	Outflow Vein
1	Distal Axillary	Ipsilateral Int. Jugular
2	Proximal Axillary	Ipsilateral Int. Jugular
3	Distal Axillary	Ipsilateral Int. Jugular
4	Cephalic	CONTRALATERAL Int. Jugular
5	Cephalic	Ipsilateral Int. Jugular
6	Cephalic	Ipsilateral Int. Jugular
7	Proximal Axillary	CONTRALATERAL Prox. Axillary
8	Distal Axillary	Ipsilateral Int. Jugular

Notes: 1. Distal axillary is lateral to pectoralis minor muscle (axillary fossa).
2. Proximal axillary is medial to pectoralis minor muscle (chest wall).

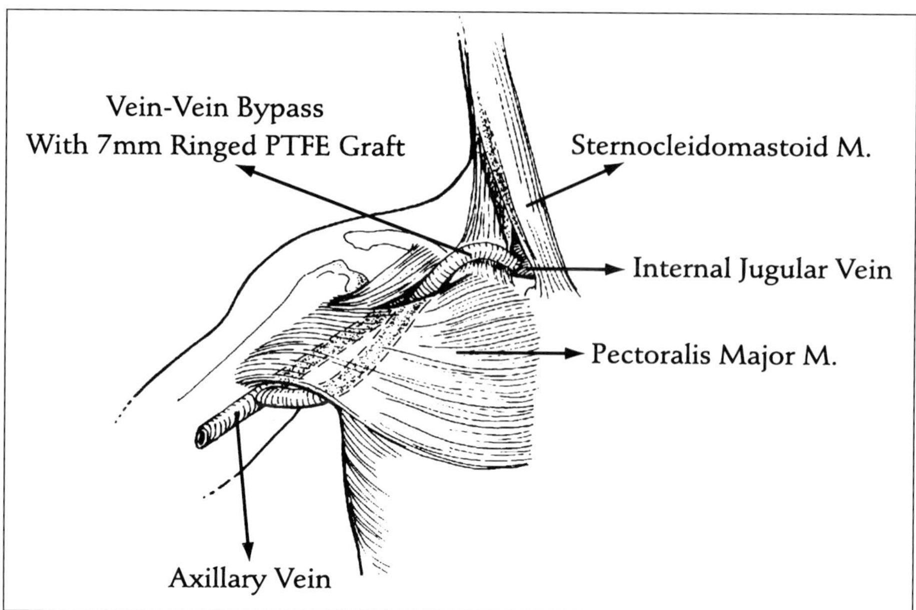

Figure 6-1. Extrathoracic veno-venous bypass of a central vein lesion. The graft extends submuscularly from the right axillary vein to the right internal jugular vein.

tunneled to the internal jugular vein, superficial to the clavicle. Anastomoses between the VVBG and native veins (proximal and distal) were constructed in an end-to-side fashion.

Cephalic-ipsilateral internal jugular veno-venous bypass. The cephalic vein outflow of the AVF or AVG was isolated in the deltopectoral groove or at the distal border of the deltoid. The infraclavicular incision was not needed. The procedure was thus accomplished with 2 incisions.

Cephalic-contralateral internal jugular veno-venous bypass. A subcutaneous tunnel was created for bypass from the cephalic vein to the contralateral internal jugular from isolated cephalic vein, extending over the deltoid, over the ipsilateral clavicle and the sternum and then to the contralateral neck. A single counterincision in the infraclavicular fossa on the side of the cephalic vein was used (3 incisions total).

Axillo-contralateral axillary veno-venous bypass. A horizontal infraclavicular incision was made and the pectoralis major was spread in the direction of its fibers. The pectoralis minor was divided in order to expose the axillary vein. A symmetric incision was accomplished on the contralateral side of the chest. The graft was tunneled between the 2 incisions, superficial to the pectoralis major, using a counterincision on the lower sternum. The ends were directed deep, through the pectoralis major. Each graft end was anastomosed to its corresponding axillary vein using a side-biting clamp.

Graft patency was followed on the grounds of the clinic. New signs or symptoms of venous hypertension were pursued with color duplex ultrasonography or venography. Kaplan-Meier statistics were used to construct primary unassisted and secondary patency curves (SPSS Inc, Chicago, IL).

Results

There were no operative complications and all postoperative courses were uneventful. All patients experienced initial improvement in upper extremity edema. Primary and secondary patencies for individual VVBG appear in table 6-4 with Kaplan-Meier curves in figures 6-2a and 6-2b. Primary (unassisted) and secondary patencies of VVBGs at 1 year using Kaplan-Meier statistics were 44% and 56%, respectively. One patient was lost to follow-up.

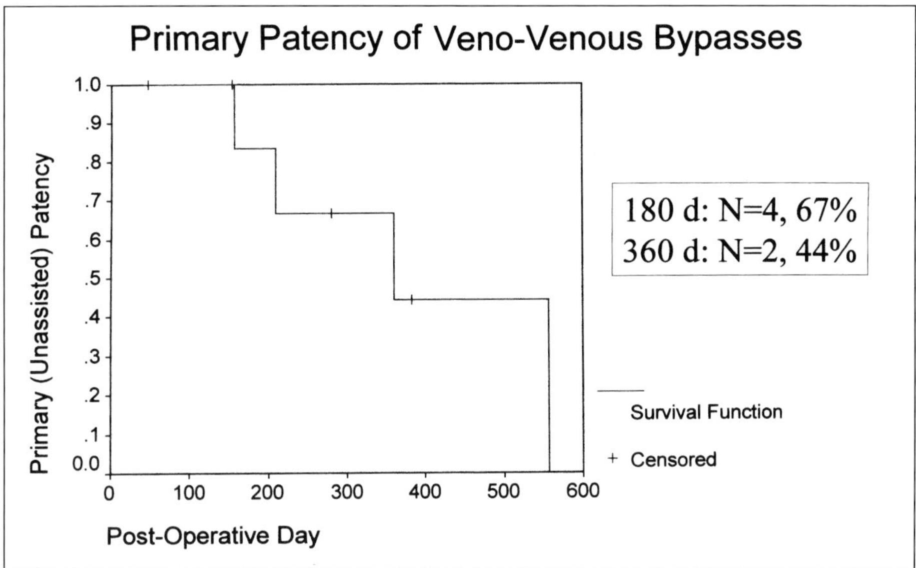

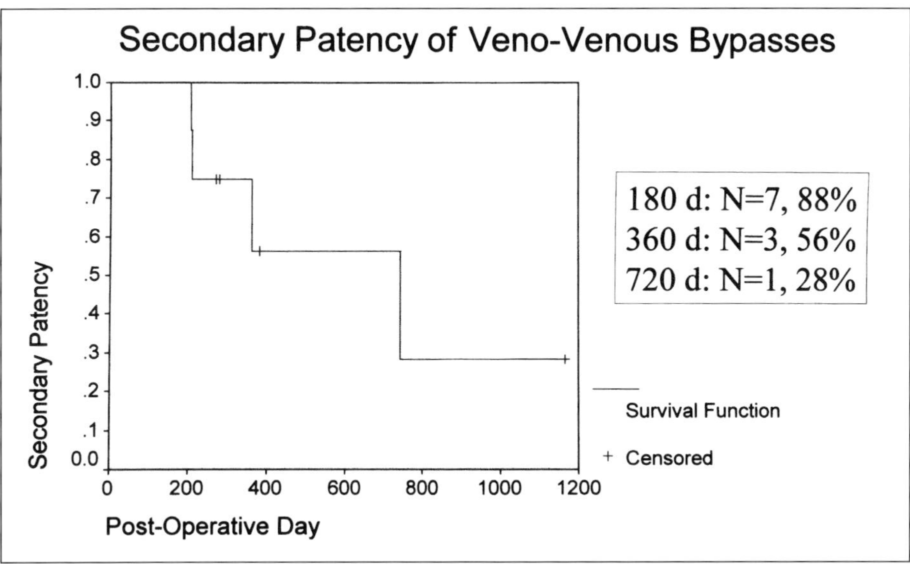

Figures 6-2a and 6-2b. Kaplan-Meier primary (2a) and secondary (2b) patency curves for veno-venous bypass grafts.

Table 6-4. Results of VVBG: raw data and graft information. Mean and median primary and secondary patencies were calculated using Kaplan-Meier statistics.

Patient Number	Primary Patency (days)	Secondary Patency (days)	Comments & Secondary Interventions
1	360	360	Thrombosed
2	154	270	PTA
3	156	204	Revision
4	382	382	Death w/ Patent Bypass
5	280	280	Lost to Follow-up
6	47	1165	Revision
7	209	209	Thrombosed
8	558	741	PTA
Mean	389	655	
Median	360	741	

Interventions to extend patency were done on 4 grafts. Patients No. 2 and No. 8 each had a single PTA, at 5 and 19 months postoperatively, respectively. Six months postoperatively, patient No. 3 had a surgical thrombectomy and endophlebectomy (ie, removal of hyperplasic tissue at the venous anastomosis) of the VVBG with simultaneous thrombectomy of the forearm. Patient No. 6 had 7 subsequent interventions (PTA on 4 occasions and surgical revision on 3 occasions), which extended the life of his graft for 37 months beyond its primary patency.

Discussion

Our initial approach to the patient with an upper extremity AVF or AVG presenting with venous hypertension is venography with PTA and stent placement, if required. Additional therapy with PTA and stenting is often required. Inelastic stenoses or complete occlusions have a worse response to stenting.[10,12] If a patient can tolerate a general anesthetic, extrathoracic VVBG is considered when a guidewire cannot cross the lesion because of near total or complete occlusion, and for endovascular failures, and for patients with anaphylactic dye allergies.

Several surgical approaches to central vein lesions have been advocated, including: a right atrial bypass (from the internal jugular, subclavian, or axillary vein), an internal jugular turndown to the subclavian vein, direct vein repair with a vein or PTFE patch, and extrathoracic veno-venous bypass using a saphenous vein or PTFE conduit.[4-6,10,11,13] We have preferred an extrathoracic approach whenever possible, using the internal jugular as a proximal target. The internal jugular itself must be patent and free of more central lesions (ie, in the superior vena cava or innominate). Unlike a right atrial bypass, which requires a median sternotomy or thoracotomy, this operation was less invasive, because the tunneling was completely extrathoracic. The subpectoral graft position helped to prevent skin erosion over the graft. Using a PTFE conduit, rather than an autogenous vein (ie, internal jugular turndown or saphenous vein), required less operative dissection, no division of the clavicle, and probably less operative time.

As demonstrated in table 6-2, four of the VVBGs in this series were placed to preserve a patient's initial AVF or AVG. We believe that systematically exhausting all access possibilities in a given extremity will ultimately extend the time a patient may undergo hemodialysis. When VVBGs are failing or fail, attempts to salvage them were made, as with any AVF or AVG. This contrasts with surgical procedures done only as a final effort after alternative sites have been depleted.[13]

There are various approaches for anticoagulation of patients who have undergone reconstruction for central vein lesions. Rather than prescribe anticoagulants, we have relied on the inherent platelet dysfunction in this group of patients as a means to help facilitate patency. Other factors that may contribute to higher than expected patencies for grafts in the venous system include a functioning, distal AVF or AVG, and the large size of the inflow and outflow veins.

In conclusion, veno-venous bypass grafting is an effective approach for treating venous hypertension and extending the patency of existing AVFs with minimal morbidity. When the internal jugular and those veins proximal to it are patent, extrathoracic VVBG to the internal jugular or contralateral axillary vein avoids a median sternotomy. VVBG should be considered for patients who have failed endovascular interventions or central vein occlusions.

References

1. Schwab SJ, Quarles D, Middleton JP, et al. Hemodialysis-associated subclavian vein stenosis. Kidney Int 1988; 33:1156-59.
2. Surratt RS, Picus D, Hicks ME, et al. The importance of preoperative evaluation of the subclavian vein in dialysis access planning. Am J Roentgenol 1991; 156:623-25.
3. Spinowitz BS, Galler M, Golden RA, et al. Subclavian vein stenosis as complication of subclavian vein catheterization for hemodialysis. Arch Intern Med 1987; 147:305-07.
4. Gradman WS, Bressman P, Sernaque JD. Subclavian vein repair in patients with an ipsilateral arteriovenous fistula. Ann Vasc Surg 1994; 8:549-56.
5. Fulks KD, Hyde GL. Jugular-axillary vein bypass for salvage of arteriovenous access. J Vasc Surg 1988; 8:169-71.
6. Gloviczki P, Pairolero PC, Toomey BJ, et al. Reconstruction of large veins for nonmalignant venous occlusive disease. J Vasc Surg 1992; 16:750-61.
7. Shoenfeld R, Hermans H, Novick A, et al. Stenting of proximal venous obstructions to maintain hemodialysis access. J Vasc Surg 1994; 19:532-39.

8. Glanz S, Gordon DH, Lipkowitz GS, et al. Axillary and subclavian vein stenosis: Percutaneous angioplasty. Radiology 1988; 168:371-73.
9. Landwehr P, Lackner K, Gotz R. Dilation and balloon-expandable stents for the treatment of central venous stenosis in dialysis patients. Rofo. Fortschritte auf dem Gebiete der Rontgenstrahlen und der Neuen Bildgebenden Verfahren 1990; 153:239-45.
10. Bhatia DS, Money SR, Ochsner JL, et al. Comparison of surgical bypass and percutaneous balloon dilatation with primary stent placement in the treatment of central venous obstruction in the dialysis patient: One-year follow-up. Ann Vasc Surg 1996; 10:452-55.
11. Wisselink W, Money SR, Becker MO, et al. Comparison of operative reconstruction and percutaneous balloon dilatation for central venous obstruction. Am J Surg 1993; 166:200-05.
12. Kovalik EC, Newman GE, Suhocki P, et al. Correction of central venous stenoses: Use of angioplasty and vascular Wallstents. Kidney Int 1994; 45:1177-81.
13. El-Sabrout RA, Duncan JM. Right atrial bypass grafting for central venous obstruction associated with dialysis access: Another treatment option. J Vasc Surg 1999; 29:472-78.

DISCUSSION

Moderator:
Mitchell L. Henry, M.D.
Panelists:
Francisco S. Escobar III, M.D.
David E. Morris, M.D.

Discussant: What about some of the technical features? I guess I have never used a ring PTFE graft to the contralateral internal jugular vein. Do you want to tell us how you have done that?

Dr. Morris: That was done similarly to the slide that I put up earlier, except that instead of using the counter-incision on the ipsilateral side inferior to the clavicle, it was actually placed on the contralateral side inferior to the clavicle. Again, it was tunneled subcutaneously across and then up to the contralateral IJ. That same incision between the heads of the sternomastoid was made, only again, that was on the contralateral side.

Discussant: I was just wondering if this procedure interferes in any way with the patient's functionality of their, say, arm or use of the pectoral muscle?

Dr. Morris: It has not, no.

Dr. Henry: How do you handle the superior end of the jugular vein? Do you ligate it?

Dr. Escobar: We have left that open for the jugular turn down procedure that I referred to earlier. That is usually ligated as high up as it can be, but we have not had much experience in doing that.

Dr. Henry: No problems with the intracranial pressure changes such as headaches or other symptoms?

Dr. Escobar: Not as of yet. That is a good point though. It is a good thought.

Discussant: Mitch, can I just comment on that? We have done about 10 of these and we never ligated the internal jugular vein, and I am not aware that anyone has had any symptoms.

7

TREATMENT OF FAILING AND FAILED IMMATURE FISTULAE BY INTERVENTIONAL RADIOLOGY: MIDTERM FOLLOW-UP

Luc A. Turmel-Rodrigues, M.D.

Recent U.S. publications have reported apparently conflicting results of attempts to create more forearm fistulae, the first choice for hemodialysis access recommended by the National Kidney Foundation-Dialysis Outcomes Quality Initiative guidelines.[1] Silva et al. reported an excellent 84% 1-year primary patency rate, and Ascher et al. reported an honorable 75% rate[2,3], whereas Miller et al. reported 34% at 6 months.[4] This apparent discrepancy can be explained by differing populations and a more aggressive approach attempting creation of fistulae in more marginal cases by the latter team. Like the vast majority of surgical articles, however, these 3 articles did not clearly define policy for exploration and treatment of insufficiently developing fistulae; furthermore, only 1 article mentioned even a small role for interventional radiology, probably because it has long been believed that an immature fistula is a contraindication to any endovascular approach.

In centers working with an actual team approach, surgeons and nephrologists are now aware, and have been convinced for many years, of the potential benefits of interventional radiology alternatives. Thus, they have referred immature fistulae to radiologists. The aim of this article is to report the 8-year experience of a single radiological center in the angiographic evaluation and endovascular treatment of forearm fistulae that failed to mature spontaneously.

Subjects and Methods

The definition of an immature fistula used in this study is either a fistula created less than 3 months earlier or a fistula created more than 3 months earlier but used for less than 1 month for dialysis because of difficulty due to small vessel size.

Sixty patients with immature fistula dysfunction were treated from 1992 to March 2000; 60% were men, 25% had diabetes, and only 1 was black. The mean age was 62.0 years, with 40% of patients older than 65 years and 20% older than 75 years. Forty-four fistulae were still patent, and 16 were thrombosed. The mean age of the fistulae was 10.07 weeks. Patients were referred to the radiologist by 6 hemodialysis centers, comprising 18 nephrologists and 3 surgeons. The less numerous cases of immature upper arm fistulae treated during the same period were not included in this study because recent studies have shown different long-term outcomes in forearm and upper arm fistulae.[5,6]

All radiological interventions were outpatient procedures. There were no contraindications to angiography. Diluted iodine or carbon dioxide was used in patients who had not previously been hemodialyzed, and either carbon dioxide or gadolinium (the contrast medium used in magnetic resonance imaging) was used with patients who were allergic to iodine. The contraindications to dilation were local infection and anastomotic stenosis in fistulae created less than 6 weeks earlier (because of risk of disruption of the anastomosis). Contraindications to declotting were local infection and fistulae that had not been successfully used at least once for dialysis.

Treatment of patent fistulae. Angiography was performed in all cases after cannulation of the brachial artery at the elbow with an 18-gauge needle and placement of a short 3 French catheter over a 0.035-inch straight guidewire. Angiography of the forearm arteries was performed by digital subtraction angiography at a rate of 6 images per second, with an iodine injection rate of 5 mL/s for 1 second. Iodine diluted to one third of normal strength or carbon dioxide[7,8] was used in patients who had not previously been hemodialized, and the number of injections was limited as much as possible.

The initial large angiography field was centered on the anastomotic area, which was studied in supination, and then in pronation or in profile when necessary to show the arteriovenous anastomosis at its best view. The vascularization status of the hand was sytematically checked, as was patency of the palmar arch and the antegrade or retrograde filling of the distal segment of the artery (radial or ulnar) feeding the fistula.

The outflow veins were then studied at the elbow and upper arm, as well as in the thorax, basically in supination, with additional studies when necessary in cases of superimposition. If the whole fistula appeared angiographically normal, a 4 French catheter was then pushed up to the subclavian artery to rule out a subclavian, axillary, or brachial artery stenosis.

Once the stenosis or stenoses had been diagnosed, dilation was performed by cannulation of the fistula itself. Both clinical examination and angiography aided in the choice of the best cannulation site.

For stenoses located on the artery or at the anastomosis, a retrograde approach was used from the vein in the upper third of the forearm or from the elbow. Small injections of contrast medium into the brachial artery facilitated cannulation under fluoroscopy when the thrill was too weak. Retrograde catheterization of the anastomosis for treatment of stenoses of the feeding artery was performed with the help of an angled 4 or 5 French catheter(selective internal mammary type). If this retrograde approach was unsuccessful, the arterial stenosis was treated by antegrade cannulation of the brachial artery at the elbow and selective catheterization of the feeding artery.

In contrast, antegrade cannulation of the fistula close to the anastomosis was performed for stenoses located on the vein far from the anastomosis. Gentle cannulation was performed with a 16- or 18-gauge needle, and either a Bentson or hydrophilic guidewire was pushed through the stenosis.

After placement of a 5 or 6 French introducer sheath, a dilation balloon no smaller than 5 mm in diameter was used for venous stenoses, and a balloon no smaller than 4 mm in diameter was used for arterial or anastomotic stenoses. High-pressure balloons inflatable up to 25 atm (Blue Max [Medi-Tech, Natick, MA]; Centurion [Bard, Covington, GA]) were used when necessary to eliminate waste of the stenosis on the balloon, a key to a good clinical result. The balloon was left inflated for 3 minutes, and no heparin was injected. The final result was assessed both clinically and angiographically. When the introducer sheath used for dilation caused a stenosis at its entry point, it was necessary to recannulate the fistula in the opposite direction to reopen the lumen of the vein at the level of the introducer sheath by local dilation.

In cases of dilation-induced rupture of the vein, the dilation balloon was first reinflated locally at low pressure (2-4 atm) for a period of 10 minutes. If the leakage persisted in spite of 30 minutes of balloon tamponade, stent placement was the only way to save the fistula. The best stent for this indication was the Passager (Boston Scientific Europe, La Garennes-Colombes, France), a wide-mesh nitinol stent covered with Dacron, available in Europe but not in the United States. The Dacron coat stopped the leakage in all cases, and the wide mesh then made the stent routinely puncturable for dialysis.

Treatment of thrombosed fistulae. The declotting of thrombosed native fistulae has been discussed by Turmel-Rodrigues et al.[9] The major technical problem with immature fistulae was cannulation of the vessel and placement of the first guidewire into the lumen, which occasionally took more than 1 hour. It was often necessary to place a tourniquet at the elbow to cause the nonthrombosed segment to swell and make it puncturable or to perform antegrade cannulation of the feeding artery from the brachial artery at the elbow to gain access to the fistula. Once a guidewire had been successfully pushed into both the arterial inflow and the venous outflow, the success of the procedure was predictable, because the clot burden was always very small owing to the small vein diameter. Furthermore, removal of the thrombus was never a problem. Sufficient dilation of the underlying stenosis was the only requirement for success.

Statistics. The results are reported according to the Kaplan-Meier life table method. Success was defined as the ability to perform at least 1 full dialysis treatment after either dilation or declotting. Major complications were defined as complications with clinical consequences necessitating an additional intervention or inpatient hospitalization.

Primary patency was considered to begin on the day of the first radiological procedure and to end on the day of access failure or further reintervention (radiological or surgical). Secondary patency included all further radiological therapy (dilation, stent placement, and declotting) but ended with any surgical intervention. Death and renal transplantation with a patent fistula were considered to be the end of follow-up.

Results

An underlying stenosis was diagnosed in all cases. It was located on the feeding artery far from the anastomosis in 8% of cases, in the anastomotic area (artery or vein) in 47% of cases, in the cannulation segment in 35% of cases, and at the elbow level in 10% of cases.

The overall radiological success rate was 96% (100% for the thrombosed fistula subgroup). Failures were attributable to the inability to traverse tight stenoses. There was 1 significant complication (1.6%) in the form of severe bacteremia resulting from an overlooked infection of an 8-week-old anastomotic scar. Two acute ruptures in cannulation areas were controlled by placement of a Passager stent. They were then routinely cannulated for 10 months in 1 case and 24 months in the other.

Primary patency rates were 70%, 47%, 35%, and 24% at 3, 6, 12, and 24 months, respectively. Secondary patency rates were 86%, 80%, 80%, and 76%, respectively, with an average of 1.2 reinterventions per year. Thrombosed fistulae did not fare worse than patent fistulae.

Discussion

Radiology and surgery. Surgery can save immature fistulae only when the stenosis is located near the anastomosis at the wrist; a new anastomosis can be created a few centimeters above and does not sacrifice a long segment of vein. However, interventional radiology has the great advantage of being able to treat all types of stenoses in any location and is therefore more effective as a first approach.

Although the results reported here originate from a single radiological center, there is no doubt that the vast majority of immature fistulae can be salvaged radiologically and that the availability of stents covered with wide mesh, which are puncturable, is extremely helpful to optimize the results where complications arise.

Although there is no doubt that when delayed maturation becomes obvious, interventional radiology must be performed from the second month either to save the fistula or have it ready for dialysis, the future of this radiologically salvaged immature fistula must then be analyzed in a multidisciplinary fashion. In cases of early recurrence of stenosis (eg, within 3 months) what is the best strategy: redilation or creation of a new fistula?

In cases of early restenosis close to the anastomosis, the surgical creation of a new anastomosis a few centimeters above is obviously the solution. In all other circumstances, each patient should be assessed on a case-by-case basis. If, according to preoperative venous mapping, there is a good chance that the creation of a new native fistula in the opposite forearm would be more successful, the surgical alternative is obviously preferable to redilation every 3 months or even every 6 months, although redilation must nevertheless be performed as long as the new fistula is not usable. In contrast, if the only alternative surgery available is placement of a prosthetic graft, it is likely that preservation of the native fistula might be preferable from a strategic point of view, even with redilation every 3 months, because we know that secondary failures of grafts are frequent and can necessitate reintervention every 3 months.

If the surgical alternative is the creation of an upper arm fistula, the age or life expectancy of the patient is probably a major consideration. A young patient is likely to undergo renal transplantation, and the forearm fistula can be maintained by interventional radiology until this transplantation occurs, usually within some months, thus preserving the upper arm veins for the future. In contrast, the upper arm veins can be arterialized immediately in older patients, in whom long-term venous preservation is less vital. Finally, the patient's choice must also be borne in mind.

The potential of interventional radiology can also influence the overall vascular access strategy and encourage surgeons to intervene in more marginal cases and be less exigent in analyzing the quality of both arteries and veins before the creation of a native fistula, especially in young patients. For example, Ascher et al.[2] achieved a 100% primary success rate at 3 months in the creation of forearm fistulae, but only by arterializing cephalic veins larger than 3 mm in diameter, which was a very restrictive positive selection bias. Similarly, Silva et al.[3] reported a low 8% failure rate using only cephalic veins larger than 2.5 mm at the wrist. If cephalic veins smaller than 2.5 mm were inappropriate for fistula creation, it would not be possible to create such fistulae in children; however, they are routinely created, but in such cases microsurgery is mandatory.[10]

Iodine or no iodine? Iodine injection is a concern in patients who have not been previously hemodialyzed. Our team hoped to have found the solution by the injection of carbon dioxide; the imaging quality was poor, but there were no renal implications.[7,8,11] Unfortunately, inadvertent reflux of carbon dioxide up to the right carotid artery of a patient treated for stenosis on a dialysis graft led to the patient's death in September 1999 after 3 weeks of coma with left-sided hemiplegia. The lethal risk of carbon dioxide was then demonstrated for the first time, according to the existing literature, and we prohibited its further use in upper limb vascular access.

Some teams proposed using gadolinium (the contrast medium for magnetic resonance imaging) instead of iodine.[8,12] Unfortunately, gadolinium is at least 10 times more expensive than iodine and is $3^1/_2$ times less radiopaque than iodine. It has not been demonstrated that gadolinium is sufficiently less nephrotoxic than iodine diluted to one-third normal strength to warrant this expense. We therefore reserve gadolinium for use in patients with a history of severe allergy to iodine, and we treat immature fistulae in patients who have not undergone hemodialysis with diluted iodine, with no consequences for renal function to date. This small risk cannot be ignored, however, and the decision depends on the nephrologist. Ultrasonographic screening of such patients can help differentiate those who can undergo direct surgical repair (short stenoses close to the anastomosis) from those who need contrast injection for the endovascular approach (either long stenoses or stenoses far from the anastomosis).

Opposition to Beathard's approach. The findings and techniques described here contradict those of the only previously published article on this topic, written in 1999 by Beathard et al.[13] In my experience as a vascular radiologist, there has never been a native fistula failure without underlying tight stenosis. I am therefore extremely skeptical about the value of both the technique and the interpretation of the angiograms in the article by Beathard et al., because the article described an underlying stenosis in only 21 of 63 cases of fistulae with delayed maturation. Beathard et al. considered collateral, or accessory veins visualized to be a cause of delayed maturation and reported a technique of selective ligation of these veins. All vascular radiologists know that there is no opacification of venous collaterals without underlying stenosis of the main outflow vein and that these collaterals are not the cause, but a clinical sign, of delayed maturation due to stenosis of the main outflow vein.

The general rule is that whenever possible, it is usually more effective to treat the cause of a problem than its consequences. In immature fistulae, the appropriate angiography technique (ie, puncture of the brachial artery at the elbow rather than puncture of the fistula itself, as described by Beathard et al.) allows physiological opacification and shows in all cases a stenosis somewhere from the feeding artery to the superior vena cava. If there are collaterals, a stenosis or occlusion is localized in all cases on the main outflow vein somewhere downstream from the ostia of the collaterals.

The technique of accessory vein ligation and/or main vein banding described by Beathard et al., furthermore, appears unusual because stenosis reduces the blood flow of any arteriovenous access[1], while fistula flow should increase with maturation. The ligation performed by Beathard et al. can act as a local permanent tourniquet, but in no case will it change the outcome of the vein if the underlying stenosis is not treated.

The apparently good results of Beathard et al. (75% secondary patency rate at 1 year) may be influenced by several biases within their population. The mean age of the fistulae at the time of treatment was 5 months (versus 2½ months in our series), which means that the vast majority of patients had passed the most dangerous stage of the first 3 months. Beathard et al. did not treat thrombosed fistulae, fistulae that failed but were salvageable, according to our study. Lesions in the feeding arteries were not diagnosed, and therefore not treated, in their study. None of the fistulae was used for dialysis before treatment, which means that these fistulae could not be properly evaluated for dialysis use.

Conclusions

Systematic clinical examination of forearm native fistulae should be scheduled every month after creation until the initiation of dialysis, and either ultrasonographic or angiographic evaluation should be requested if there are any doubts from the second month, because the vast majority of immature fistulae can be salvaged through interventional radiology. Multidisciplinary reevaluation of the patient must nevertheless be performed after endovascular salvaging of the fistula to determine whether it should undergo redilation in cases of early recurrence of stenosis after dilation or if a new fistula should be created.

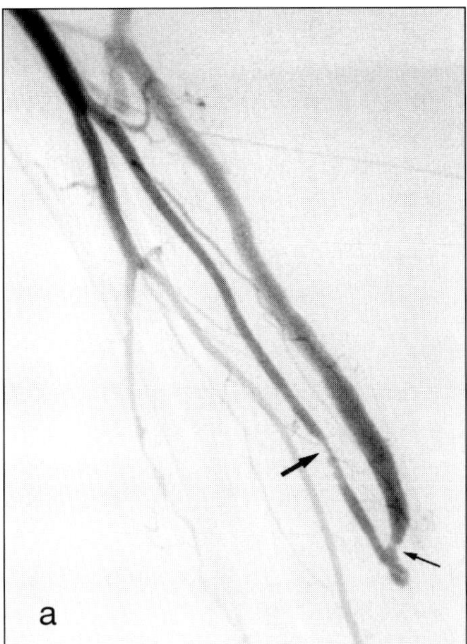

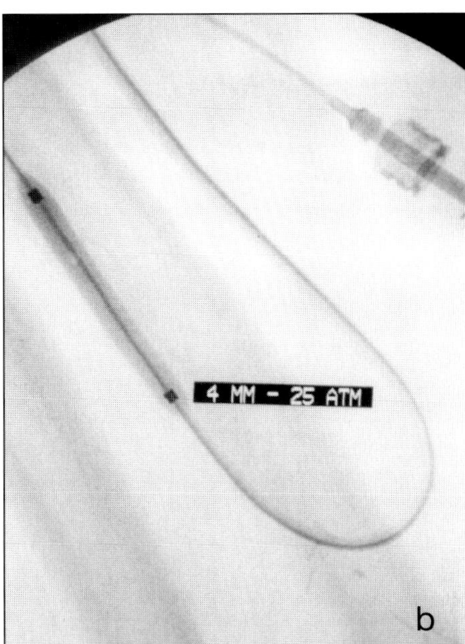

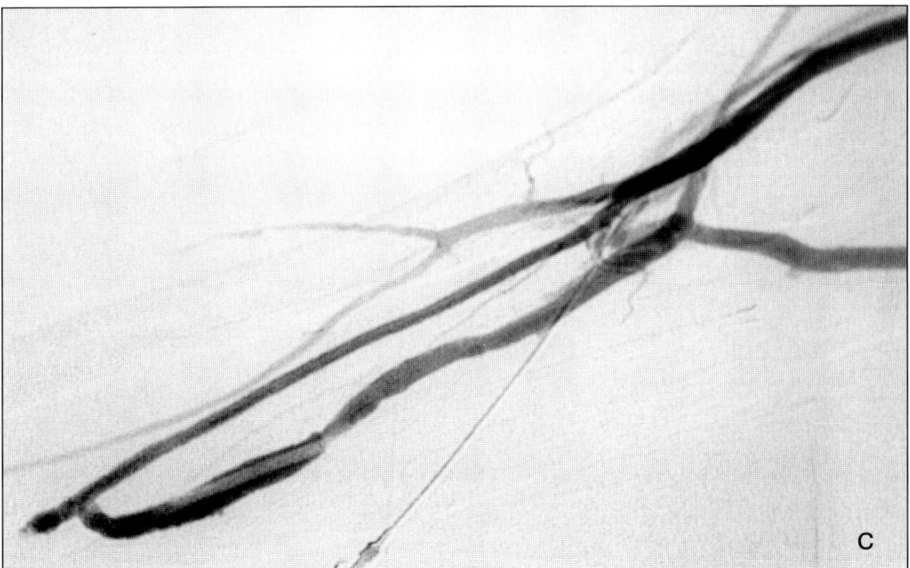

Figure 7-1. a) Insufficient inflow in this radiocephalic fistula of a patient with diabetes is mainly due to a stenosis of the feeding artery located 3 cm above the anastomosis (thick arrow). There is also a short postanastomotic stenosis of the vein (thin arrow).
b) Dilation is performed by retrograde catheterization of the fistula itself, and a 4-mm high-pressure balloon inflated to 25 atm is necessary to efface the waist.
c) After dilation, the result is so good that it is impossible to say where the initial arterial stenosis was located. This fistula has been used for 4 months with no reintervention.

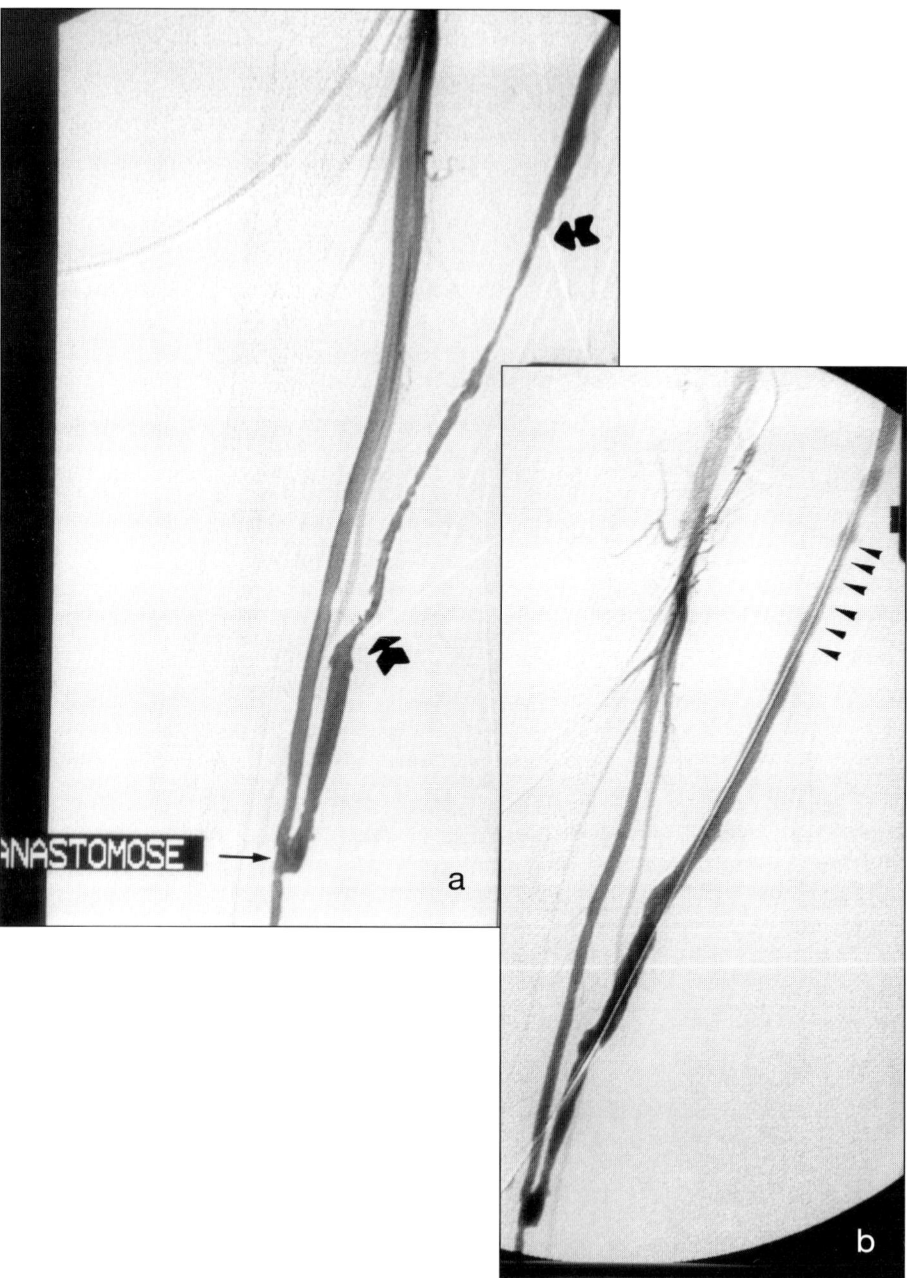

Figure 7-2. a) Delayed maturation of this radiocephalic fistula is due to a long stenosis of the vein, starting 3 cm above the anastomosis (between the 2 big arrows).
b) Dilation to 6 mm by the antegrade approach from the relatively well developed postanastomotic venous segment achieved an excellent clinical result despite transient spasm in the upper part of the vein (arrowheads). Redilation to 7 mm was performed 3 months later, and this fistula has been used for 9 months.

References

1. Schwab S, Besarab A, Beathard G, et al. NKF-DOQI clinical practice guidelines for vascular access. New York: National Kidney Foundation; 1997.
2. Silva M, Hobson R, Pappas P, et al. A strategy for increasing use of autogenous hemodialysis access procedures: Impact of preoperative noninvasive evaluation. J Vasc Surg 1998; 27:302-08.
3. Ascher E, Hingorani A, Mazzariol F, Gunduz Y, Fodera M, Yorkovich W. Changes in the practice of angioaccess surgery: Impact of dialysis outcome and quality initiative recommendations. J Vasc Surg 2000; 31:84-92.
4. Miller P, Tolwani A, Luscy C, et al. Predictors of adequacy of arteriovenous fistulas in hemodialysis patients. Kidney Int 1999; 56:275-80.
5. Rodriguez J, Armadans L, Ferrer E, et al. The function of permanent vascular access. Nephrol Dial Transplant 2000; 15:402-08.
6. Turmel-Rodrigues L, Pengloan J, Baudin S, et al. Treatment of stenosis and thrombosis in haemodialysis fistulas and grafts by interventional radiology. Nephrol Dial Transplant 2000; 15:2029-36.
7. Ehrman K, Taber T, Gaylord G, Brown P, Hage J. Comparison of diagnostic accuracy with carbon dioxide versus iodinated contrast material in the imaging of hemodialysis access fistulas. J Vasc Interv Radiol 1994; 5:771-75.
8. Spinosa D, Angle F, Hagspiel K, Schenk W, Matsumoto A. CO2 and gadopentetate dimeglumine as alternative contrast agents for malfunctioning dialysis grafts and fistulas. Kidney Int 1998; 54:945-50.
9. Turmel-Rodrigues L, Pengloan J, Baudin S, et al. Treatment of failed native arterio-venous fistulae for hemodialysis by interventional radiology. Kidney Int 2000; 57:1124-40.
10. Bourquelot P, Cussenot O, Corbi P, et al. Microsurgical creation and follow-up of arteriovenous fistulae for chronic hemodialysis in children. Pediatr Nephrol 1990; 4:156-59.
11. Hawkins I, Caridi J. Carbon dioxide (CO2) digital subtraction angiography: 26-year experience at the University of Florida. Eur Radiol 1998; 8:391-402.
12. Hammer F, Goffette P, Malaise J, Mathurin P. Gadolinium dimeglumine: An alternative contrast agent for digital subtraction angiography. Eur Radiol 1999; 9:128-36.
13. Beathard G, Settle S, Shields M. Salvage of the nonfunctioning arteriovenous fistula. Am J Kidney Dis 1999; 5:910-16.

DISCUSSION

Moderator:
Mitchell L. Henry, M.D.
Panelist:
Luc A. Turmel-Rodrigues, M.D.

Discussant: I have noticed with your brachial artery approach, you then have a second access to dilate the venous outflows. Have you tried and found unsuccessful to do a retrograde access of the vein and compression to allow it to reflux up the artery to visualize that?

Dr. Turmel-Rodrigues: What do you mean, the diagnostic stage or the intervention stage? The diagnostic stage must always be performed by puncture of the brachial artery and only puncture of the brachial artery. For the dilation stage, you must try to puncture and cannulate the vein under angiographic control. If you have some difficulties, you can use the retrograde arterial approach.

Discussant: Okay, so you have had success because your arterial puncture appeared to be retrograde in the artery. So from that, are you able to get around the anastomosis?

Dr. Turmel-Rodrigues: No, I said in most cases I try to dilate using a direct approach from the fistula. If there is need for intervention, it is only in the rare cases when you can not cannulate the fistula. It is very rough, but sometimes you can use an antegrade arterial approach.

Discussant: My question is, why do you only use the brachial artery for diagnosis when you can at time reflux contrast in a retrograde fashion?

Dr. Turmel-Rodrigues: This is the only way to be sure to have a good evaluation of all the arterial inflow including from the subclavian artery. It is like I explained earlier, that sometimes the failure of the fistula can be explained only by a very proximal artery stenoses. This is the only way to be sure to get the anastomosis. If you puncture the fistula, even with the compression, you can miss the anastomosis or you have a variation of the feeding artery.

Discussant: I agree. What is the number of re-intraventions that you have had to do on these fistulas an average?

Dr. Turmel-Rodrigues: About every 11 months. You have good fistulas and you have the very poor fistula. With the poor fistulas, of course, the surgeons have to do something. We are just here to try to avoid temporary central catheters.

Dr. Henry: I offer my congratulations on your excellent work, as usual. My real question is, at what length of that venous outflow segment that stenosed would you not try to attempt to dilate out?

Dr. Turmel-Rodrigues: The venous outflow stenosis is always an indication because the only thing that you can do is to create a much more proximal anastomosis. So in all cases I try to dilate and I wait and see. Sometimes the outcomes are very good and sometimes we have problems.

Dr. Henry: In your usual approach, you would just be very aggressive and see which one if it works or not?

Dr. Turmel-Rodrigues: Yes, I always try such things. Especially because they are a very poor surgical subject.

Discussant: I keep listening to your talks. I wonder when you get time to do all of this excellent work back in France. I agree 100% with what you are doing to get this fistula going and I am interested personally. I am a surgeon and I place a lot of fistulas. But I have never seen this work reproduced by any interventional person in this country. Do you have any idea why it is so hard and if an interventionalist can tell me why this cannot be done here?

Dr. Turmel-Rodrigues: Unfortunately, for the radiologist they have a very poor experience with AV fistula because the surgeons have not created enough of them. But they are going to improve.

Discussant: That is why I said that. I disagree because we do place fistulas. In fact, I have checked my experience in the last 2 years and my fistula placement rate for de novo access creation is over 60%.

Dr. Michael Levine: Yes, very good talk. You were trashing the concept of side branches, saying that they are a manifestation of stenosis and not the cause. I agree with that. You have not encountered the case where there is a significant side branch or side branches, that if you ligate that side branch you will improve the function of the fistula?

Dr. Turmel-Rodrigues: I think that the ligation of side branches is a waste of time and money. It has no positive effect on the long-term outcome.

Discussant: There is no question, but what you say is wrong. We can debate the issue for quite a while as long as you understand before we start that you are wrong. You have to distinguish between collateral vessels in normal anatomy. I think sometimes you have difficulty being sure that you have collateral vessels obviously related to stenosis. Normal anatomy has multiple branches, not stenosis. If you look at any anatomy texts and if you look at any patient you have them, there is just no question. What you say is partially correct, but not totally correct.

Dr. Turmel-Rodrigues: No, you have no significant side branches without stenosis on the main outflow vein. There is no question but what in those circumstances ligating those can render a fistula that is not usable can render it usable. No, no, I am certain. You have not randomized ligation of collaterals. In your article about fistulas, your age of the fistulas was 5 months. In my experience it was 2 months and a half. I recall that you never treated the stenosis on the arterial inflow, which is a mistake according to me, and you do not declot the fistulas when they thrombose.

Dr. Bethard: We do declot them when they thrombose.

Dr. Turmel-Rodrigues: No, not in your article.

Dr. Bethard: There are many things that were not in the article because that was not the subject of the article.

Discussant: This is not a question but a comment, I think this problem will help them solve the problem they are having between them. At the same time I agree that side branches do steel blood in certain patients. The problem is, what is the blood flow in the fistula. Regardless of having a normal anatomy, if you are not able to get the blood flow adequate for dialysis in the fistula, if by ligating the side branches you are not going to get that fistula matured. Unfortunately, so far, no one has written up about checking the blood flow in the fistula in a systematic fashion. But if there are 2 branches and you have 200 cc of blood, definitely part of that blood is going to go in a branch by ligating 1 branch.

SECTION III

8

COMBINATION OF ELEPHANT TRUNK ANASTOMOSIS AND VASCULAR CLIPS FOR THE VENOUS END OF DIALYSIS GRAFTS

Alan S. Coulson, M.D., Ph.D.

Neointimal hyperplasia (NIH) continues to be a significant problem in the hemodialysis population. The condition progressively blocks off the venous end of polytetrafluoroethylene (PTFE) grafts as a result of the centripetal migration of vascular smooth muscle cells (SMCs).

There has been considerable speculation regarding the etiology of NIH. Stimulation of SMCs and foreign body reaction to the graft material have been the suggested causes of NIH.[1] With a conventional sutured anastomosis, the circular zone of venous tissue immediately around the anastomosis of the PTFE graft is uniquely located at the convergence of 2 types of ongoing noxious stimulation. Each individually contributes to the stimulation of SMCs and the development of NIH.

First, there is constant barrage of mechanical stimuli from the temblor-like vibration of the graft itself and from the stress arising from the blood flow as it exits the graft. Secondly, local production of a dangerous cocktail of growth factors results from the trauma incurred during the suturing of the graft to the vein and the associated platelet deposition and activation.

In the past, when Scribner shunts were used for dialysis access, NIH development was not as frequent. One of the shunts' protective features may have been the surgical exclusion of the venotomy site as a result of the Tevdek tie around the vein. A second feature was that at the venous end of the shunt, the Teflon tip inserted inside the vein, and was separated by about 2 cm from the venotomy. This distance was a barrier to any migration of SMCs. A third feature was that the flow of blood exiting from the shunt entered the center of the vein, dissipating kinetic energy downstream in a more laminar fashion.

An attempt has been made to maintain these protective features in the currently described modification of the venous end of the dialysis graft. The PTFE graft inserted inside the vein, and the venotomy was isolated from the vein's lumen. This technique is described as an elephant trunk because it resembles the technique used in aortic surgery in which the distal end of the prosthesis inserts inside the descending thoracic aorta. This procedure probably introduces the arterial blood flow into the venous side of the circulation in such a way that it reduces the mixing, and enhances the smooth collinear flow, of both re-entrant and venous blood (personal communication, G.M. Homsy, Ph.D., April 1999).

Vascular clips (U.S. Surgical, Norwalk, CT) are used to effect the anastomosis between the venotomy and the plastic ring on the PTFE graft to isolate the cut edge of the endothelium from the bloodstream. Pressure of the vascular clips on the vein wall leads to the formation of significant amounts of hydroxypyridinium in hours instead of months.

Hydroxypyridinium is believed to act as a signal for the completion of the first stage of wound healing and to contribute to the inhibition of SMC migration.[2] Vascular clips reduce some of the other risk factors that may contribute to hyperplasia, such as endothelial trauma, mural ischemia, and platelet deposition.[3]

Materials and Methods

In the period between January 1998 and April 2000, a total of 152 vascular access procedures were performed by the author at Dameron Hospital, Stockton, California, a local community hospital. About two thirds were new grafts and one third consisted of repairs or revisions of existing PTFE grafts. In 13 cases (8.5%) the axillary vein, brachial vein, or cephalic vein was found to be big enough to permit the insertion of the graft inside the vein. The graft used was a Gore-Tex RD06007050L, 6 mm in diameter, 50 cm in length, with 7 cm of eccentrically placed rings (W.L. Gore and Associates, Medical Products Division, Flagstaff, AZ). The recommended vein diameter that will easily accept such a graft is about 15 mm. The surgical technique has been described in detail.[4,5] It consists of exposing the axillary vein with a minimum amount of trauma (figure 8-1). An area large enough to accommodate the graft insertion is cleaned on the surface of the vein (figure 8-2). A methylene blue ring is made using the end of the graft as a template (figures 8-3 and 8-4). A polypropylene pursestring is then made outside the blue ring using a 5-0 suture. Care is taken to avoid penetration of the lumen of the vein, which would cause endothelium trauma (figure 8-5). An incision is then made to permit the insertion of a vascular punch (Medtronic, Minneapolis, MN), and a circular piece of vein is removed (figures 8-6 and 8-7). It is helpful to allow the vein to distend prior to operating the punch to avoid cutting outside the blue ring.

The PTFE graft is cut at a 45-degree angle at the level of the 11th plastic ring to facilitate insertion into the venotomy (figure 8-8). The graft is then loaded onto a urethral dilator (van Buren sound, Codman, Boston, MA; see figure 8-9). A small amount of lubrication facilitates loading onto the van Buren sound and insertion into the vein. The graft is then inserted inside the vein until the last plastic ring is about 2 mm below the venotomy (figure 8-10). The pursestring is pulled tight and tied to

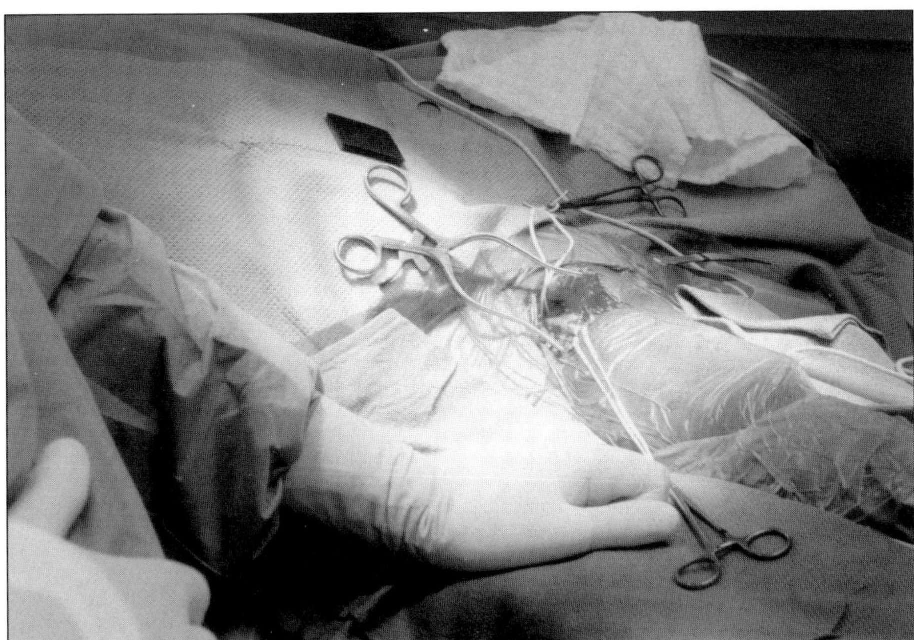

Figure 8-1. General appearance of the operative site. The patient's head is to the top right-hand corner of the picture. The left axilla is exposed with Silastic tapes around the brachial vein.

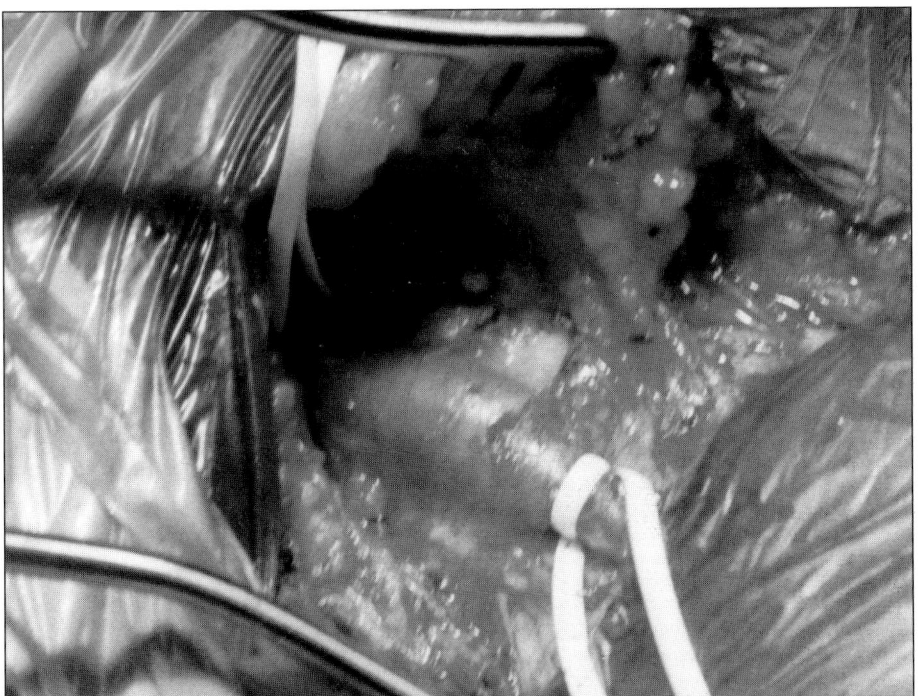

Figure 8-2. An area large enough to accommodate the graft insertion is cleaned on the surface of the vein.

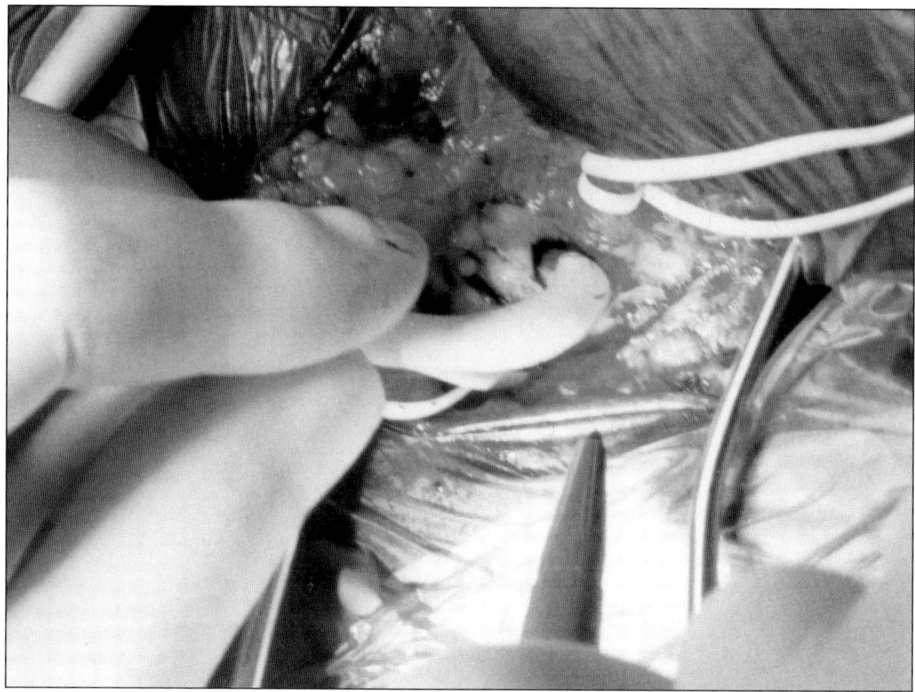

Figure 8-3. A methylene blue ring is made on the surface of the vein, using the end of the graft as a template.

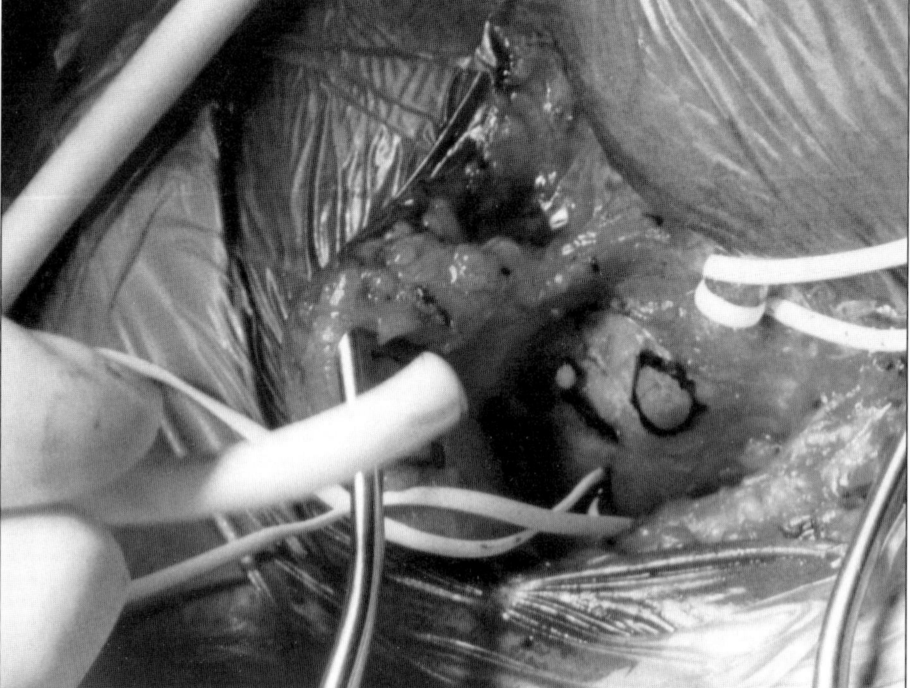

Figure 8-4. The methylene blue ring is completed.

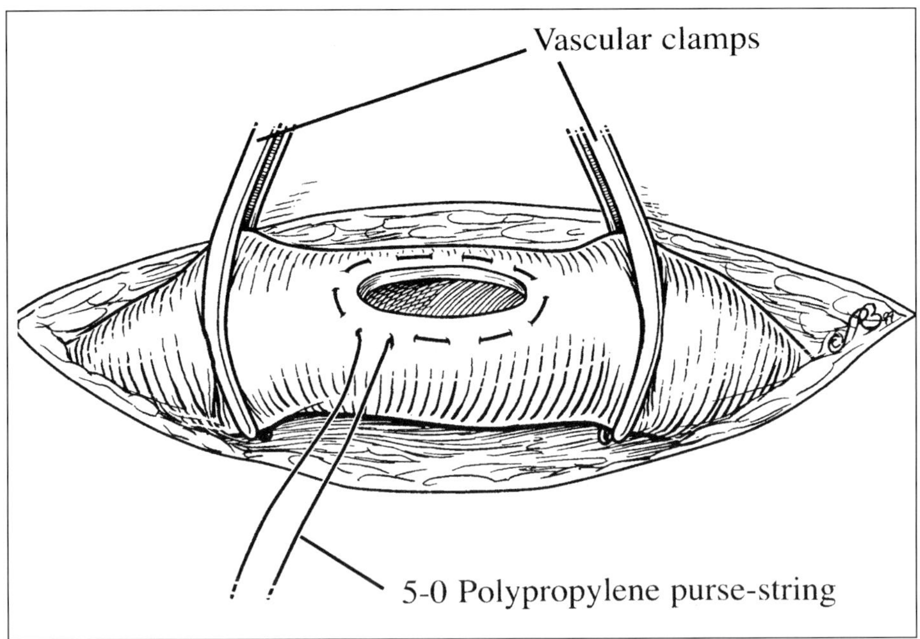

Figure 8-5. A 5-0 polypropylene pursestring suture is placed around the blue ring.

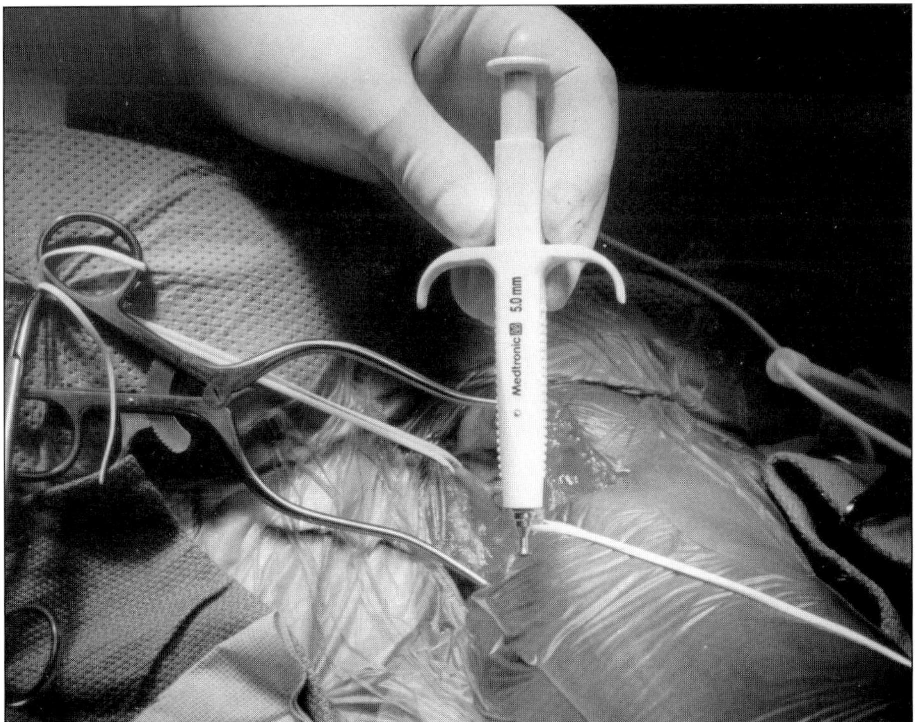

Figure 8-6. A Medtronic punch is used to cut out a circular piece of vein inside the blue ring.

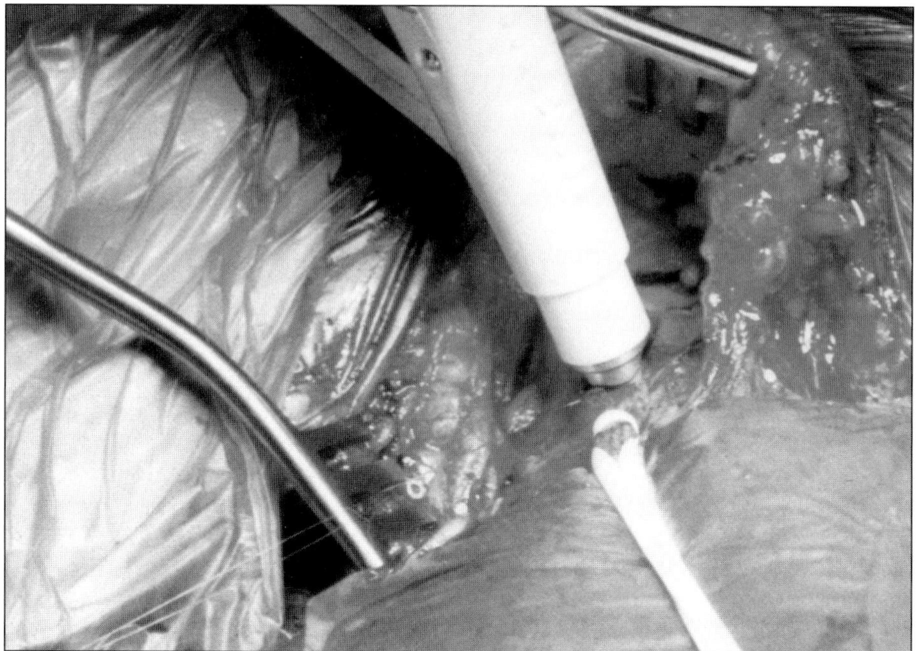

Figure 8-7. The punch is seen in the vein. The vein should be distended prior to operating the punch to avoid cutting too much vein wall. The 5-0 polypropylene sutures are evident coming from the pursestring.

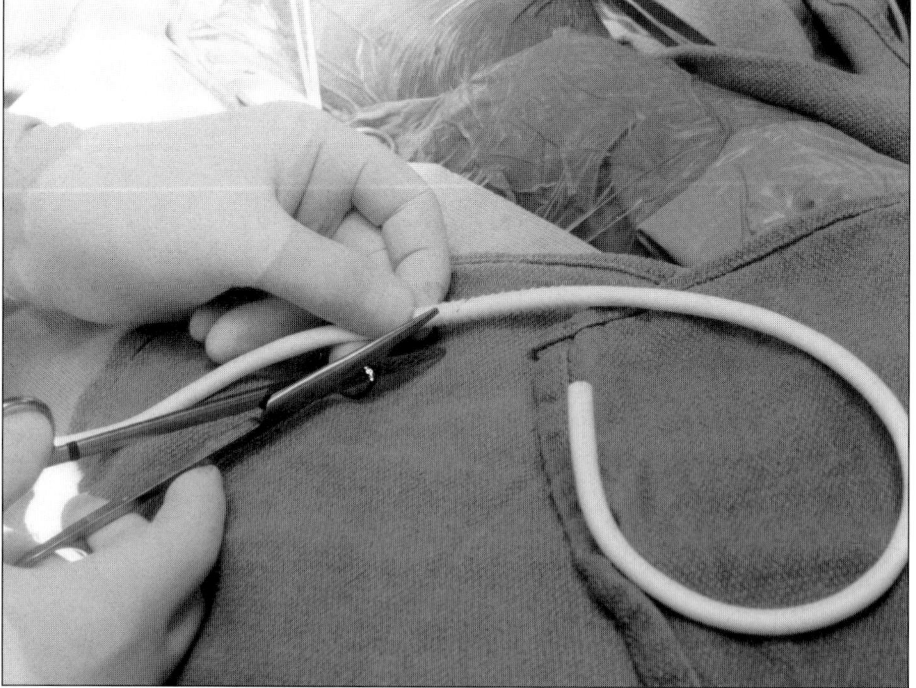

Figure 8-8. The PTFE graft is cut at a 45-degree angle at the 11th plastic ring.

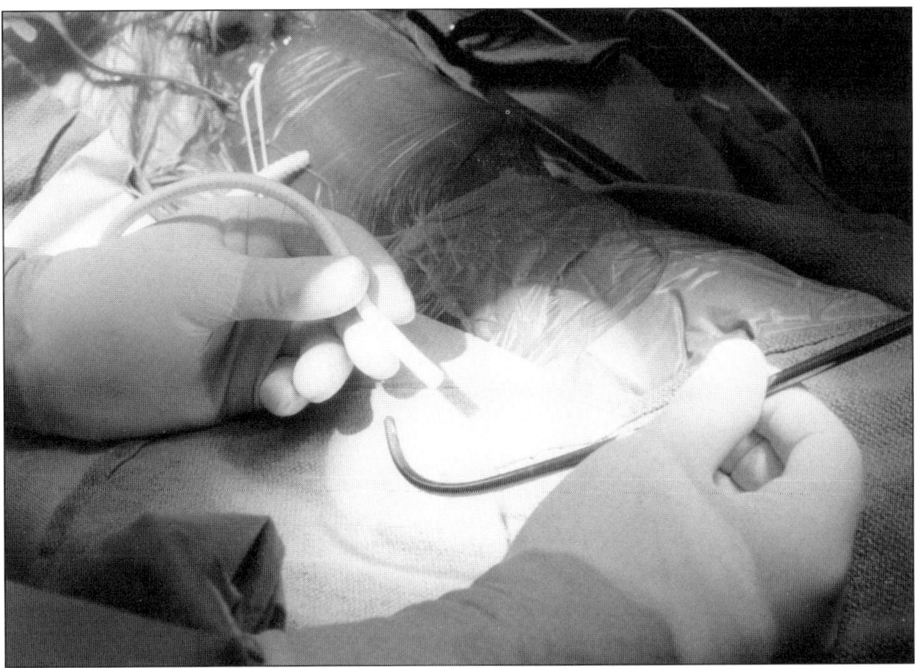

Figure 8-9. The graft is lubricated and loaded on a van Buren sound.

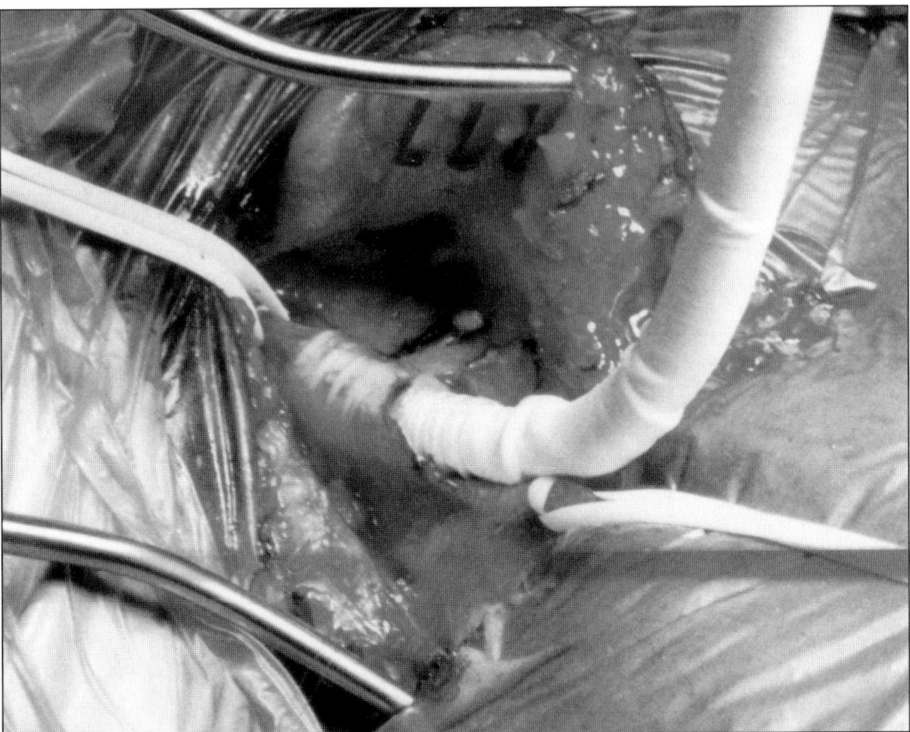

Figure 8-10. The graft and dilator are inserted inside the venotomy.

obtain hemostasis. This also effectively isolates the venotomy from the lumen of the vein and everts the venotomy incision. A collar of vein below the venotomy margin is anastomosed to the first plastic ring of the graft. Vascular clips are used to cinch the vein wall around the plastic ring in the manner of a circular mortise-and-tenon joint (figures 8-11 and 8-12). The vein thus grasps the first plastic ring of the graft, which acts like an O ring (figure 8-13). In this way, the cut endothelium does not make contact with the bloodstream. The other end of the PTFE graft is attached to the arterial inflow in the usual fashion.

Depending on the situation, the native artery may be used for a first-time surgery, or the arterial end of an old, established graft may be used, provided it is free of disease and the blood flow is satisfactory.

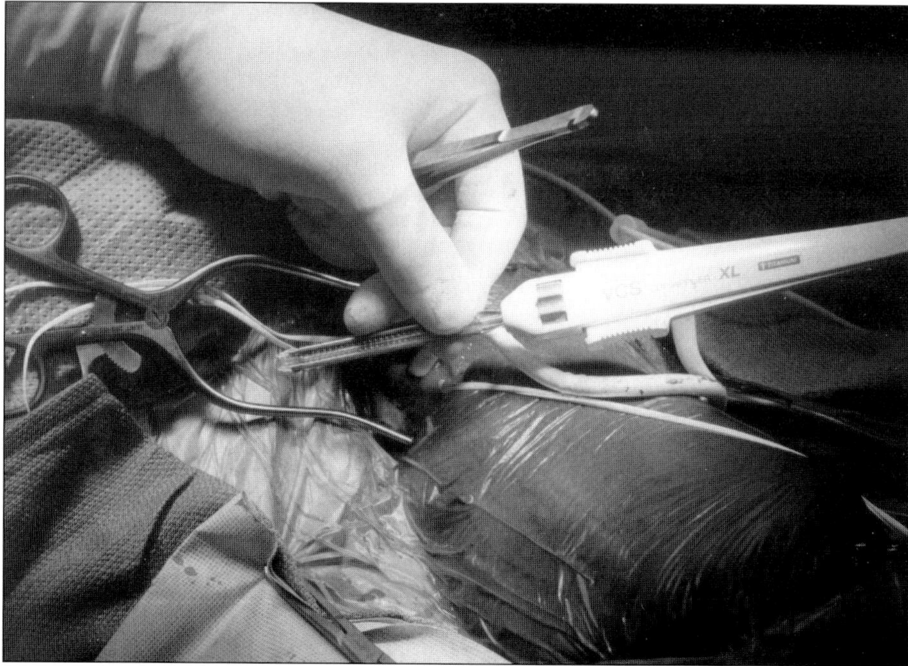

Figure 8-11. A surgical clip applier of extra large size is used to secure the vein wall to the topmost plastic ring. The graft and dilator are inserted inside the venotomy.

Results

Between February 1998 and April 2000, 13 patients (7 men and 6 women) received elephant trunk grafts. The average age was 55 years, with a range of 43 to 77 years.

The etiology of renal failure was diabetes in 7 cases, hypertension in 3 cases, and various other causes in 3 cases. The comorbidities are detailed in table 8-1. In 6 cases, the grafts were new and in 7 cases they were revisions. Most of the surgery was performed in the left upper arm.

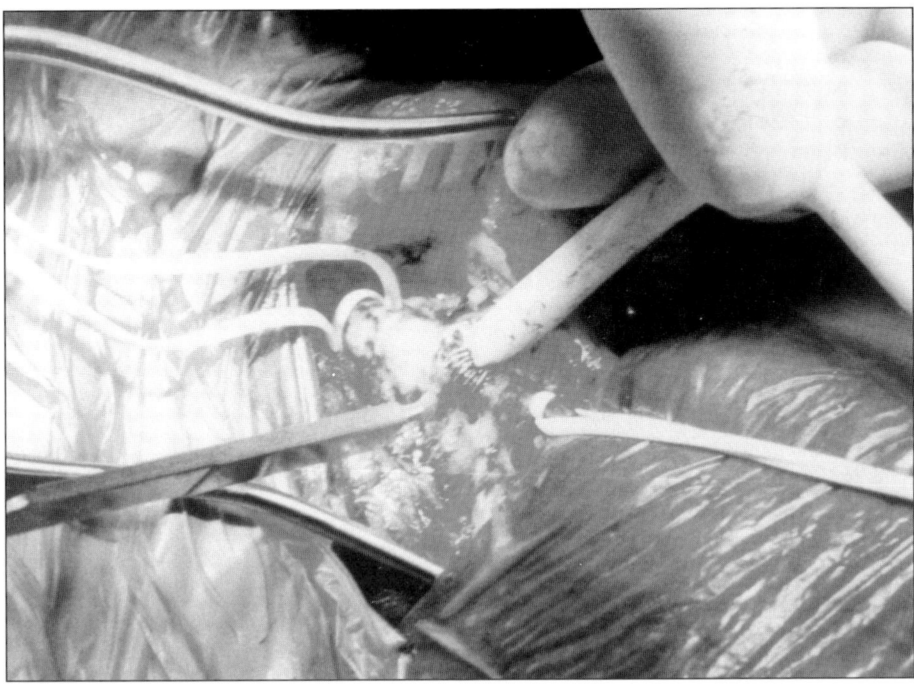

Figure 8-12. The vascular clips should be started at the heel of the anastomosis first.

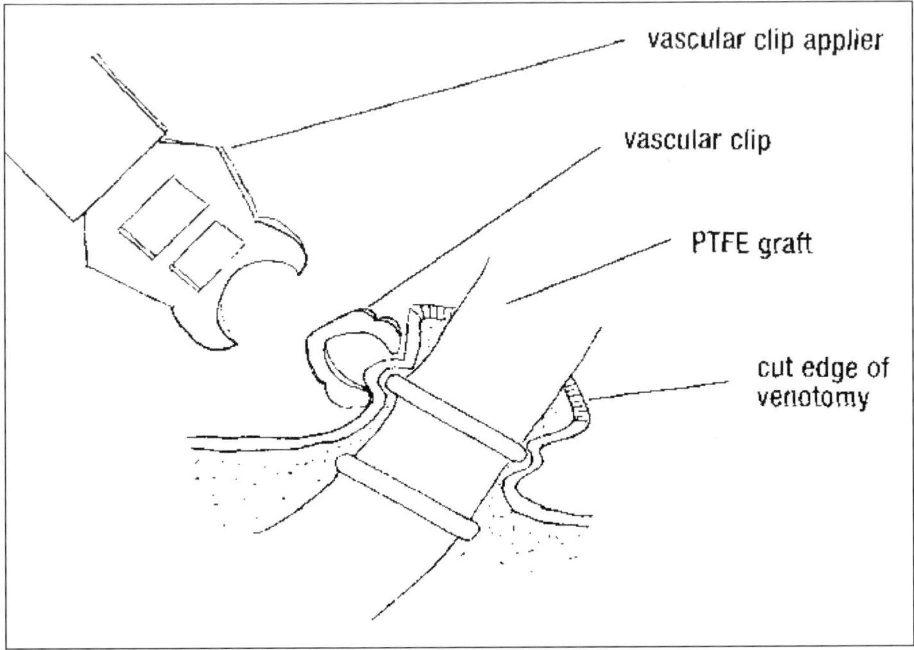

Figure 8-13. The vein grasps the first plastic ring of the graft, which acts like an O ring. The cut edge of the venotomy is everted so it does not make contact with the interior of the vein.

Table 8-1: Characteristics and comorbidities of the hemodialysis patients (N=13) in whom modification of venous end of the vascular access graft was employed.

Patient No.	Age in Years	Sex	ESRF Etiology	Comorbidities							Date of Surgery	New Graft or Revision	Site of Graft
				DM	HTN	CAD	CABG	COPD	CHF	Others			
1	77	F	Heart surgery	–	+	+	+	+	–	Anemia, hip replacement	Feb. 98	Revision	Left forearm
2	65	M	DM	+	–	+	+	–	+	CVA, osteomyelitis	Apr. 98	New	Left upper arm
3	48	M	DM	+	+	+	–	–	+	Morbid obesity, cardiomegaly, steal syndrome from graft in right arm	Oct. 98	New	Left upper arm
4	66	M	DM	+	+	+	–	–	–	GI bleeding, previous graft angioplasty	Jan. 99	Revision	Left upper arm
5	50	M	Cryoglo-bulinemia	–	+	–	–	+	–	Percardial tamponade, pneumonia, pul-monary edema	Jan. 99	New	Right upper arm
6	64	F	DM	+	–	–	–	–	+	Retinopathy, anemia, PVD	Aug. 99	New	Left upper arm
7	49	M	HTN	–	+	–	–	–	–	Hepatitis C, kidney stones	Sep. 99	New	Left upper arm
8	70	M	IgA nephropathy	–	+	–	–	–	–	Cholecystectomy, anemia previous graft angioplasty	Dec. 99	Revision	Left upper arm

Table 8-1: Characteristics and comorbidities of the hemodialysis patients (N=13) in whom modification of venous end of the vascular access graft was employed. *(continued)*

Patient No.	Age in Years	Sex	ESRF Etiology	Comorbidities							Date of Surgery	New Graft or Revision	Site of Graft
				DM	HTN	CAD	CABG	COPD	CHF	Others			
9	59	F	DM	+	+	–	–	+	–	Respiratory failure, pulmonary embolism, retroperitoneal bleeding, osteomyelitis, CVA, tuberculosis	Jan. 00	New	Left upper arm
10	66	F	HTN	–	+	–	–	–	–	Arrythmias, asthma, PUD, pancreatitis, kidney stones	Feb. 00	RTevision	left upper arm
11	74	F	HTN	–	+	+	+	–	–	Angioplasty of graft PVD, BKA, anemia	Mar. 00	Revision	Left upper arm
12	61	F	DM	+	+	–	–	–	–	Infected Hickman theter, amputations of fingers, myasthenia gravis, Leriche syndrome, bilateral AKA, pericardial infussion, GI bleeding	Apr. 00	Revision	Left upper arm
13	43	M	DM	+	+	+	++	+	+	PVD< CVA, bilateral AKA, blindness, pancreatitis, hepatitis, previous graft stenting	Apr. 00	Revision	Left upper arm

AKA=Above-knee amputation; BKA=Below-knee amputation; CABG=Coronary artery bypass grafting; CAD=Coronary artery disease; COPD=Chronic obstructive pulmonary disease; CHF=Congestive heart failure; CVA=Cerebrovascular accident; DM=Diabetes mellitus; ESRF=End-stage renal failure; GI=Gastrointestinal; HTN=Hypertension; PUD=Peptic ulcer disease, PVD=peripheral vascular disease.

Table 8-2: Dialysis related data obtained from 1 to 24 months after graft insertion using modified anastomotic technique.

	1 Month After Surgery			3 Months After Surgery			6 Months After Surgery			12 Months After Surgery			15 Months After Surgery			18 Months Post Surgery			21 Months After Surgery			24 Months After Surgery		
No.	Flow	VP	Kt/V	Flow	VP	Kt/V	Flow	VP	Kt/V	Flow	VP	Kt/V	Flow	VP	Kt/V	Flow	VP	Kt/V	Flow	VP	Kt/V	Flow	VP	Kt/V
1	500	216	1.78	500	272	1.77	500	276	1.71	500	272	1.84	500	260	1.72	450	212	1.6	500	216	1.48	500	240	1.21
2	300	112	1.54	400	204	1.47	400	176	1.56	400	190	1.54	450	232	1.50	450	244	1.21	400	200	1.38	400	228	NA
3	400	250	1.40	400	250	1.36	480	260	1.16	480	280	1.41	480	232	1.40	480	244	1.43						
4	200	192	1.42	400	236	1.40	Patient died																	
5	300	184	1.43	450	212	1.48	400	196	1.42	400	224	1.40	400	201	1.16									
6	200	200	0.91	450	260	1.49	450	340	1.26															
7	400	268	NA	Patient lost to follow-up																				
8	Patient died																							
9	400	208	NA	500	228	1.41																		
10	400	228	1.32																					
11	400	207	1.31																					

Flow is cc/minute. VP (venous pressure) is mm Hg (millimeters of mercury). Kt/V is a measure of the efficiency of dialysis, and it is derived from the patient's body water, urea clearance, and protein metabolism, N/A is not available.

There were no intraoperative mortalities. There was 1 mortality within 30 days as a result of myocardial infarction (MI), and there was 1 intraoperative complication of bleeding due to a tear in the vein, which resulted in an enlarged anastomotic annulus. There were no other complications as a result of the surgery. Specifically, there was no edema of the arm or the hand, or evidence of any steal syndrome or venous obstruction. There was 1 late death in the series. Patient No. 4 died of an MI 6 months postoperatively. One patient has been lost to follow-up, and the grafts are in use and free of complications in all other patients (n=10) as of April 2000, the time of this writing.

In the period after surgery (range 1 to 24 months), graft function was checked in a retrospective fashion to evaluate venous pressure, flow rate, and Kt/V in all surviving patients. All values have remained within a satisfactory range (table 8-2). Initial Kt/V ranged from 0.91 to 1.78 with an average of 1.39 (n=8). By 3 months, the average was 1.48 (n=7). At 1 year, it was 1.55 (n=4), and at 21 months it was 1.43 (n=2; see figure 8-14). The ultrasound graft of patient No. 11, which showed turbulence, was studied a few days after the surgery (figure 8-15). Figure 8-16 shows the graft of patient No. 2, 24 months after his surgery. It displays no evidence of extensive NIH migration down the outside, but there is evidence of some filling of the angle between the interior of the vein and the graft. The flow appears laminar.

Discussion

The etiology of NIH has been investigated since the introduction of PTFE as a material for AV grafts for hemodialysis in 1973. From a biochemical viewpoint, the

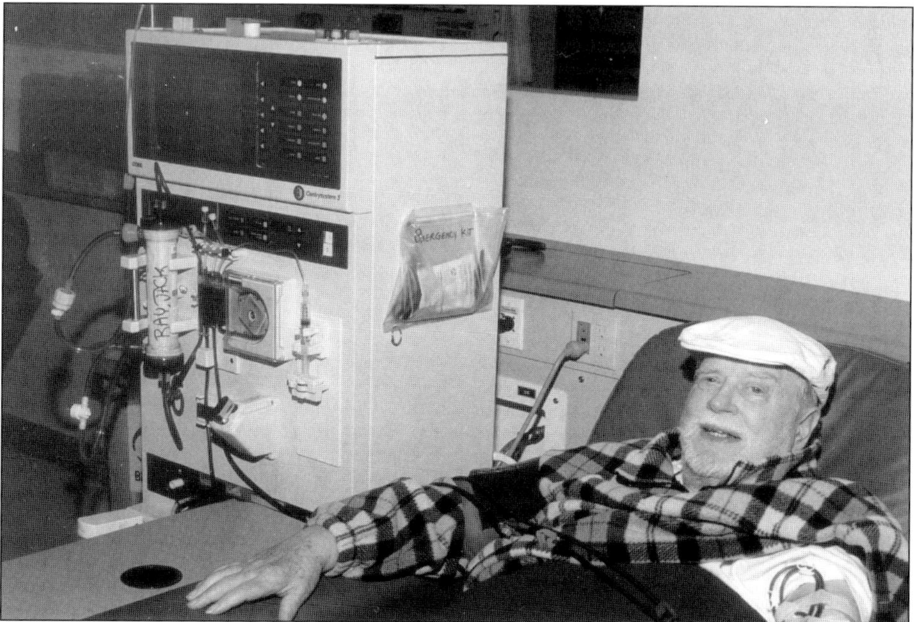

Figure 8-14. Patient No. 2 on dialysis 2 years after graft insertion.

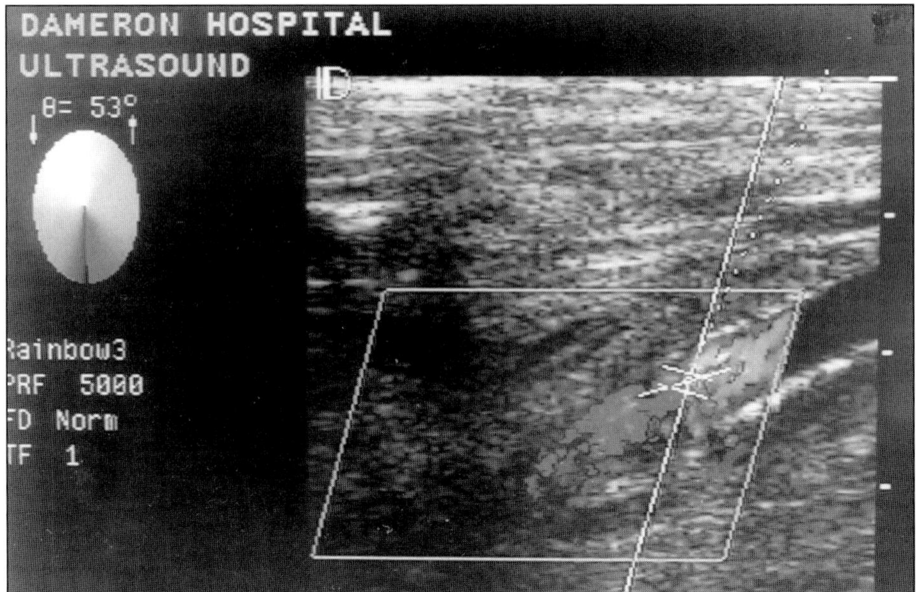

Figure 8-15. Ultrasound appearance of patient No. 11 a few days after graft insertion. There is more collinear flow in the vein compared to the conventional anastomosis, but some turbulence is still evident.

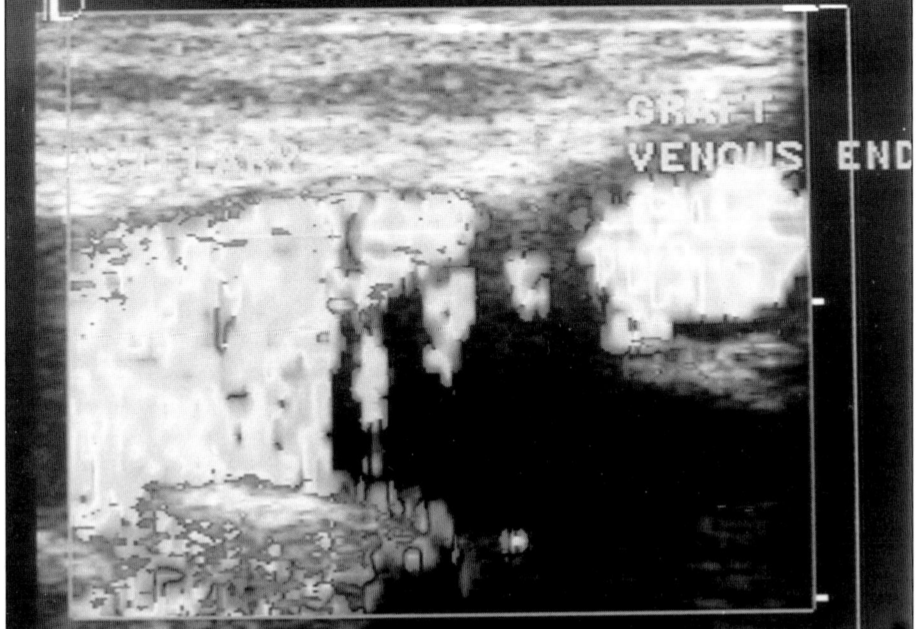

Figure 8-16. Appearance of the graft of patient No. 2 two years after its insertion. There is minimal evidence of NIH migration down the PTFE graft that lies in the lumen of the vein. There is evidence of some filling of the angle between the interior of the vein and the exterior of the graft. The flow appears more laminar.

area around the anastomosis is a hotbed of stimulatory factors that have been implicated in the stimulation of NIH (figure 8-17). On the other hand, some researchers favor a physical basis for the SMC stimulation, invoking the presence of mechanoreceptors on the SMCs and sheer stress receptors on endothelial cells (figure 8-18). Back and White reported that, by purely mechanical means, blood flow rate and corresponding wall sheer stress along the graft can influence platelet aggregation and thus determine the thickness of neointima.[1]

Another area of research has focused on the maelstrom effect resulting from the arterial blood's impacting into the side of the slow moving venous laminar flow. In this regard, Kerns wrote: "Of the hemodynamic variables measured, turbulence had the strongest correlation with anastomotic venous intimal-medial thickening."[6]

The technique described in this paper involves the insertion of the graft inside the vein and advancing it a short distance. Thus, the blood exit annulus is topographically separated from the anastomosis annulus (figure 8-19). In addition, the venotomy is isolated from the interior of the vein. This creates a barrier, making it difficult for the SMCs to migrate from the venotomy, enter the vein, migrate down the outside of the PTFE graft, and clear the plastic ring hurdles en route to the blood exit annulus.

The elephant trunk technique minimizes mechanical stimulation as a possible etiologic factor by creating a more laminar flow and diverting some of the physical forces from the area around the anastomosis annulus to the column of blood in the lumen of the vein (figure 8-20). By avoiding endothelial trauma, vascular clips also avoid triggering platelet accumulation and set in motion a cascade of events resulting from the release of platelet-derived growth factor.

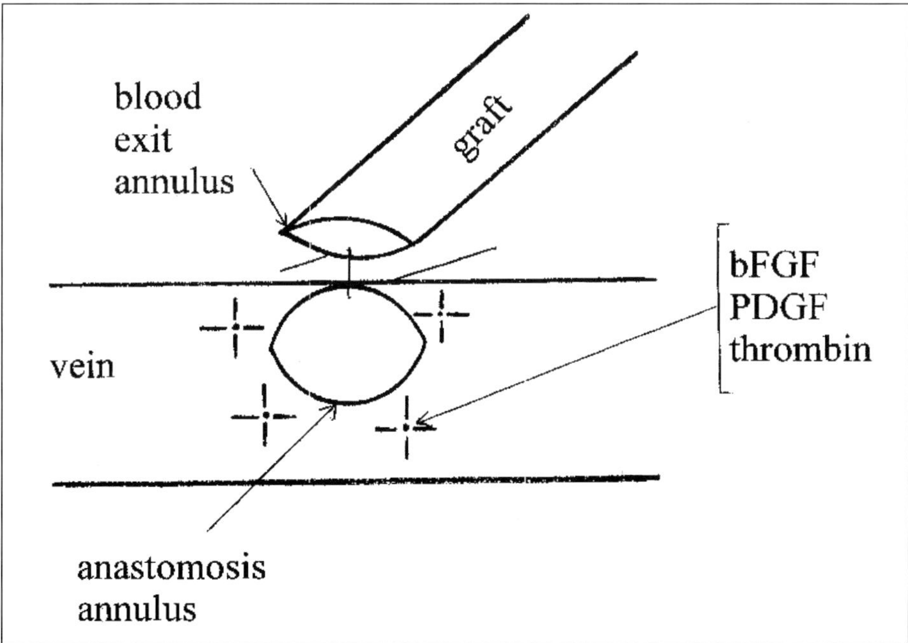

Figure 8-17. The production of biochemical stimulatory factors in the area of the vein around the anastomosis. These include bFGF (basic fibroblast growth factor), PDGF (platelet-derived growth factor) and thrombin, all of which can stimulate smooth muscle cells.

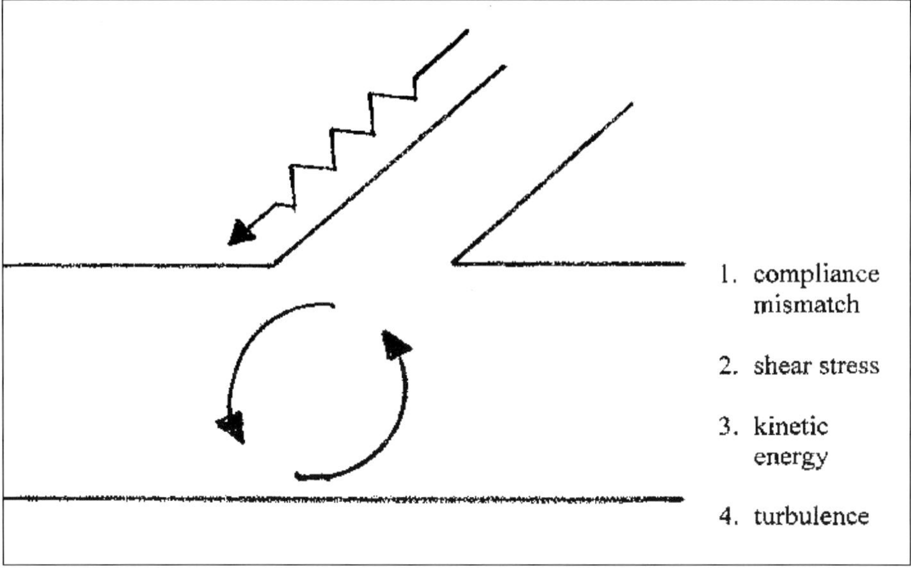

Figure 8-18. Some of the physical factors that may contribute to the production of neointimal hyperplasia include compliance mismatch, sheer stress, transmission of kinetic energy, and turbulence within the lumen of the vein.

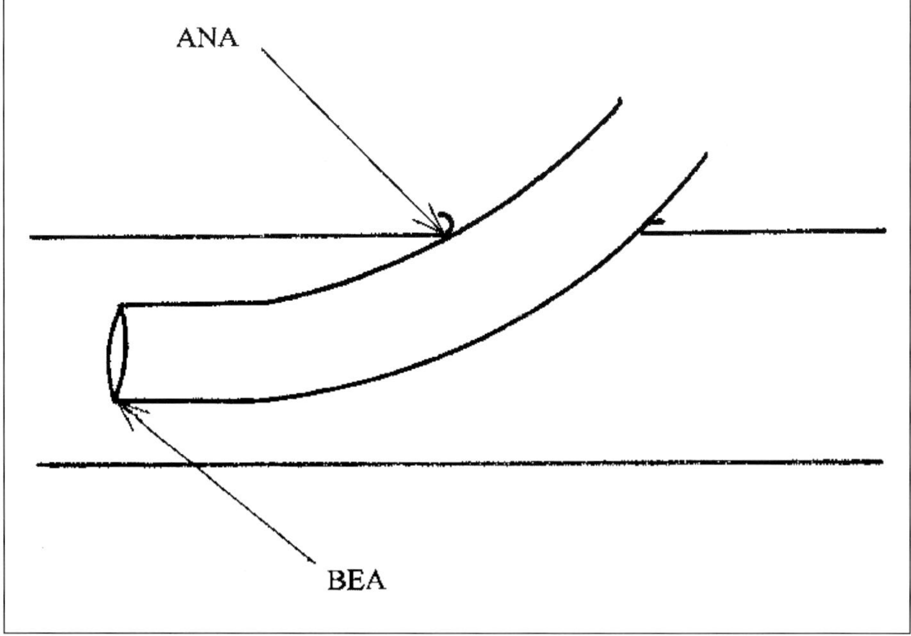

Figure 8-19. The blood exit annulus (BEA) is separated from the anastomosis annulus (ANA) in the elephant trunk technique. In addition, the edges of the venotomy are everted so the cut edges of the vein do not make contact with the lumen of the vein.

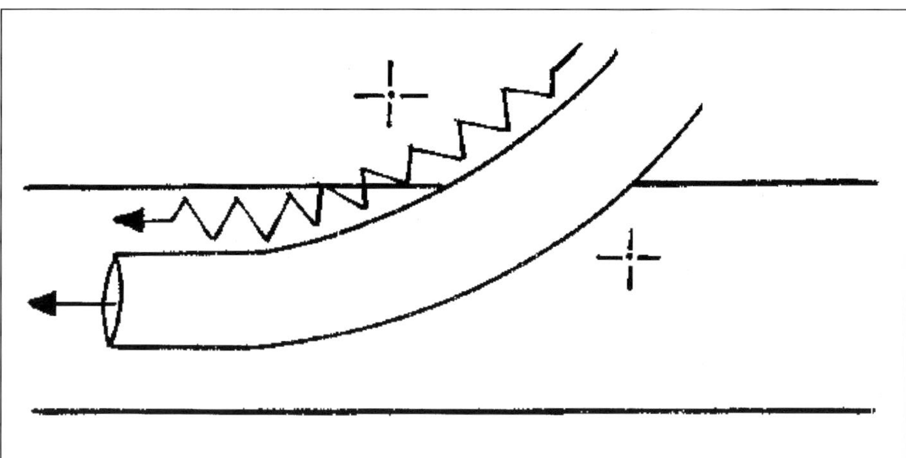

Figure 8-20. Diversion of some of the physical forces from the anastomosis annulus and the venous tissue around the anastomosis area to the column of blood in the lumen of the vein.

The problem with growth factors arising inside the PTFE graft or hemodialysis machine that stimulate SMC is reduced by diverting the flow away from the venotomy area and dispersing the factors downstream. With the elephant trunk arrangement, the arterial and the venous flows are made parallel, which makes the momentum vectors of both streams collinear and reduces mixing and separation phenomenon. Further discussion of the theoretical advantages of the elephant trunk technique has been outlined in an article in *Surgical Rounds*.[4]

Conclusion

This paper documents 13 chronic hemodialysis patients with the new elephant trunk technique. Surviving patients (n=10) are now up to 24 months postoperative and are free of NIH complications. The average Kt/V values have stayed fairly constant with the passage of time. This type of surgery is limited by the need for a big vein to accommodate insertion of the graft. Though this study retrospectively analyzed small numbers of patients over a relatively short time, the results seem to be promising.

Acknowledgements

The author would like to express his gratitude and appreciation to the following for reviewing the original research and for their helpful comments: Professor J.T. Brandt, Professor R.R. Gray, Professor M.L. Henry, Professor W.M. Kirsch, and

Professor A.F. Schild. The author is also deeply indebted to Professor G.M. Homsy and Professor S. Shakerin for their advice on the fluid mechanics of the elephant trunk technique and for comparing the fluid mechanics of the conventional anastomosis between the PTFE graft and vein.

References

1. Back MR, White RA. The biologic response of prosthetic dialysis grafts. In: Wilson SE, ed. Vascular access: Principles and practices, third edition. St. Louis, MO: C.V. Mosby Company, 1996; 137-49.
2. Kirsch WM. What's new in vascular clipping: The one-shot device and the effects of clipping on intimal hyperplasia. Paper presented at: 25th Annual Current Clinical Problems, New Horizons and Techniques in Vascular and Endovascular Surgery; November 19-22, 1998; New York City, NY.
3. Leppaniemi AK, Wherry D, Pikoulis E, et al. Arterial and venous repair with vascular clips: Comparison with suture closure. J Vasc Surg 1997; 26:24-28.
4. Coulson AS, Quarnstrom J, Moshirnia J. A combination of the elephant trunk anastomosis and vascular clips for dialysis grafts. Surg Rounds 1999; 22:596-608.
5. Coulson AS, Singh J, Moya JC. Modification of venous end of dialysis grafts: An attempt to reduce neointimal hyperplasia. Dial Transplantation 2000; 29:10-18.
6. Kerns DB, Fillinger MF. Compliance mismatch, hemodynamics of hyperplasia in arteriovenous grafts [syllabus]. The Fifth Biannual Symposium on Dialysis Access. Tuscon, AZ; 1996:31.

9

A NOVEL USE FOR AN "UNUSABLE" BRESCIA FISTULA

David D. Oakes, M.D., F.A.C.S., Gregg A. Adams, M.D., and John P. Sherck, M.D., F.A.C.S.

We present the case of a 56-year-old woman whose Brescia fistula was patent but unusable 1 year after creation due to an occlusion of the main cephalic vein in the mid-forearm. Only about 4 cm of dilated vein was available for cannulation, which was not enough for adequate separation of inflow and outflow needles. Rather than simply abandoning the fistula, however, we reasoned that because the runoff had been adequate to keep the fistula patent, it should also be adequate to provide venous drainage for an arteriovenous graft. The dilated venous segment was, therefore, anastomosed to a bovine graft based upon the brachial artery in the proximal forearm. The vein was ligated distally to prevent competing flow from the original anastomosis. The graft functioned well. Aided by a single angioplasty, it provided uninterrupted dialysis access until the patient received a renal transplant approximately 10½ months later.

Case Report

On December 8, 1997, a 55-year-old woman with a history of polycystic kidney disease presented to our institution with fatigue and malaise. Laboratory studies revealed a blood urea nitrogen (BUN) of 85 mg/dL and a creatinine of 9.5 mg/dL. She was not overtly uremic, and dialysis was determined to be imminent but not urgent. On December 11, 1997, a Brescia fistula was created at her left wrist. Her symptoms progressed, and on December 19, 1997, hemodialysis was instituted, using a PermCath® (Kendall Sherwood Davis & Geck, St. Louis, MO) cuffed central venous dialysis catheter introduced via her right internal jugular vein. She was evaluated for renal transplantation and determined to be a good candidate.

The patient's Brescia fistula remained patent but was slow to develop. A fistulogram on April 17, 1998, (figure 9-1) revealed a focal area of narrowing just distal to the anastomotic site. Angioplasty was planned for April 23, 1998, but on that day no definite narrowing could be demonstrated (figure 9-2). The fistula remained open but failed to develop a dominant vein in the forearm. On August 3, 1998, a right Brescia fistula was created, but it failed to develop.

Both fistulae remained patent, but by October the left was noted to have an unusual venous pattern. A fistulogram on November 6, 1998, demonstrated the presence of a normal anastomosis and juxta-anastomotic vein, but a long, severe stenosis of the main cephalic vein in the mid-forearm (figure 9-3). The vein was occluded near the site of puncture from the attempted angioplasty of April 23, 1998, suggesting that the vessel may have been damaged during that procedure.

At this point, it was apparent that the left Brescia fistula was not likely to develop a sufficiently long segment to permit dual cannulation. We were, however, reluctant to abandon the 4 cm segment of vein that had dilated and matured near the anastomosis. At that point, we reasoned that, because the venous runoff had been adequate to keep the fistula patent for 12 months, it should also be adequate to provide enough outflow to sustain an arteriovenous graft.

On December 3, 1998, a bovine graft was anastomosed to the distal left brachial artery in the proximal forearm. The graft was tunneled along the ulnar aspect of the

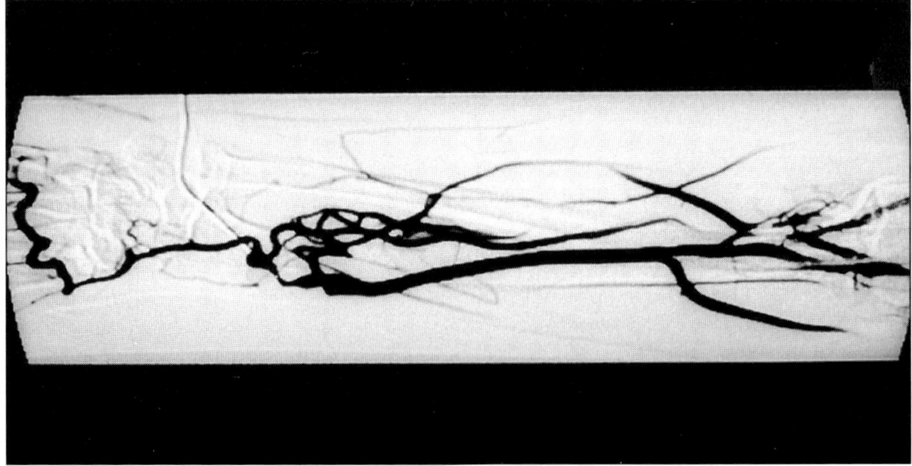

Figure 9-1. This angiogram was performed on April 17, 1998, approximately 4 months after the patient's Brescia fistula had been created. It was done because the fistula was not yet ready for cannulation, and we wished to see if there were any anatomic problems. There appeared to be a tight focal stenosis of the vein just beyond the anastomosis to the radial artery. An angioplasty was planned.

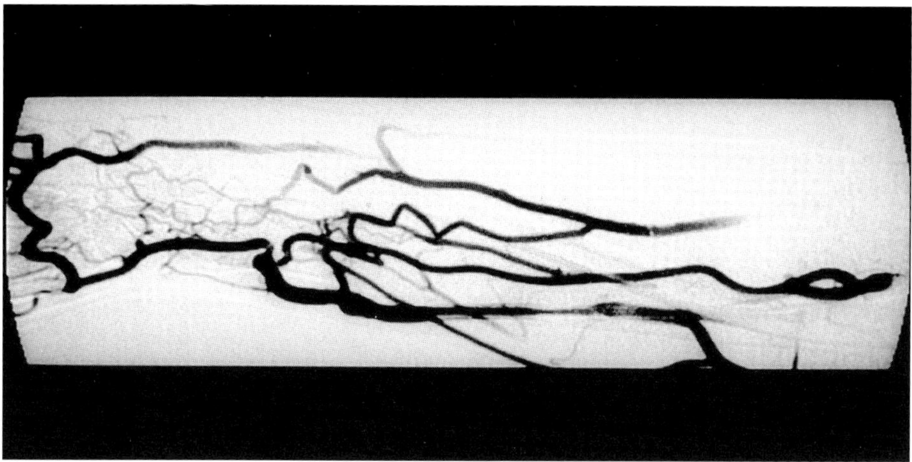

Figure 9-2. An angiogram performed on April 23, 1998 at the time of proposed angioplasty. The previously noted stenotic area could no longer be seen and was presumably some type of artifact.

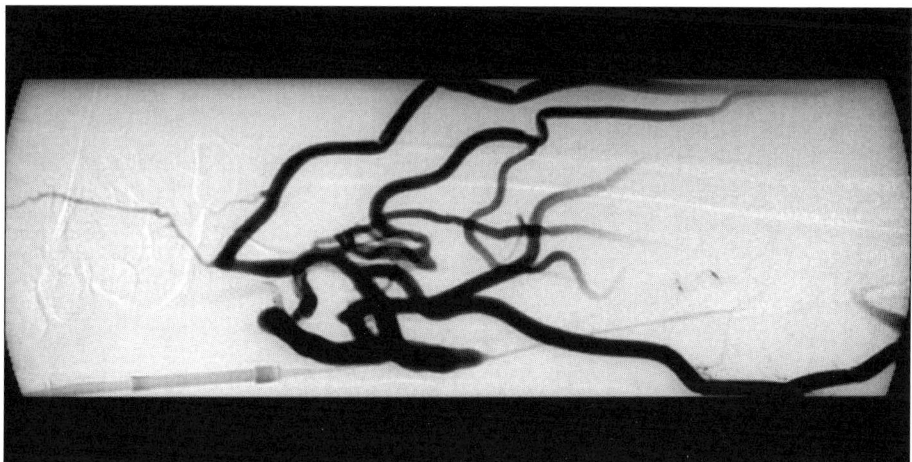

Figure 9-3. This angiogram was performed on November 6, 1998, 11 months after the Brescia fistula had been created. At this time, the patient was noted to have an unusual venous pattern involving her distal forearm. She did not appear to have a dominant cephalic vein extending to the antecubital space. The angiogram shows occlusion of the main cephalic vein in the mid-forearm. The location of the occlusion suggests that the vessel may have been damaged at the site of cannulation on April 23, 1998.

forearm and sewn to the dilated, matured venous segment of the Brescia fistula, just beyond the original anastomosis. The vein was ligated distally, disconnecting it from the radial artery to prevent competing flow. There was an excellent thrill, with most of the outflow passing into the deep venous system (figures 9-4 to 9-6). After the graft had healed into the subcutaneous tunnel, it was easily cannulated and provided excellent flow. The central venous catheter was removed on January

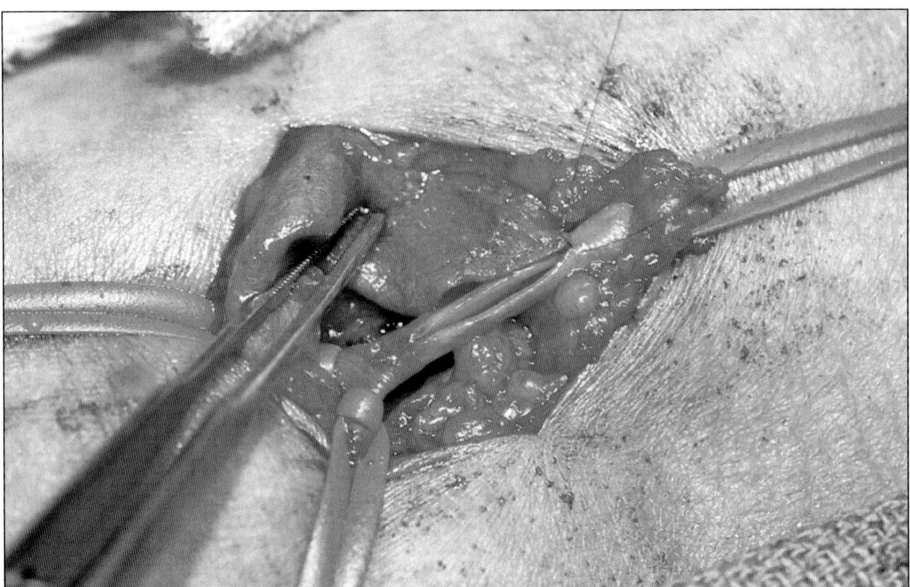

Figure 9-4. This intraoperative photograph shows an 8-mm bovine graft being anastomosed to the distal brachial artery in the antecubital space.

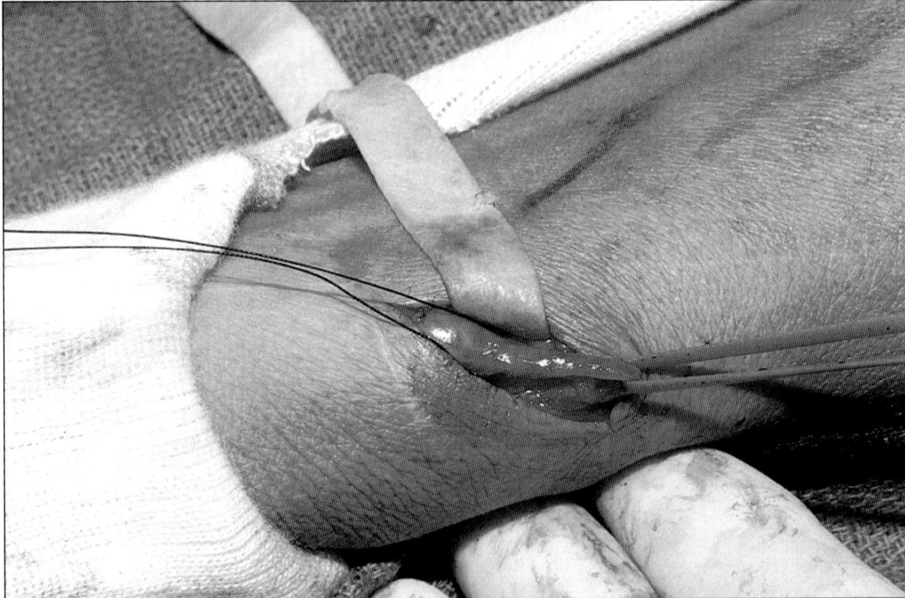

Figure 9-5. Here the bovine graft is being placed in a gently curving tunnel, passing from the antecubital incision toward the ulnar aspect of the forearm before curving back to join the dilated venous segment of the Brescia fistula at the wrist. The graft was passed in this fashion so that a second limb could be added in the future, converting the access to a forearm loop, if and when the venous outflow at the wrist became inadequate.

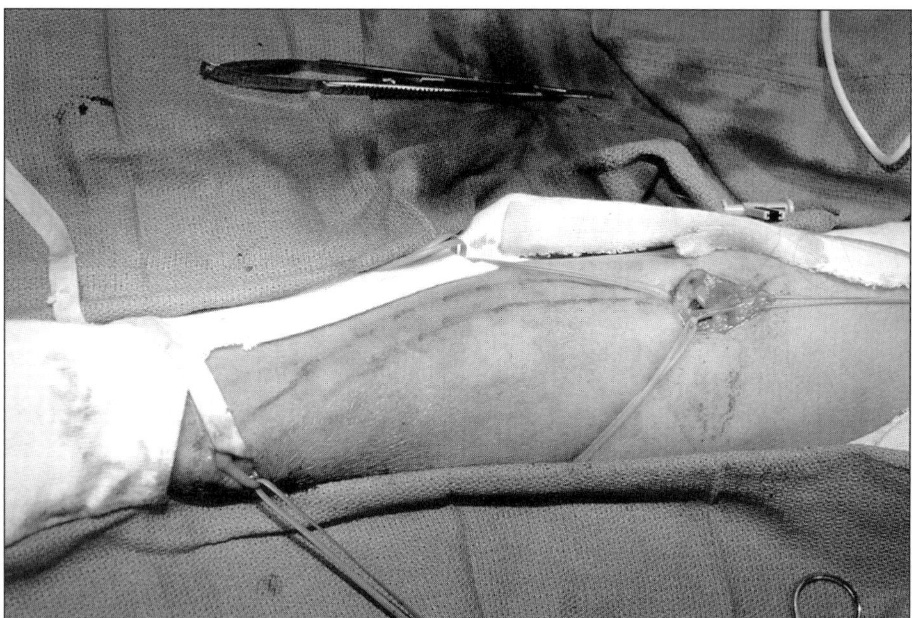

Figure 9-6. In this figure, the dilated portion of the Brescia fistula was being prepared for anastomosis to the bovine graft. Note that the vein has been ligated distally with a 3-0 silk suture to disconnect it from the previous anastomosis to the radial artery, thus preventing competing flow.

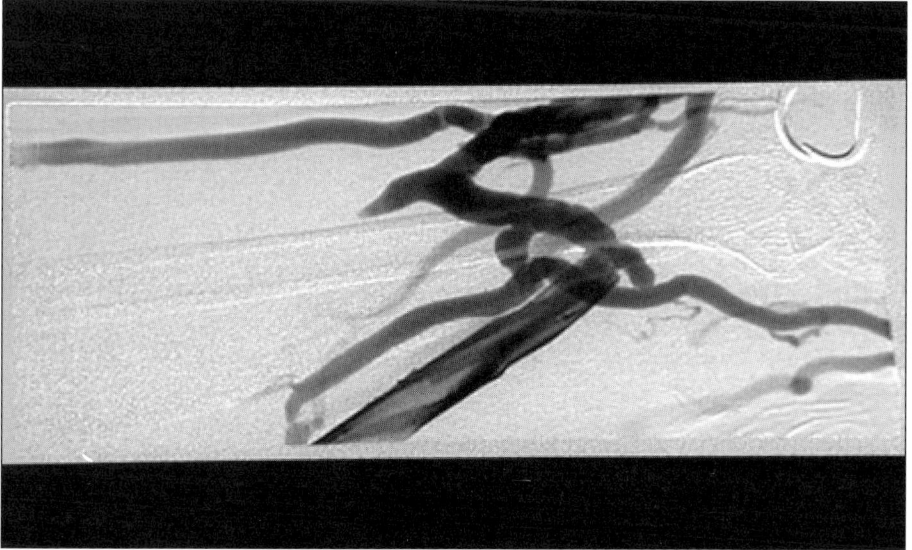

Figure 9-7. A fistulogram performed May 23, 1999 revealed a narrowing at the bovine-venous anastomosis. This was successfully angioplastied with a 5-mm balloon. The graft functioned well without further interventions for 5 additional months until the patient was successfully transplanted.

27, 1999. Because of rising venous pressures, a fistulogram was performed on May 23, 1999. A narrowing was noted at the venous anastomosis, so an angioplasty was performed with a 5-mm balloon (figure 9-7). With this single intervention, the graft functioned well until the patient received a renal transplant in October 1999.

Discussion

Since its first description in 1966, the Brescia-Cimino fistula has been recognized as the best available form of vascular access for hemodialysis.[1,2] Once developed, these autologous fistulae are remarkably durable and free from complications.[3] Unfortunately, not all patients have favorable forearm vasculature, and 1-year failure rates between 24% and 71% have been reported.[4,5] Some fistulae thrombose and fail completely. Others remain patent but, for various reasons, are not usable for hemodialysis.

In our patient, the dilated venous segment was too short to permit reliable dual cannulation. In the past, we simply abandoned such fistulae or used them for arterial inflow for a straight forearm graft between the wrist and the antecubital space. This may or may not have been preferable to a direct anastomosis between the graft and the radial artery, but in any case, it required the use of an antecubital vein. The theoretical advantage of the procedure that we are now reporting is that, by utilizing the wrist veins for outflow, more proximal veins are preserved for future access procedures.

Several points are worth noting. We believe the brachial artery should be exposed through a longitudinal incision in the proximal forearm. A transverse incision might damage antecubital veins by direct injury or by later scar formation if the vessels need to be dissected free and retracted out of the way during exposure of the artery. The graft should be tunneled toward the ulnar aspect of the volar forearm before curving back to the radial side to join the wrist incision. This gentle curve will facilitate conversion of the graft to a loop if venous outflow is no longer adequate at the wrist. It is essential to ligate the vein between the new anastomosis and the original anastomosis to prevent competing flow from the radial artery. Finally, it is important to communicate with the dialysis technicians, explaining that flow in this type of access is opposite to that in conventional straight forearm grafts.

Encouraged by our experience with the patient presented above, we have continued to study the use of this procedure. As of December 1, 1999, we performed the operation in 13 patients. Although follow-up was short, our early results are encouraging. Six of 7 patients followed more than 5 months had functioning grafts, with patencies ranging from 5 to 10½ months (mean patency 8.3 months). The single early failure was a graft lost because of infection. This represents a technical problem rather than a failure of the operative concept per se. A primary access failure of 8% satisfies the published guidelines of the National Kidney Foundation-Dialysis Outcomes Quality Initiative for forearm grafts.[6]

In summary, we present a new operation that utilizes patent, but unusable, Brescia fistulae in such a way as to preserve more proximal veins for future access procedures. Our early experience is encouraging and justifies further study of this operation in selected patients.

References

1. Brescia MJ, Cimino JE, Appel K, Hurwich BJ. Chronic hemodialysis using venipuncture and a surgically created arteriovenous fistula. N Engl J Med 1966; 275:1089-92.
2. Ryan JJ, Dennis MJ. Radiocephalic fistula in vascular access. Brit J Surg 1990; 77:1321-23.
3. Kumpe DA, Cohen MA. Angioplasty/thrombolytic treatment of failing and failed hemodialysis access sites: Comparison with surgical treatment. Prog Cardiovasc Dis 1992; 34:263-78.
4. Palder SB, Kirkman RL, Whittemore AD, Hakim RM, Lazarus JM, Tilney NL. Vascular access for hemodialysis: Patency rates and results of revision. Ann Surg 1985; 202:235-39.
5. Ballard JL, Bunt TJ, Malone JM. Major complications of angioaccess surgery. Am J Surg 1992; 164:229-32.
6. Schwab S, Besarab A, Beathard G, et al. NKF-DOQI clinical practice guidelines for vascular access. New York: National Kidney Foundation; 1997.

10

A TECHNIQUE TO SALVAGE THE END-TO-SIDE RADIOCEPHALIC ARTERIOVENOUS FISTULA FOR CHRONIC HEMODIALYSIS

John Raheb, D.O., Robert Esterl, Jr., M.D., William Washburn, M.D., Francisco Cigarroa, M.D., and Glenn Halff, M.D.

The end-to-side radiocephalic arteriovenous fistula (AVF) has become the preferred technique for vascular access for chronic hemodialysis. When compared with polytetrafluoroethylene (PTFE) grafts, the AVF has superior patency rates and fewer complications. The most frequent complication after AVF is early failure (25% of complications), and thrombosis remains the most common cause of early failure. In rare cases, early failure is due to venous stenosis at or just beyond the arteriovenous anastomosis. Fistulography may be helpful in such cases to define the location and extent of the venous stenosis.

Management of the venous stenosis has included transluminal angioplasty, anastomotic revision, segmental venous resection with primary repair, and conversion to an end-to-end anastomosis. In this retrospective study, the authors describe a useful technique to salvage AVFs that fail secondary to anastomotic stenosis/thrombosis or distal cephalic vein stenosis (within 8 cm of the anastomosis) with an otherwise patent cephalic vein. This technique involves ligation of the cephalic vein and creation of a more proximal anastomosis between the matured cephalic vein and the radial artery.

Subjects and Methods

Between August 1992 and October 1999, 173 patients underwent placement of a primary forearm AVF at the University of Texas Health Science Center at San

Antonio, Texas. Twenty-two patients (12.7%) developed anastomotic stenosis, thrombosis, or distal cephalic vein stenosis within 8 cm of the anastomosis. All 22 patients demonstrated a patent proximal cephalic vein. These 22 patients consisted of 7 women and 15 men with a mean age of 49 years of age (median 49 years and a range 29 to 69 years of age). There were 19 Hispanic and 3 black patients. The causes of renal failure were diabetes mellitus (14 patients), essential hypertension (4 patients), IgA nephropathy (2 patients), systemic lupus erythematosis (1 patient), and focal segmental glomerulosclerosis (1 patient).

Each AVF was initially constructed as an end-to-side radiocephalic AVF in the distal forearm under local anesthesia (0.5% to 1% lidocaine). The mean diameter of the cephalic vein was 3.71 mm (range 2.5 to 5 mm) in 12 patients. The mean length of operation was 1.53 hours (range 0.92 to 2.17 hours). All AVFs were performed by surgical residents under the supervision of 2 faculty surgeons.

The 22 patients in the study included 14 patients who developed low flow in the AVF as a cause of failure (mean 463 days, range 92 to 1170 days), and 8 patients who developed thrombosis as a cause of failure (mean 74 days, range 6 to 344 days). All 14 patients with low flow underwent fistulography that demonstrated distal cephalic vein stenosis (9 patients), anastomotic stenosis (1 patient), both anastomotic and distal cephalic vein stenosis (3 patients), and proximal arterial stenosis (1 patient). All 8 patients with thrombosis demonstrated no flow in the fistula with an otherwise patent proximal cephalic vein. Only 1 of the 8 patients underwent fistulography, which demonstrated occlusion at the arteriovenous anastomosis and a patent cephalic vein.

All 22 patients underwent revision of the AVF in the operative suite under local anesthesia (figure 10-1). The revisions were performed by surgical residents under the supervision of the same 2 faculty surgeons. All patients received preoperative intravenous antibiotics. In this technique, a transverse incision was made in the anterolateral forearm proximal to the venous stenosis or anastomotic stenosis/thrombosis. The radial artery and cephalic vein were exposed proximally to the venous stenosis or anastomotic stenosis/thrombosis. The distal cephalic vein was ligated and transected just proximal to the venous stenosis or arteriovenous stenosis/thrombosis. The cephalic vein was flushed with heparinized saline and serially dilated to 4 mm in diameter. After control of the radial artery with vessel loops, an arteriotomy was made on the anterior radial artery with a No. 11 scalpel. The proximal and distal radial artery was flushed with heparinized saline (1:1000 U). An end-to-side radiocephalic AVF was constructed with continuous 6-0 polypropylene suture. The subcutaneous and cutaneous layers were reapproximated with interrupted 3-0 polyglycolic and 4-0 nylon sutures, respectively.

Results

All 22 patients utilized the AVF immediately after revision. Sixteen (73%) of 22 patients had functional AVFs at a mean 992 days (median 873 days, range 570 to 1719 days) after revision. Five (23%) patients underwent renal transplants, and 4 (80%) of 5 recipients have functional AVFs to date. Five (22%) patients developed

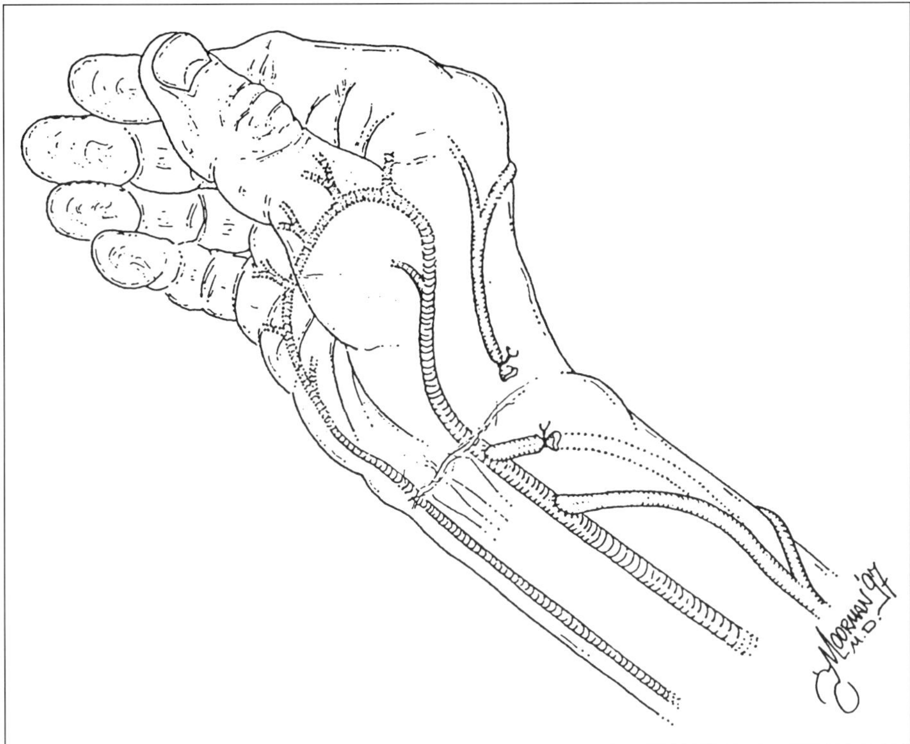

Figure 10-1. Revision of forearm primary AVF.

AVF failure at a mean 519 days (median 98 days, range 41 to 1220 days) after revision, and required placement of forearm PTFE loops grafts. One recipient required ligation of the AVF for an expanding pseudoaneurysm 1604 days after revision. One patient died from a CVA but the AVF was functional 1089 days after revision. One patient developed low flow in the AVF 198 days after revision. This patient underwent balloon angioplasty of the arteriovenous anastomosis and the cephalic vein, and this AVF was still functional 1719 days after revision. The only complication after revision of the AVF was temporary paresthesia of the cutaneous branch of the radial nerve in 3 patients (13.7%).

Discussion

The end-to-side radiocephalic AVF is the preferred method of permanent hemodialysis with superior patency and fewer complications compared with PTFE grafts. The most common complication after construction of the AVF is early failure, and thrombosis of a significant length of ccphalic vein remains the most common cause of early failure. In fewer than 5% of cases, the AVF slowly fails, due to the development of an anastomotic stenosis or from distal cephalic vein stenosis that presents as low flow in the AVF. With low flow rates, AVF fistulography may be important in defining the exact location and extent of stenosis. Fistulography identifies the location on the forearm to make an appropriate incision for revision. In rare cases the AVF fails from thrombosis at the anastomosis but the cephalic vein remains patent from venous collateral blood supply on the forearm proximal to the anastomosis. In this series, the authors describe a technique to salvage AVFs that fail from anastomotic stenosis/thrombosis or from cephalic vein stenosis within 8 cm of the anastomosis when a patent proximal cephalic vein was present.

Many authors suggest that construction of a PTFE graft in the ipsilateral lower or upper arm is the next procedure of choice for permanent hemodialysis after failure of the radiocephalic AVF. We believe that our technique of revision of the AVF provides several potential benefits in selected patients. First, the technique preserves future access sites in the ipsilateral lower and upper arm. Second, this technique avoids placement of a PTFE graft in the ipsilateral arm, which will likely have poorer patency and greater complications than an AVF. Third, the patency of the revised AVF should be excellent because the radial artery and cephalic vein have greater caliber in the proximal forearm. There is every reason to believe that the patency of the revised AVF should be similar to or better than the patency of the primary AVF. Finally, the cephalic vein in most cases is mature and can be accessed immediately for hemodialysis. Immediate access to the cephalic vein avoids placement of a temporary hemodialysis catheter with its inherent complications.

Thirteen percent of patients developed transient neuropathy of the posterolateral hand after revision of the AVF. Cautious dissection of the proximal forearm is necessary to avoid injury to the cutaneous branch of the radial nerve as it pierces the brachioradialis muscle to supply the posterolateral forearm.

Preliminary results are encouraging for this technique for revision of the radiocephalic AVF. Seventy-three percent of patients have a functional AVF at a mean follow up of 992 days. Salvage of the AVF by a proximal revision provides a durable access with excellent long term patency and few complications. This technique provides the surgeon with another alternative for a failing or clotted radiocephalic AVF.

11

CLINICAL OUTCOMES OF FOUR HEMODIALYSIS PATIENTS IMPLANTED WITH THE LIFESITE® HEMODIALYSIS ACCESS SYSTEM: A NOVEL APPROACH FOR VASCULAR ACCESS

John R. Ross, M.D.

The advent of the Quinton-Scribner arteriovenous (AV) shunt in 1960 made prolonged hemodialysis possible for patients suffering end-stage renal disease (ESRD), though its attendant infection and thrombosis rates made it an imperfect solution.[1,2] After the development of the AV shunt, Cimino and Brescia described their native arteriovenous fistula (AVF) in 1966[3], and their surgical innovation quickly became the ideal for hemodialysis vascular access. Unfortunately, despite the benefits of their autogenous approach, it soon became apparent that patients with certain comorbidities were unable to form a satisfactory fistula for dialysis.[4-6] As a result, variations on the AVF technique evolved in the 1970s and 1980s-including the employment of grafts made of expanded polytetrafluoroethylene (ePTFE), Dacron velour, human umbilical vein, and even bovine carotid artery-all aimed at addressing the shortcomings of the native AV fistula.[6-13]

Still, vascular access remains the biggest challenge for hemodialysis.[14] The high rate of comorbidities in the US ESRD population, coupled with late presentation by patients and late referrals by their doctors, has forced hemodialysis caregivers to use access modalities that emphasize expedience rather than efficacy and safety.[6,15-19] Physicians with no other options have gravitated toward lesser alternatives with outcomes that fall short of patient care ideals.[6,19-21] Given the trend that patients are presenting with ESRD when they are older and sicker, the disparity between the Dialysis Outcomes Quality Initiative (DOQI) goal for native fistulae placement (50%) and the actual use of fistulae will grow. Already, excessive reliance on ePTFE grafts and an alarming trend toward implanting transcutaneous central venous catheters (CVCs) as permanent devices have elevated the access portion of annual ESRD costs to 30% of the total.[15-17]

Our efforts to overcome the high complication rates associated with access technologies in common use have led to the study of a new, subcutaneous hemodialysis access device. The LifeSite® Hemodialysis Access System (Vasca Inc., Tewksbury, MA) consists of two identical titanium valves with attached single lumen cannulae (figure 11-1). The valve is implanted in a subcutaneous pocket below the clavicle, with the cannula tunneled to a central vein. Two systems are implanted, 1 for draw and 1 for return. LifeSite® has an internal pinch clamp that is actuated with a 14-gauge dialysis needle (Medisystems Corp., Seatle, WA). As the needle is inserted, an internal pinch clamp opens to allow fluid flow. When the needle is removed, the clamp closes and flow stops (figures 11-2 and 11-3). Access to the LifeSite® System is obtained utilizing the buttonhole technique, with the advantages of simple and quick cannulation, less pain, and reduced scarring. The device has a high degree of patient compliance and seems poised to greatly improve patient outcomes for North America's ESRD population.

We discuss here our experiences with the device.

Materials and Methods

Implantation was performed with the patient under conscious sedation. The preferred cannula implantation location was the right internal jugular vein, with the

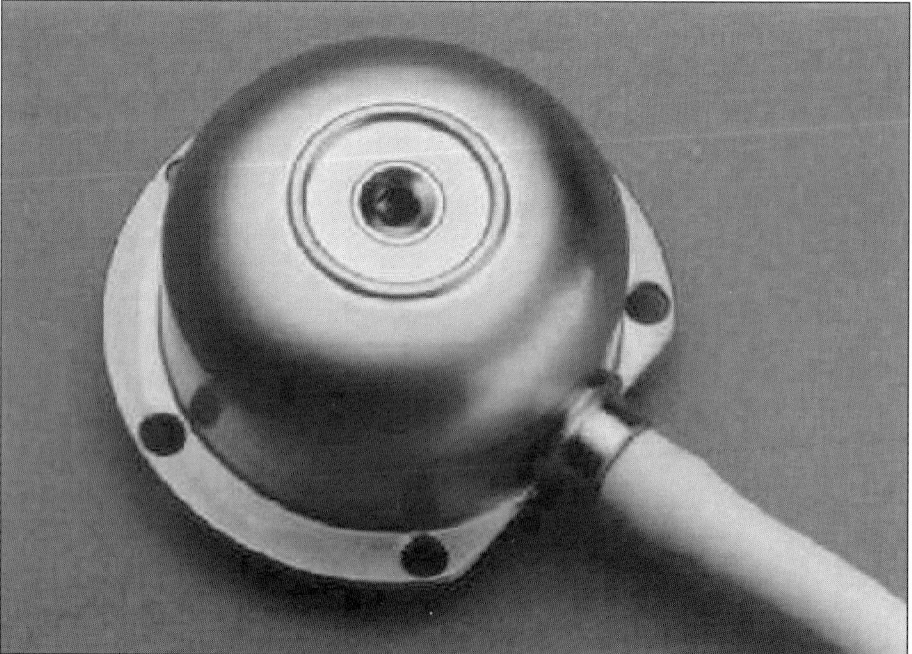

Figure 11-1. The LifeSite® Hemodialysis Access System

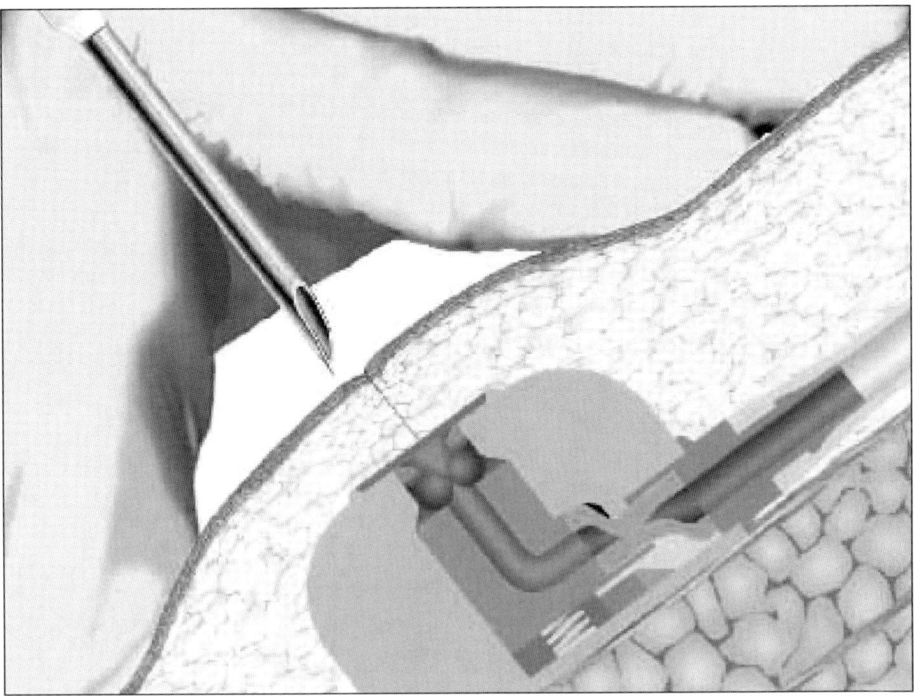

Figure 11-2. The LifeSite® internal pinch clamp is in the closed position before the needle is inserted.

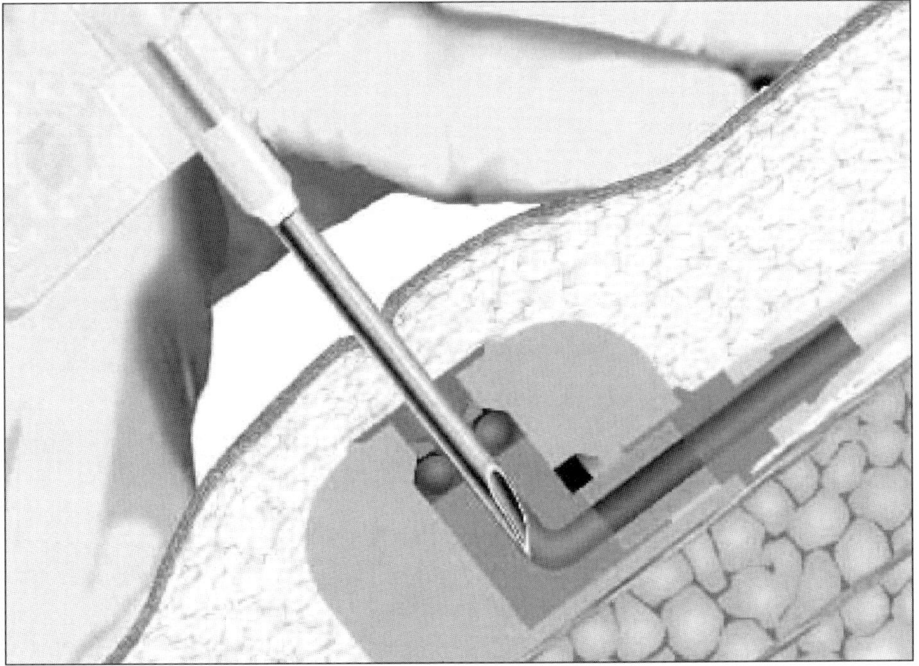

Figure 11-3. The LifeSite® internal pinch clamp opens to allow fluid flow as the needle is inserted.

subclavian vein a possible, though less desired alternative. The valve itself was placed with the upper surface of the devices between 10 and 15 mm below the skin surface.

After site selection, the right internal jugular vein was identified for size, position, patency, and then cannulated-all under sonographic guidance (figure 11-4). Next, a 0.035 inch floppy tip guidewire was passed under fluoroscopic guidance through the superior vena cava (SVC) into the right atrium and parked in the inferior vena cava (IVC). A separate, identical cannulation was performed with the second 0.35 guidewire parallel to the first, as shown in figure 11-5. A No. 11 scalpel blade then performed an incision to connect the skin cannulation puncture sites; a "tiny" hemostat was inserted and used to develop a catheter pocket. This pocket allowed ample space for the split sheath introducers and provided an expansion space that prevented kinks in the catheters (figure 11-6). A split sheath introducer was passed over the guidewire into the SVC from the right side under radiographic observation, as shown in figure 11-7. Next, the catheter was placed over the guidewire through the split sheath into the distal atrium. The split sheath could then be divided or simply retracted over the catheter and guidewire, with the second cannula placed identically as the first (figure 11-8).

Subcutaneous pockets for the valves were developed over the chest wall at a 10- to 15-mm depth. The pockets were sized to allow a snug fit for the LifeSite® valves (figure 11-9). A trochar tunneler was placed from the valve pocket to the catheter

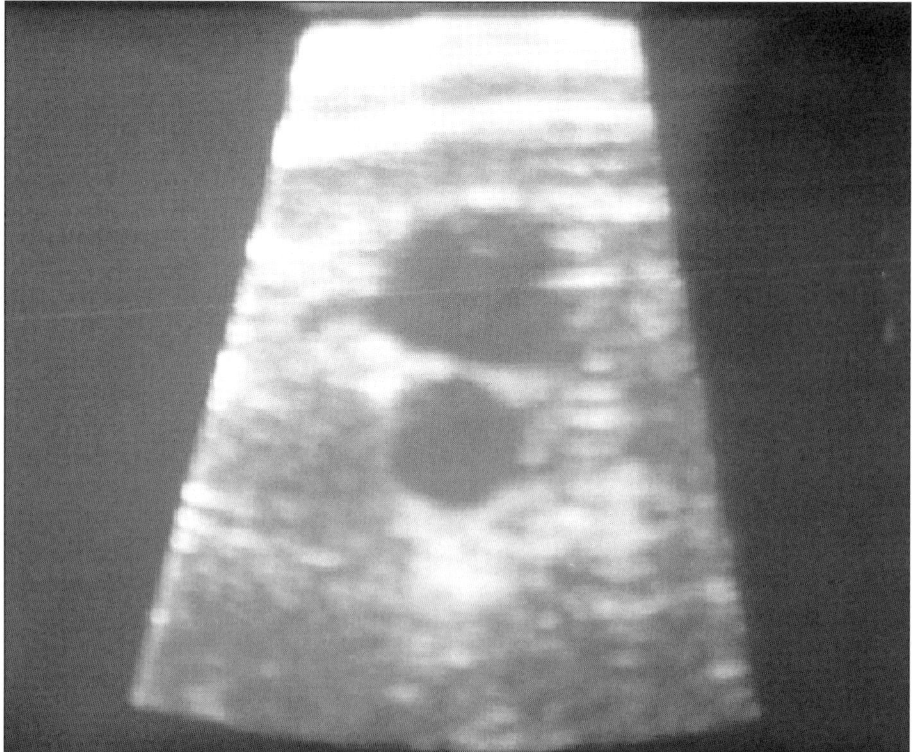

Figure 11-4. A sonographic guidance allowed evaluation of the right internal jugular vein.

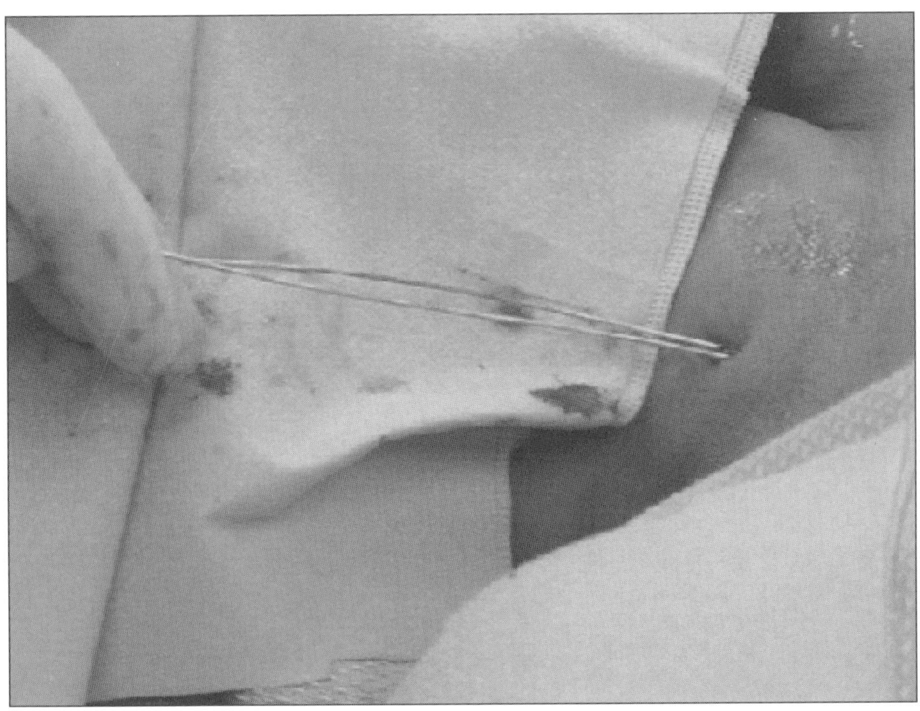

Figure 11-5. Two identical cannulations were performed with parallel 0.35 guidewires.

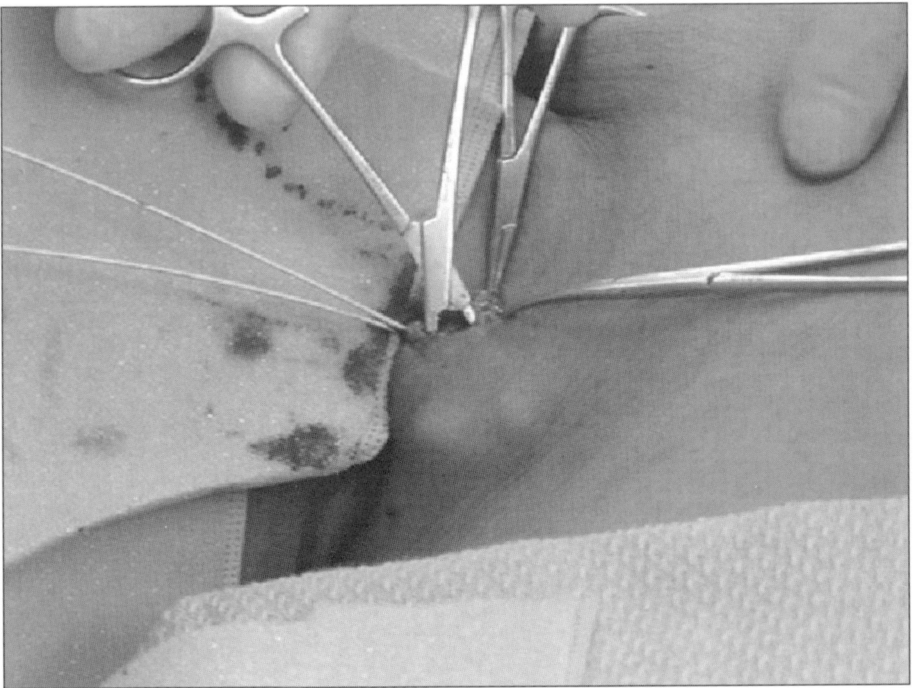

Figure 11-6. A hemostat was inserted and used to develop a catheter pocket.

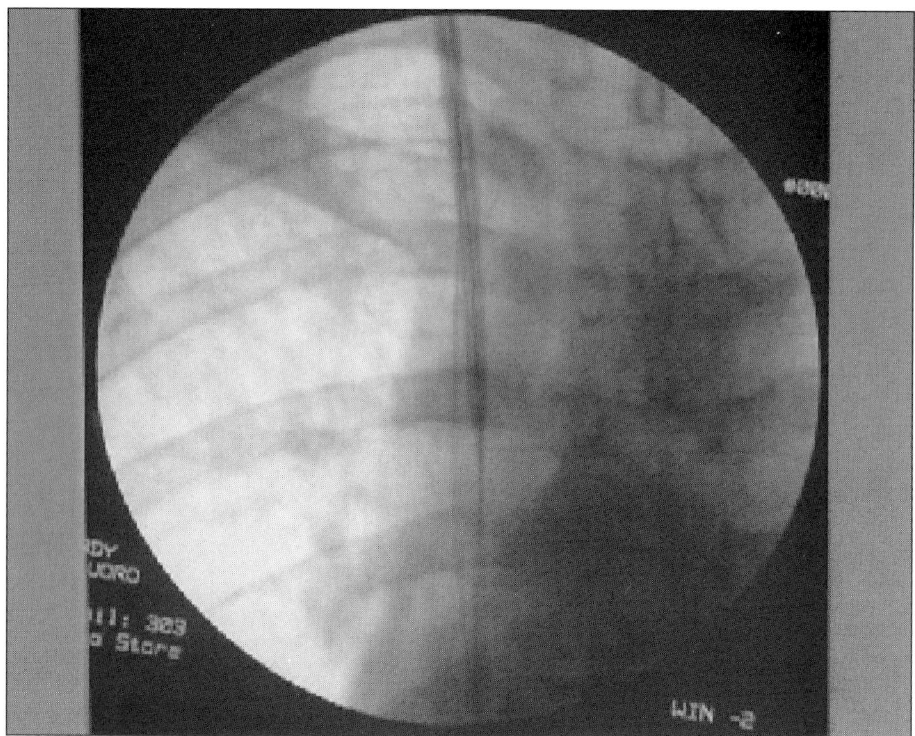

Figure 11-7. Radiographic observation directed placement of the split sheath introducer.

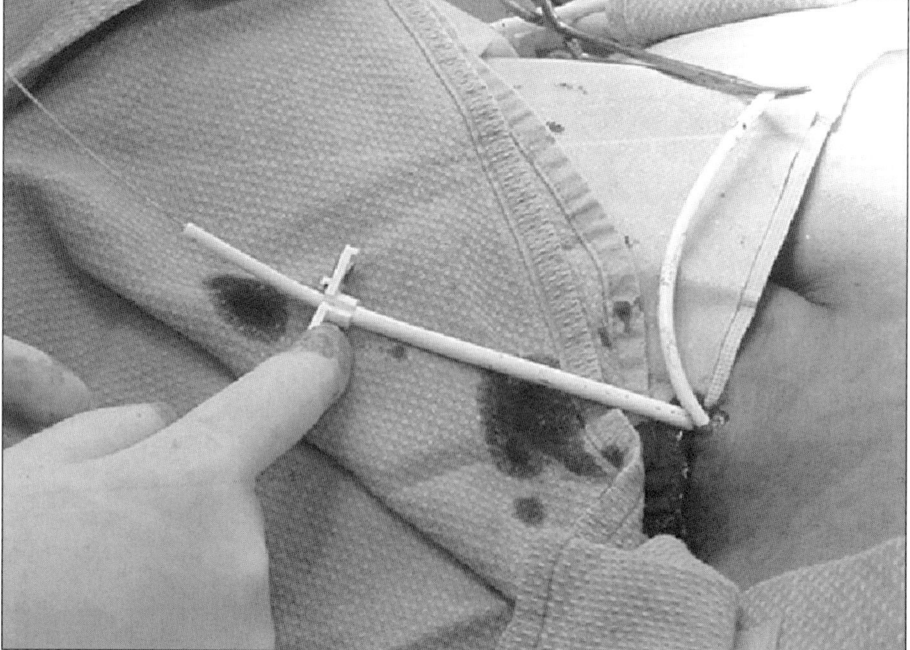

Figure 11-8. The second cannula was placed identically as the first.

pocket. Following attachment of the tunneler to the catheter, a simple pull-through of the catheter was performed. Again, an identical maneuver was performed for pulling the second catheter to the second pocket (figure 11-10).

Positioning of the catheters under fluoroscopic control is then performed. The tips were placed in the right atrium with a separation of 2 cm. Observation under fluoroscopy was then performed to assure that there were no kinks in the catheters in the neck area (figures 11-11 and 11-12).

Stay sutures were placed in the valve pocket for fixation of the valve. Connection of the catheters to the valves was done following fixation of the valves in the pockets. Confirmation of flow was performed utilizing 14-gauge fistula needles attached to 20 cc syringes (figure 11-13). Upon confirmation of flow, the pockets were closed, followed by a heparin and saline lock of the devices upon completion of the procedure.

On procedure. The design of the LifeSite® facilitates irrigation with an antimicrobial solution both pre- and postdialysis. This innovation, along with its pinch clamp valve and tapered seat seal, set it apart from chemotherapy ports and other technologies.

The procedure is quick, simple, and well accepted by patients and nursing staff. Any initial cannulation pain is due mainly to postsurgical trauma from the creation of the valve pockets, and rapidly disappears.

The dialysis caregiver first locates the LifeSite® valve by palpation. Following a 30-second scrub with 4% chlorhexidene, the nurse irrigates the valve, sinus pocket, and buttonhole tissue tract with 70% isopropyl alcohol utilizing a 3 mL syringe attached to a 25-gauge needle (figure 11-14). The small diameter of the irrigation

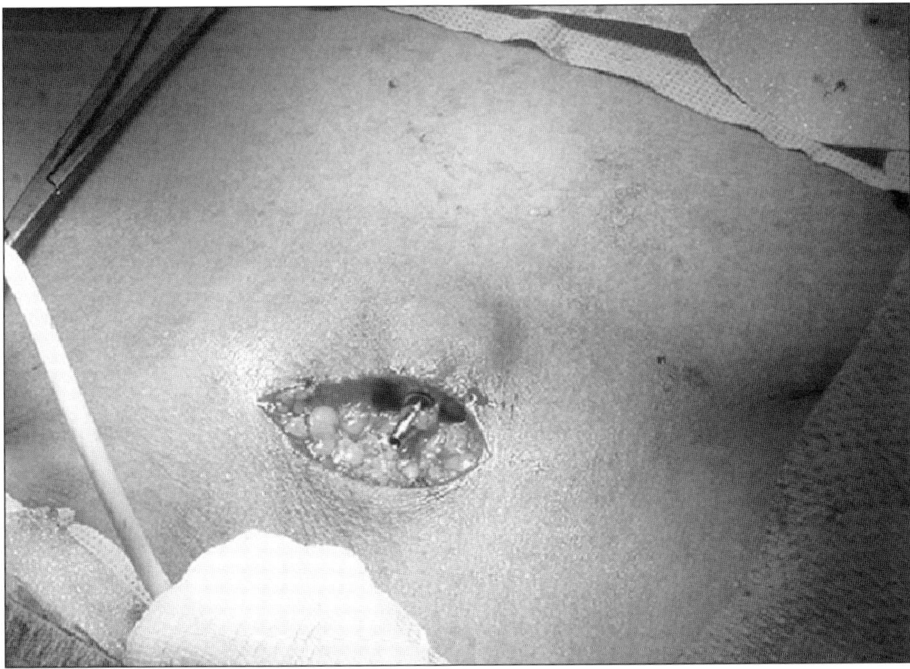

Figure 11-9. Subcutaneous pockets were sized to allow a snug fit for LifeSite® valves.

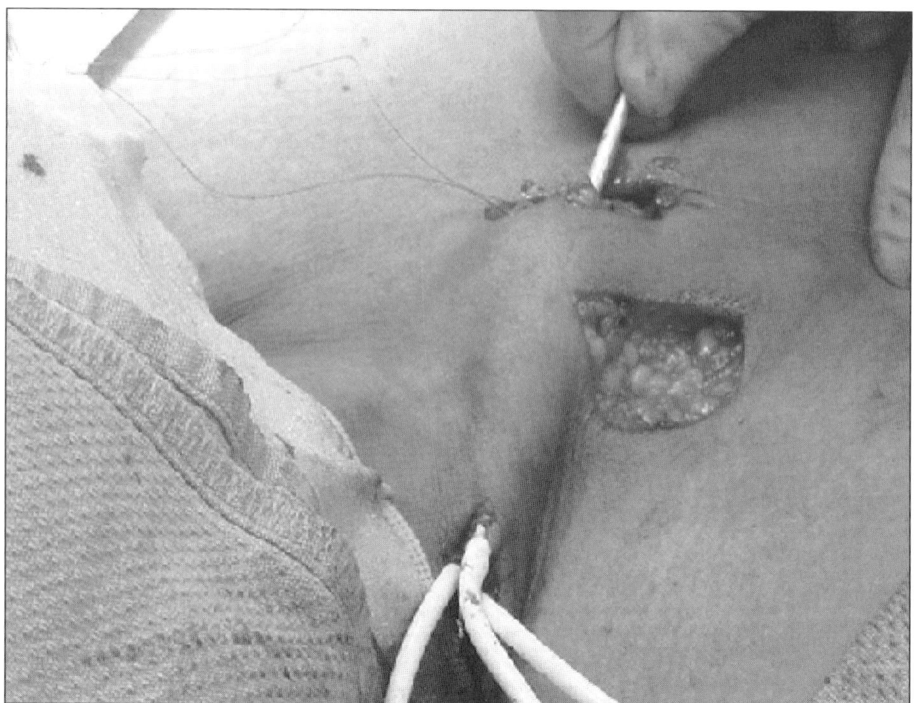

Figure 11-10. The second catheter was placed into the second pocket the same way the first catheter was placed.

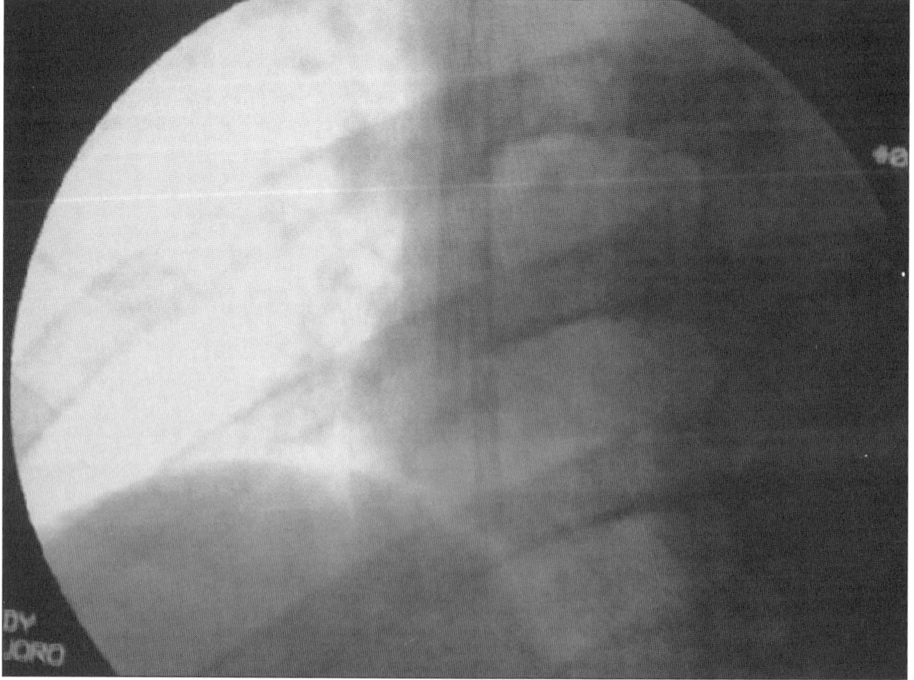

Figure 11-11. Fluoroscopy confirmed the lack of kinks in the catheters.

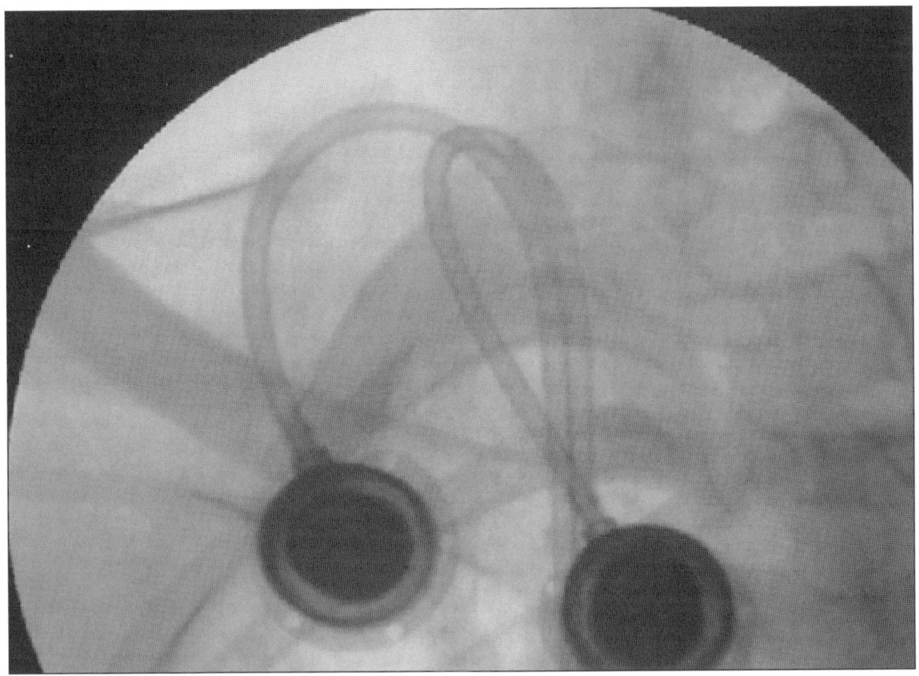

Figure 11-12. Fluoroscopic observation of the LifeSite® system showed no kinks in the neck area.

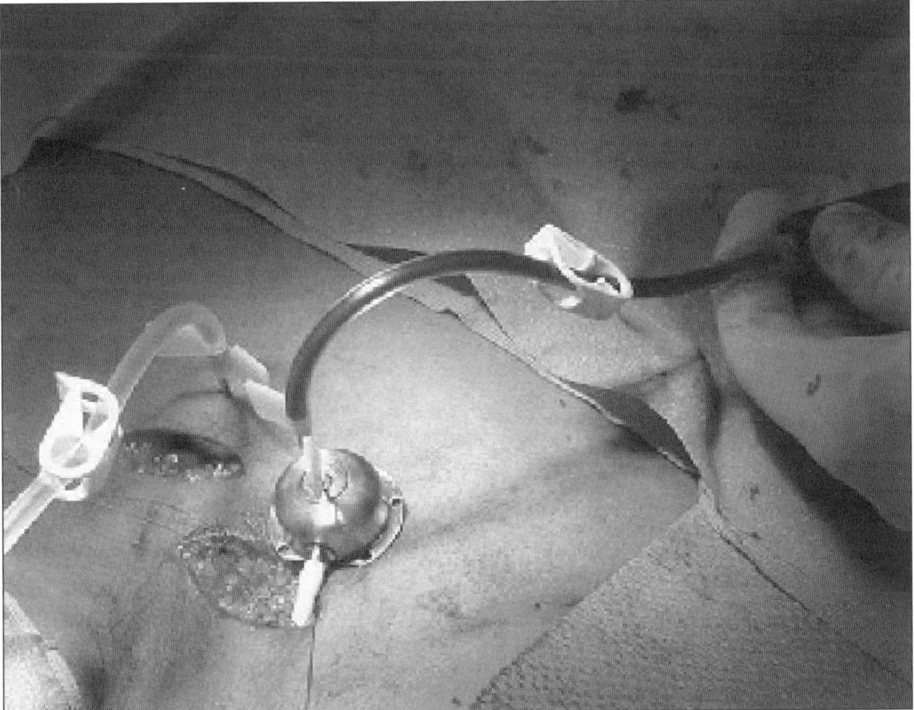

Figure 11-13. A 14-gauge fistula needle confirmed blood flow.

needle cannot activate the valve's pinch clamp mechanism, thereby precluding the antimicrobial solution from entering the bloodstream (figure 11-15).

After irrigation, the health care professional performs valve cannulation utilizing a standard 14-gauge fistula needle. The needle is held in the caregiver's dominant hand and inserted at a 90° angle to the device with a slight twisting motion as the needle reaches the tapered seat near the final one third of the valve. This push and twist motion, when combined with the malleable nature of large bore dialysis needles, achieves an exceptionally secure blood path seal that prevents accidental disconnection. The 14-gauge needle actuates a plunger and pinch clamp mechanism. The clamp, normally inclined when closed, opens when the 14-gauge needle is properly seated, making the valve open to the patient's vasculature.

Next the caregiver aspirates a 5-mL volume to remove the previous heparin lock along with any clots that may have formed. The large inner diameter (ID) of each cannula (12 French) is believed responsible for the LifeSite®'s reported 100% secondary patency rate (figure 11-15).

Off procedure. After the prescribed dialysis treatment, the caregiver follows the unit protocol on rinsing back the patient's blood, stops the blood pump, and instills a heparin lock of approximately 1.7 mL. The LifeSite® valves are then disconnected by holding the valve between the thumb and forefinger and giving the needle a quarter turn to break the taper seal, then withdrawing the fistula needle.

The isopropyl alcohol irrigation procedure is repeated and a nonocclusive dressing applied. Postdialysis bleeding times are reduced to almost nil because of the valve's unique design.

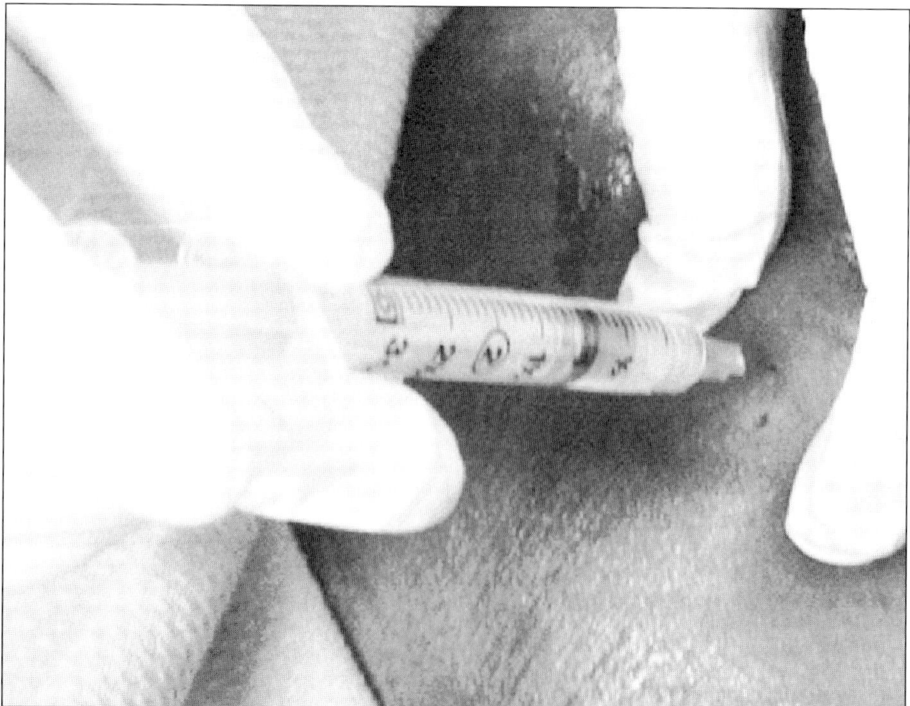

Figure 11-14. The nurse irrigated the valve using 70% isopropyl alcohol.

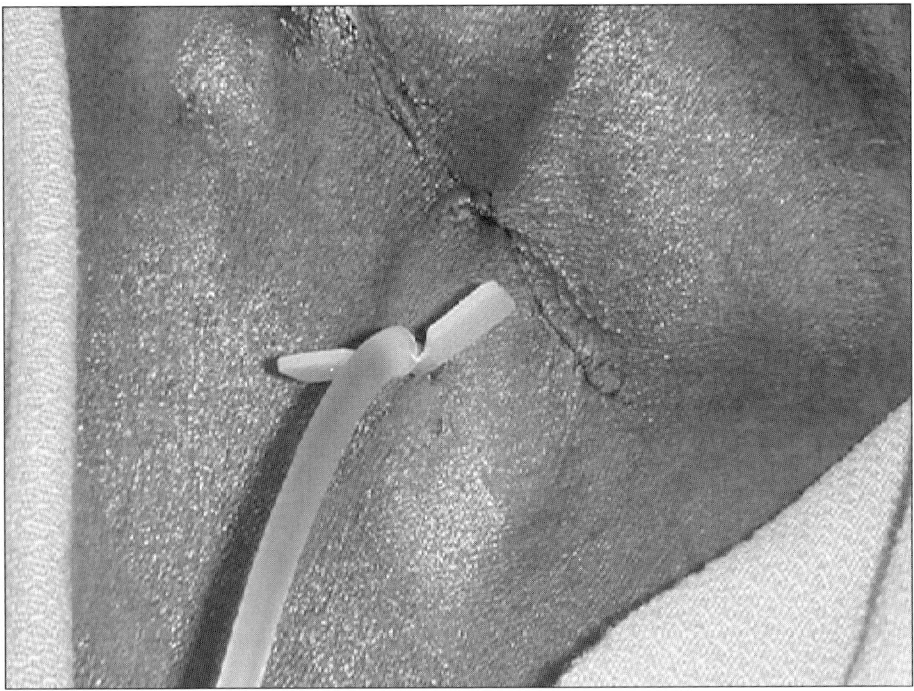

Figure 11-15. The antimicrobial solution cannot enter the bloodstream because of the small diameter of the irrigation needle.

Patients may resume normal activities, such as showering and even swimming, once the implantation sites have healed.

Results

LifeSite® devices were implanted in 4 hemodialysis patients with previous failed vascular accesses and substantial comorbidities. The valves provided access for adequate dialysis for a total of 15.4 months with only 1 episode of infection; a rate of 2.1 infections per 1000 patient days.

Discussion

Despite nearly 40 years of experience with vascular access, hemodialysis access remains a difficult medical challenge, requiring surgical placement or construction with frequent interventions. The initial experience with LifeSite® devices obtained with these 4 patients suggests a promising new alternative for vascular access. The subcutaneous device provided vascular access for adequate dialysis in a patient group with a history of failed access and comorbidities. The infection rate observed in these patients rivals that reported for dialysis catheters.[16] These clinical experiences validate the use of this device as an access for hemodialysis. It is easily implanted, easily used, provides safe and effective dialysis, and is well tolerated by patients.

References

1. Quinton WE, Dillard D, Scribner BH. Cannulation of blood vessels for prolonged hemodialysis. Trans Am Soc Artif Intern Organs 1960; 6:104-13.
2. Bell PRF, Veitch PS. Vascular access for hemodialysis. In: Nissenson AR, Fine RN, Gentile DE, eds. Clinical dialysis. New York: Appleton Century Crofts; 1990:26-43.
3. Brescia MJ, Cimino JE, Appel K, Hurwich BJ. Chronic hemodialysis using venipuncture and a surgically created arteriovenous fistula. N Engl J Med 1966; 275:1089-92.
4. Kapoian T, Sherman RA. A brief history of vascular access for hemodialysis: An unfinished story. Semin Nephrol 1997; 17:239-45.
5. Hodges TC, Fillinger MF, Zwolak RM, Walsh DB, Bech F, Cronenwett JL. Longitudinal comparison of dialysis access methods: Risk factors for failure. J Vasc Surg 1997; 26:1009-19.
6. NKF-DOQI Clinical Practice Guidelines for Vascular Access. National Kidney Foundation-Dialysis Outcomes Quality Initiative. Am J Kidney Dis 1997; 30:S150-91.
7. Baker LD Jr, Johnson JM, Goldfarb D. Expanded polytetrafluoroethylene (PTFE) subcutaneous arteriovenous conduit: An improved vascular access for chronic hemodialysis. Trans Am Soc Artif Intern Organs 1976; 22:382-87.
8. Brems J, Castenada M, Garvin PJ. A five year experience with the bovine heterograft for vascular access. Arch Surg 1986; 121:941-44.
9. Giacchino JL, Geis WP, Buckingham JM, Vertuno LL, Bansal VK. Vascular access: Long term results, new techniques. Arch Surg 1979; 114:403-09.
10. Kherlakian GM, Roedersheimer LR, Arbaugh JJ, Newmark KJ, King LR. Comparison of autogenous fistula versus expanded polytetrafluoroethylene graft fistula for angioaccess in hemodialysis. Am J Surg 1986; 152:238-43.
11. Munda R, First R, Alexander JW, Linneman CC, Fidler JP, Kittur D. Polytetrafluoroethylene graft survival in hemodialysis. JAMA 1983; 249:219-22.
12. Rapaport A, Noon GP, McCollum CH. Polytetrafluoroethylene (PTFE) grafts for haemodialysis in chronic renal failure: Assessment of durability and function at three years. Aust N Z J Surg 1981; 51:562-67.
13. Veith FJ, Wilson SE, Hobson RW, Rosenthal JJ, Tellis VA, Dagher FJ. Vascular access complications and new methods. Trans Am Soc Artif Intern Organs 1982; 28:647-57.
14. Hakim R, Himmelfarb J. Hemodialysis access failure: A call to action. Kidney Int 1998; 54:1029-40.

15. U.S. Renal Data System 1999 Annual Report: U.S. Renal Data System, 1999.
16. Schwab SJ, Beathard G. The hemodialysis catheter conundrum: Hate living with them, but can't live without them. Kidney Int 1999; 56:1-17.
17. U.S. Renal Data System. The economic cost of ESRD, vascular access procedures, and Medicare spending for alternative modalities of treatment. Am J Kidney Dis 1997; 30:S160-77.
18. Committee on Quality of Health Care in America. Nursing in the dialysis unit: Technological enframing and declining art, or an imperative for caring. J Adv Nurs 1999; 27:730-36.
19. Schwab SJ. Hemodialysis vascular access: Entering a new era. Am J Kidney Dis 1999; 34: xxxviii-xi.
20. Lenz BJ, Veldenz HC, Dennis JW, Khansarinia S, Atteberry LR. A three-year follow-up on standard versus thin wall ePTFE grafts for hemodialysis. J Vasc Surg 1998; 28:464-70.
21. Feldman HI, Kobrin S, Wasserstein A. Hemodialysis vascular access morbidity. J Am Soc Nephrol 1996; 7:523-35.

SECTION IV

12

VASCULAR ACCESS INFECTIONS

Timothy Lane Pruett, M.D.

Infection is the second leading cause of death in patients who have end-stage renal disease (ESRD) and require dialysis therapy. The permanent access site for dialysis serves as a point of entry for bacteria and a major source of infection. Each of the hemodialysis access routes, (native fistula, polytetrafluoroethylene [PTFE] or bovine arteriovenous [AV] fistula, permanent or temporary venous catheter) is at variable risk for infection. It is the goal of the surgical procedure to produce a reliable and durable access site for the life-sustaining dialysis procedure. Owing to the fact that there are only a limited number of access sites on any 1 patient, eradication of the access route infection while preserving the access site is desirable. The principles in the treatment of vascular access infections with maintenance of function are addressed in this discussion.

The ESRD patient and surgical infections. The patient referred for vascular access is usually older and has more comorbid conditions than the typical surgical patient. The skin flora of the average person's upper extremity and chest contains *Staphylococcus epidermidis* as the predominant species. The ESRD patient is very likely to be colonized predominantly with *Staphylococcus aureus (S aureus).*[1] As a consequence, it is of no surprise that this species is most prevalent (>80%) of the organisms commonly isolated from vascular access infections.

Of the various skin preparations for surgical procedures, a regimen including chlorhexidine may be the most efficacious for controlling *S aureus* organisms.[2] Antibiotic therapy directed at *S aureus* perioperatively has been associated with a wound infection rate reduction from 6% to 1%.[3] In this era of pathologic organisms being resistant to multiple antibiotics, it is crucial to tailor therapy to the antibiotic sensitivity patterns found in the local community. Increasingly, it has been shown that methicillin-resistant *Staphylococcus aureus* (MRSA) is recoverable in the community, especially from nursing home residents, and the strains can persist for a considerable length of time after discharge in patients with nosocomial colonization contracted during a hospitalization.

Vascular access infection. Taylor et al. described their experience from a single center, with regard to the incidence and treatment of vascular access infections.[4] Operations for purposes of remediation of infection accounted for 6% of the graft operations and 9% of the operations for graft revision. This excellent review appropriately recognizes that access infection may be related to the surgical wound or to the practice of repetitive puncture. Of the 263 procedures performed for infection remediation, 144 were for wound-related problems (127 wound infections, 14 abscesses, and 3 occult), while 119 procedures were for puncture-related problems (10 erosions, 97 puncture-site infections, and 12 puncture abscesses). Further description of these characteristics is shown in table 12-1.

Care of the patient with an infected graft focuses on resolution of the infection and, if possible, maintenance of vascular access function. Graft salvage may be defined as continued fistula function and successful wound healing without infection at the site for more than 30 days. Clinical judgment is key to discern whether an attempt should be made to salvage a graft or the graft should be removed.

Wound-related infections. The primary surgical strategy should be preventing further infection of the access site. By definition, owing to the presence of existing infection, this is termed a surgically clean procedure, (as opposed to a sterile procedure), and has controllable infectious complications. The lowest risk for wound infection is after the creation of autogenous upper extremity fistulae (<1%). However, not all patients have accessible or viable anatomy or tissue that is amenable to such constructions. With appropriate antistaphylococcal antimicrobial agents and appropriate surgical site preparation and technique, a surgical site infection rate of approximately 2% can be expected with PTFE or bovine venous grafts. Meticulous attention to hemostasis is crucial, as postoperative bleeding has been associated with a surgical-site infection rate of more than 10%.[4]

Wound healing complications induced by venous hypertension may result in secondary complications of wound necrosis with accompanying graft exposure and infection. Employing methods to minimize tissue edema may help decrease the risk

Table 12-1. Characteristics of vascular access infections.

Characteristics	Description
Wound-related	
Wound	Incision breakdown
Abscess	Cavity involving wound and graft
Occult	Positive blood cultures, normal looking wound
Puncture-related	
Erosion	Exposed graft, no gross purulence
Puncture infection	Localized inflammation (with/without graft exposed)
Abscess	Definite cavity around graft

of secondary surgical-site infections. Lower extremity vascular access sites have higher rates of wound infection (18% in 1 series[5]) than sites in the upper extremities. Although not reported through clinical studies, one may expect to see a higher frequency of enteric pathogen colonization from infections in access sites placed below the umbilicus.

If an early infection of the graft tunnel occurs, graft removal is anticipated. The early development of a localized abscess involving the arterial suture line may lead one to consider removing the graft, but the mere presence of a localized abscess does not necessarily preclude graft salvage. Combination therapy, including drainage, debridement, antibiotics, and rotational flap coverage may result in salvage of a significant numbers of grafts. Delayed wound infection (more than 30 days from the operation date) may account for approximately one half of the surgical site infections. Concern for, and prevention of disruption of vascular anastomoses must be of paramount consideration.

Puncture infections. The cumulative rate of puncture infections is about 5% per year.[4] These access sites have a high salvage rate, either through the use of local drainage and antibiotics, or via bypass of the infected segment by placing a new segment of graft in an uninfected field. In cases of localized infection or graft erosion, salvage of the arterial and venous anastomoses usually occurs with efforts to maintain access function. In the event that a segment of graft is bypassed, the bypassed section should be removed to prevent the formation of a continued nonhealing sinus. A variety of flap rotations to cover the eroded PTFE fistula have been described.[6,7] These typically involve excision of the erosion ulcer, with a modification of a V-Y flap advancement. One must assess the integrity of the superior surface of the graft, as it is often not amenable to mobilization for rotation flaps.

Approximately 50% of bacteremias in the dialysis patient originate from the vascular access site.[8] The relative risk ratio for early septicemia (6 months after start of dialysis) is 1.00 for native fistula, 1.63 PTFE or bovine, 2.38 permanent subclavian and 2.26 for a temporary catheter. The RR for late septicemia (after 6 months) is 1.00 for the native fistula and 1.38 with PTFE or bovine grafts.[9] A combination of appropriate antibiotics and judicious surgical procedures can result in graft salvage and preservation of the vascular access site.

References

1. Yu VL, Goetz A, Wagener M, et al. Staphylococcus aureus nasal carriage and infection in patients on hemodialysis. N Engl J Med 1986; 315:91-96.
2. Pruett TL, Pelletier SJ, Crabtree TD. Surgical antisepsis. In: Block SS, ed. Disinfection, sterilization, and preservation, fifth edition. Philadelphia, PA: Lippincott Williams & Wilkins, 2000.
3. Zibari GB, Gadallah MF, Landreneau M, et al. Preoperative vancomycin prophylaxis decreases incidence of postoperative hemodialysis vascular access infections. Am J Kidney Dis 1997; 30:343-48.
4. Taylor B, Sigley RD, May KJ. Fate of infected and eroded hemodialysis grafts and autogenous fistulas. Am J Surg 1993; 165:632-36.

5. Taylor SM, Eaves GL, Weatherford DA, et al. Results and complications of arteriovenous access dialysis grafts in the lower extremity: A five year review. Am Surg 1996; 62:188-91.
6. Moosa HH, Peitzman AB, Thompson BR, Webster MW, Steed DL. Salvage of exposed arteriovenous hemodialysis fistulas. J Vasc Surg 1985; 2:610-12.
7. Tellis VA, Weiss P, Matas AJ, Veith FJ. Skin-flap coverage of polytetrafluoroethylene vascular access graft exposed by previous infection. Surgery 1988; 103:118-21.
8. Kessler M, Hoen B, Mayeux D, Hestin D, Fontenaille C. Bacteremia in patients on chronic hemodialysis. A multicenter prospective survey. Nephron 1993; 64:95-100.
9. Powe NR, Jaar B, Furth SL, Hermann J, Briggs W. Septicemia in dialysis patients: Incidence, risk factors and prognosis. Kidney Int 1999; 55:1081-90.

13

PRELIMINARY RESULTS OF A MULTIDISCIPLINARY APPROACH TO ARTERIOVENOUS FISTULA CREATION FOR HEMODIALYSIS ACCESS

Michael H. Gallichio, M.D., Carlton J. Young, M.D., Michelle L. Robbin, M.D., Michael Allon, M.D., and Mark H. Deierhoi, M.D.

Arteriovenous (AV) fistulae are generally considered to be the preferable conduits for hemodialysis access in patients with renal failure, due to their longevity and low complication rate compared with prosthetic grafts. The Dialysis Outcomes Quality Initiative (DOQI) guidelines recommend a 50% incidence of fistula placement in new dialysis patients for optimal long-term access patency and complication rate.[1] In the past, the incidence of fistula placement at our institution has been as low as 32% in new patients presenting for the initiation of dialysis. An aggressive approach to fistula creation based solely on preoperative physical examination resulted in an increase in the frequency of fistula creation, but an unacceptably high rate of failure of fistulae to mature.[2]

In 1998, ultrasound vascular mapping was included in the preoperative assessment of dialysis patients. A prospective trial was performed to evaluate the effects of vein mapping on surgical decision making.[3] In this trial, the choice of surgical procedure was changed 32% of the time based on the results of vein mapping. Fistula creation was achieved in 58% of the patients and the rate of negative exploration decreased from 11% to 0%.

Ultrasound mapping has subsequently been included in the preoperative assessment of all patients presenting for new vascular access procedures. The preliminary results of vascular access surgery with preoperative vascular mapping have been included in this report.

Materials and Methods

We collected data on all patients undergoing surgery on the vascular access service from January 1, 1999 to December 31, 1999. All new fistula and graft placements were identified and categorized as either the patient's first access procedure or subsequent conduit creation. In addition, we identified all secondary procedures performed on patients who had fistulae created or grafts placed. We also identified all second access placement procedures in which the primary procedure performed in 1999 had failed.

The techniques for preoperative vascular mapping have been described previously.[3] Briefly, all superficial vessels in an extremity are mapped, including the cephalic, basilic, and deep brachial veins. The caliber of these vessels is recorded at the usual sites for anastomosis in the mid-forearm and mid-upper arm. Arterial assessment of the brachial, radial, and ulnar arteries includes measurement of diameter. Tourniquets are placed if vein caliber appears inadequate to maximally distend the vein.

The parameters that are used for determining suitability of vessels for fistulae include a minimal vein diameter of 0.25 mm and a minimal arterial diameter of 0.2 mm. In addition, areas of proximal vein stenoses and arterial calcification were identified and were included in the decision making process. Ultrasound assessment was followed by physical examination and subsequent surgical access placement.

Results

A total of 609 procedures were performed on the vascular access service in 1999. There were 238 primary procedures, of which 107 (45%) were the first placement of permanent access for a given patient. Of the 107 first-time procedures, 82 (77%) were fistula creations. Of the secondary and subsequent procedures, there were 32 fistulae and 99 graft placements. Both first-time and subsequent procedures are detailed in table 13-1. Sixteen percent of the patients receiving a fistula as their first procedure required a secondary procedure. Secondary procedures included ligation of tributary veins, revision of the anastomosis, superficialization of the vein to make it more accessible for cannulation, and conversion to a prosthetic graft, as illustrated in table 13-2. Six (7%) of the fistulae thrombosed.

Discussion

There is great variability in the actual incidence of fistula creation in different regions of the country[4], even though AV fistulae are acknowledged to be the preferred conduits for hemodialysis by way of vascular access. In fact, an actual decline in the overall incidence of fistula creation has been reported over the last 10 years.[5]

Table 13-1. Vascular access procedures for fistula and graft placement.

	Primary[1]	Secondary[2]
Fistula		
Radiocephalic	47 (57%)	0
Brochiocephalic	29 (35%)	23 (72%)
Basilic vein transposition	6 (7%)	9 (28%)
	82	32
Graft		
Forearm	15 (60%)	10 (10%)
Upper arm	10 (10%)	72 (72%)
Thigh	0	17 (17%)
	25	99

[1]First permanent access procedure

[2]Second or subsequent procedure

Table 13-2. Primary fistula revisions.

	(N=82)
Vein superficialization/transposition	2 (2%)
Ligation of tributary veins	3 (4%)
Anastomotic revision	6 (7%)
Conversion with prosthetic graft interposition	2 (2%)
Total	13 (15%)

Prior to the formulation of the DOQI guidelines for vascular access management, the incidence of fistula creation as the first permanent access procedure in a new dialysis patient at our center was 32%. Initial efforts at aggressive surgical management to improve this rate were successful, and the incidence of fistula creation increased to over 50%. Unfortunately, certain patient groups and access sites, such as older diabetic women with radiocephalic fistulae, recorded an unacceptably high rate of failure.

Several reports have demonstrated the efficacy of ultrasound assessment preoperatively in improving the incidence of fistula placement.[6,7] These studies resulted in our decision to undertake a prospective trial and subsequently incorporate ultrasound assessment routinely in the preoperative evaluation of patients.

The introduction of ultrasound vascular mapping for preoperative evaluation has led to a significant increase in the creation of AV fistulae as first-time access procedures for hemodialysis patients. In our institution the rate was 58%, and when applying ultrasound studies to all patients requiring new access procedures, the rate of fistula creation increased to 76%. We observed a low thrombosis rate of 7%, and the percentage of patients requiring completely new procedures at a different site was similarly low, based on early results. Fifteen percent of patients required some secondary procedure to modify the fistula to promote maturation and accessibility for cannulation. These results are preliminary, however, and most patients had a follow-up of less than 1 year. A several year follow-up will be necessary to determine if the use of ultrasound mapping has resulted in a significant improvement in conduit patency. A number of these fistulae do not mature well, and we are still in the process of evaluating which patients, even with acceptable anatomy as determined by ultrasound, are likely to be unsuitable for fistulae. Nonetheless, a fistula creation incidence of 76% for first-time access is an encouraging improvement over our previous efforts in this area.

References

1. National Kidney Foundation-Dialysis Outcomes Quality Initiative. NKF-DOQI clinical practice guidelines for vascular access. Am J of Kidney Dis 1997; 30 (suppl) 3:S150-91.
2. Miller PE, Tolwani A, Luscy CP, et al. Predictors of adequacy of arteriovenous fistulae in hemodialysis patients. Kidney Int 1999; 56:275-80.
3. Robbin ML, Gallichio MH, Deierhoi MH, Young CJ, Weber TM, Allon M. US vascular mapping before hemodialysis access placement. Radiology 2000; 217:83-88.
4. Sehgal AR, Silver MR, Covinsky KE, Coffin R, Cain JA. Use of standardized ratios to examine variability in hemodialysis vascular access across facilities. Am J Kidney Dis 2000; 35:275-80.
5. Hirth RA, Turenne MN, Woods JD, et al. Predictors of type of vascular access in hemodialysis patients. JAMA 1996; 276:1303-08.
6. Silva MB, Hobson RW, Pappas PJ, et al. A strategy for increasing use of autogenous hemodialysis access procedures: Impact of preoperative noninvasive evaluation. J Vasc Surg 1998; 27:307-08.
7. Comeaux ME, Bryant PS, Harkrider WW. Preoperative evaluation of the renal access patient with color doppler imaging. J Vasc Tech 1993; 17:247-50.

14

TRENDS IN VASCULAR ACCESS PROCEDURES AND EXPENDITURES IN MEDICARE'S ESRD PROGRAM

Paul W. Eggers, Ph.D., and Roger Milam, M.S.

The creation and maintenance of vascular access sites for dialysis patients is not only a source of considerable morbidity within the dialysis population, but also constitutes a major cost to the Medicare ESRD program. This paper examines recent trends in vascular access procedures and compares the costs to Medicare following placement of fistula, graft, and catheter access procedures.

The Dialysis Outcomes Quality Initiative (DOQI) clinical guidelines for vascular access have a fistula placement goal of 40% in prevalent hemodialysis patients. As of 1998, only 27% of patients nationwide had a fistula, with 20% using a central venous catheter for access. Although fistula rates were higher in the Northeast, none of the ESRD networks met the DOQI guideline level. Health Care Finacing Association (HCFA) billing data however, show that fistula placement has been increasing the past few years and that more vascular procedures are performed in the outpatient setting. As a result, expenditures for vascular access are decreasing in absolute terms and as a percent of all dialysis costs.

Total Medicare per capita expenditures following access placements are \$77,600 in the first year following placement and \$54,200 in the second year. Adjusted annual costs for fistulae are \$4,500 less than for grafts and \$9,000 less than for catheters. Unmeasured patient comorbidities, however, probably account for some of these differences.

Background

The creation, maintenance, and replacement of vascular access in dialysis patients is recognized as one of the major sources of morbidity and costs of Medicare's ESRD program.[1-3] In addition, recent evidence suggests that costs may be increasing as a% of program expenditures[4-7] and that fistulae are decreasing as a% of vascular access procedures.[6,8] The importance of vascular access in the care of dialysis patients was recognized in the development of the Dialysis Outcomes Quality Initiative (DOQI) guidelines by the National Kidney Foundation.[9] All the studies listed above deal with trends prior to publication of DOQI. Post-DOQI trends have not yet been documented.

Barriers to fistula placement include a large percentage of patients with inadequate sites for creation of artery to vein anastomoses and late referrals to dialysis that prevent the opportunity for a fistula to mature.[4] However, fistulae are recommended over grafts and catheters because of their superior long-term patency. It is widely believed that the superior patency of fistulae should also be reflected in lower costs of care because fewer interventions and replacements would be necessary. The empirical evidence for this belief is largely missing. Some have argued that the implementation of DOQI guidelines may result in higher costs[10], but at least 1 study has shown that the aggressive shift from a predominantly graft-based access system to the primary use of fistulae has decreased overall costs.[11]

This study presents information on trends in vascular access in the immediate post-DOQI era. The most recent trends in vascular access procedures are examined using data collected through the HCFA Clinical Performance Measures project as well as HCFA billing data. This study also compares total Medicare expenditures following placement of fistula, graft and catheter types of access.

Methods/Data

Data for this study were obtained from 2 sources. The distribution of vascular access procedures in 1998 was taken from the Clinical Performance Measures (CPM) project. The CPM is an extension of the ESRD Core Indicators Project, started in 1994.[12] The Core Indicators Project was HCFA's first nationwide, population-based study designed to improve the care of patients with ESRD. The project has collected clinical information annually on 4 key care indicators (adequacy of dialysis, hematocrit value, nutritional status, and blood pressure control) on a national sample of adult in-center hemodialysis and peritoneal dialysis patients. The ESRD CPMs are similar to the core indicators with the addition of measures for vascular access. The 1998 sample includes 8336 dialysis patients, 1621 of whom began dialysis in 1998 and are defined as incident patients.

The expenditure analyses were taken from data from the ESRD Program Management and Medical Information System (ESRD PMMIS) maintained by the Office of Clinical Standards and Quality (OCSQ) at the HCFA. The ESRD PMMIS is a longitudinal file of patients with ESRD who are entitled to Medicare benefits.

In addition to the basic enrollment data available for all Medicare beneficiaries such as sex, race, date of birth, date of death, and entitlement dates, the PMMIS contains information unique to ESRD beneficiaries. The medical evidence form (HCFA 2728) is used to determine date and cause of renal failure. The ESRD PMMIS file used in this study was updated through November 1999. This update of the ESRD PMMIS contained over 967,000 patients, which is the complete count of Medicare ESRD patients ever entitled since 1978.

In addition to entitlement records, HCFA receives billing data on all ESRD persons served by fee-for-service providers. All billing data for ESRD beneficiaries receiving care in the fee-for-service sector were linked to individual ESRD beneficiaries. Services covered by Medicare include short stay hospitalizations, physician services, outpatient services (largely dialysis and erythropoeitin treatment), home health care, skilled nursing care, and hospice. Vascular procedures are coded by the HCFA common procedure coding system (HCPCS). The HCPCS is based on the American Medical Association Common Procedure Coding (CPT) system with additions for durable medical equipment, drugs, ambulance, and other services not provided by physicians. Vascular surgery was defined as: fistula (HCPCS=36821 and 36825), graft (HCPC=36830), and catheter (HCPC=36533).

Results

Recent trends in vascular access surgery. Vascular access results from the CPM are shown in table 14-1. In 1998, just over one quarter (27%) of hemodialysis patients had a fistula as their access site. Over one-half were using a synthetic graft (53%), and the remaining 20% were dialyzing via a catheter. Catheter use was greater (25%) for the patients who began dialysis during 1998. Use of fistulae was greater for males (36%), whites (30%), and for persons in the 18 to 44 age group (36%). Persons whose renal failure was caused by diabetes were less likely (23%) to have a fistula than were other persons. Fistula placement rates varied by region (data not shown), and were highest in the Northeast (36%) and lowest in a number of Southern States and in Southern California (20 to 21%).

Table 14-2 shows the number of fistula and graft procedures billed to Medicare for the years 1992 through 1999.† In 1992 there were almost 69,000 vascular procedures, of which 17,000, or 25%, were fistula placements. The percentage with a fistula remained largely unchanged through 1996. In 1997, 1998 and 1999, the percentage of vascular procedures that were fistulae was 29%, 32%, and 36%, respectively. The increase in fistulae coincides with the publication of the DOQI guidelines in the Spring of 1997. The promulgation of the guidelines has very likely led to more serious efforts to use fistulae for vascular access. The other notable trend evidenced in table 14-2 is the increasing tendency to perform these surgeries in the outpatient setting. In 1992, less than one fifth (19%) of vascular placements were performed in an outpatient setting. By 1999, over one half of these placements were done in the outpatient setting. This greatly reduced the costs of these procedures because the costs of an inpatient stay greatly exceed outpatient surgery.

† Catheters were not included in this table because the source of data, the part B extract and summary system (BESS), does not distinguish between ESRD and other patients. Most of the catheter implants in the Medicare population are for purposes other than dialysis access.

Table 14-1. Percent of sampled patients with different access types for incident and prevalent samples: 1998.

	1998 Incident (N=1,621)			Prevalent (N=8,336)		
Characteristic	Catheter	Fistula	Graft	Catheter	Fistula	Graft
TOTAL	27	48	25	27	53	20
Gender						
Male	19	43	24	36*	46	18
Female	34*	54	27	17	61	22
Race						
White	28	44	27	30*	49	22
African American	20	59	21	22	60	18
Age group (years)						
18 to 44	36	37	26	36*	45	19
45 to 64	31	46	24	29	53	18
65 and over	20	54	26	22	56	22
Primary ESRD cause						
Diabetes mellitus	24*	52	24	23*	57	20
Hypertension	24	51	26	27	55	18
Glomerulonephritis	36	44	20	36	47	16
Other/unknown	31	39	30	31	47	22
Duration of dialysis (years)						
0.5	N.A.	N.A.	N.A.	21*	38	40
0.5 to 0.9	N.A.	N.A.	N.A.	27	49	24
1 to 1.9	N.A.	N.A.	N.A.	28	53	19
2 or more	N.A.	N.A.	N.A.	29	58	13

Source: Vascular Access for In-Center Hemodialysis Patients: Preliminary Findings: Supplemental Report No. 1. 1999 ESRD Clinical Performance Measures Project, from www.hcfa.gov. N.A. = Not Applicable *$P<.05$

Table 14-2. Number of medicare billings for vascular access, by type of placement and site of service: 1992 to 1999.

Year	Total (N)	Graft (N)	Fistula (N)	Fistula (%)	Inpatient (N)	Outpatient (N)	Outpatient (%)
1992	68,988	51,841	17,147	25	55,964	13,024	19
1993	70,023	53,657	16,366	23	54,907	15,116	22
1994	75,021	57,520	17,501	23	56,162	18,859	25
1995	77,855	59,347	18,508	24	54,729	23,126	30
1996	80,132	60,413	19,719	25	52,118	28,014	35
1997	80,873	57,413	23,460	29	48,412	32,461	40
1998	83,638	56,560	27,078	32	45,757	37,881	45
1999	84,948	54,715	30,233	36	41,065	43,883	52

Source: Part B extract and summary system (BESS), maintained by the Office of Information Services, Health Care Financing Administration.

Hospitalization rates for vascular access are shown in table 14-3. This table represents all vascular procedures, initial placement as well as revisions, declottings and other repairs. In 1994 there were 48 hospitalizations per 100 dialysis patients for vascular procedures. The rate ranged from a low of 34 per 100 persons aged 15 to 24 years of age to a rate of 66 hospitalizations per 100 persons aged 75 years of age and over. Females had higher rates than did males (52 and 44 per 100, respectively), and rates were higher for African Americans (52 per 100) than for other races. From 1994 to 1998 vascular hospitalizations declined by 16%, to 40 per 100 persons. Declines were greater for the elderly and for white and African-American dialysis patients.

Table 14-3. Medicare ESRD dialysis patients inpatient hospitalization rates per 100 persons for vascular access: 1994 to 1998.

Age, sex, race	1994	1995	1996	1997	1998	percent change
All Persons	48	48	45	42	40	-16%
Age						
Under 15 years	40	44	37	29	33	-17
15-24 years	34	41	39	35	36	6
25-34 years	39	40	38	37	36	-7
35-44 years	38	40	39	36	36	-5
45-54 years	42	41	39	37	35	-15
55-64 years	44	44	43	38	37	-15
65-74 years	55	52	48	45	42	-23
75 years or over	66	58	53	49	46	-31
Sex						
Male	44	44	41	39	37	-16
Female	52	53	49	46	43	-16
Race						
Asian	33	32	31	31	31	-8
African American	52	53	49	46	43	-17
White	46	46	43	40	38	-18
Native American	44	51	52	43	44	1
Other/unknown	40	50	49	44	44	11

Source: HCFA ESRD Program Management and Medical Information System and National Claims History.

The impact of these declines in vascular inpatient hospitalizations on Medicare expenditures are shown in table 14-4. Per capita Medicare expenditures for inpatient hospital stays for dialysis patients in 1994 were \$17,720. This increased to \$19,828 by 1997 and then dropped slightly in 1998 to \$19,329, for an overall increase of 9%. Per capita expenditures for vascular access hospitalizations, however, dropped by almost \$500, or 12%. Expenditures increased by over 20% for circulatory, respiratory, infectious, and signs and symptoms related hospitalizations.

Medicare expenditures following access placement. This analysis was designed to compare total Medicare expenditures following placement of a native fistula, an artificial graft, and central venous catheters. The earliest date at which

Table 14-4. Medicare per capita expenditures for dialysis patients for inpatient care, by reason for stay: 1994 to 1998.

	1994	1995	1996	1997	1998	Change (%)
All Causes	$17,720	$18,464	$19,271	$19,828	$19,329	9
Vascular Access	4147	4131	4055	3908	3657	-12
Circulatory (390-459)	4333	4685	5097	5362	5273	22
Digestive (520-579)	1632	1618	1648	1698	1639	0
Genitourinary (580-629)	777	868	880	888	801	3
Endocrine/ Metabolic (240-279)	1521	1543	1551	1572	1554	2
Respiratory (460-519)	1175	1273	1375	1439	1437	22
Infectious (001-139)	796	902	1036	1093	1025	29
Signs and symptoms (780-799)	700	696	729	786	844	21
All Others	2639	2748	2899	3083		

Numbers in parentheses represent ranges of ICD-9 codes. *Source:* HCFA ESRD Program Management and Medical Information System and National Claims History.

placement (fistula, graft, or catheter) was made during 1997 was used as the starting date. Total Medicare expenditures (including the initial placement) were then calculated through the end of 1998. That is, follow-up ranged from 12 months for procedures occurring in December 1997, to 24 months for procedures occurring in January 1997. Patients were censored at either death or transplantation. Expenditures were attributed to the initial type of access placement (ie, an intent to treat fashion), regardless of changes in access type during the observation period.

Table 14-5 shows the number of initial vascular placements* in 1997 by various demographic groupings. There were a total of 75,820 initial placements, of which 20% were fistulas, 48% were grafts and 32% were catheters. Fistula placement did not vary greatly by age, but catheters were most common among persons under the age of 25 (44%) and least common among those 65 to 74 (29%). Males were much more likely to have a fistula placement than were females (25% and 15%, respectively). Fistula placement was least common among African (16%) and Asian (19%) Americans. The most common cause of renal failure for persons with fistula placement was glomerulonephritis (23%). Not surprisingly, the longer the person had been on dialysis, the less likely that he or she received a fistula. For persons whose renal failure preceded 1996, the fistula placement rate was only 14%. Conversely, for the 2,823 persons whose vascular placement preceded the start of dialysis (in

*The intial placement was defined as the first placement in 1997. Many of these patients had vascular procedures in previous years not captured in this analysis. As such, these distributions are not directly comparable to the rates shown in table 1, which represent a cross section of procedures functioning at the end of 1998.

Table 14-5. First vascular access procedure in 1997 by age, sex, race, cause of renal failure, ESRD incident year, and place of service.

	All Procedures (N)	Fistula (%)	Graft (%)	Catheter (%)
ALL	75,820	20	48	32
Age Group				
0 to 24	894	21	35	44
25 to 44	8779	21	43	35
45 to 64	20,385	18	49	33
65 to 74	24,523	22	49	29
75 +	21,239	20	48	32
Gender				
Male	37,956	25	45	29
Female	37,864	15	50	34
Race				
White	43,949	22	44	33
African American	26,665	16	53	31
Asian	1427	19	58	23
Native American	976	23	43	34
Other	2803	24	53	23
Cause of ESRD				
Diabetes	31,364	20	50	30
Hypertension	22,636	20	49	31
G. nephritis	7857	23	45	32
Other	13,963	20	42	38
Incident Year				
Pre-1994	6263	14	50	36
1994	5980	14	49	37
1995	7851	14	47	39
1996	11,863	18	48	34
1997	31,040	25	48	28
1998	2823	50	39	11
Place of Service				
Inpatient	47,363	18	48	34
Outpatient	28,457	24	48	28

Source: HCFA ESRD Program Management and Medical Information System and National Claims History.

1998), the fistula placement rate was 50%, with only 11% receiving a catheter.** Fistulae accounted for 18% of the procedures done on an inpatient basis and 24% of those done on an outpatient basis.

Table 14-6 shows Medicare expenditures for the first year following placement of a vascular access. Overall, Medicare expenditures were $77,619 per person-year,

**Note that table 1 shows functioning vascular access types in 1998. An unknown number of the fistulae in this table and the expenditure analysis failed to mature. Thus the comparison of types of access should be considered as "intent to trest."

Table 14-6. Total per capita medicare expenditures for 1st and 2nd year following 1997 access placement, by type of service.

	All Procedures	Fistula	Graft	Catheter
1st year				
Total	$77,619	$68,002	$75,611	$86,927
Inpatient	35,037	29,069	32,980	42,108
Outpatient	22,877	22,599	23,528	22,014
Physician	14,304	12,449	13,900	16,126
Home Health	2649	1836	2687	3104
Skilled Nursing	2681	1997	2459	3468
Hospice	71	52	56	107
2nd year				
Total	54,206	49,689	54,555	57,178
Inpatient	19,535	17,067	19,181	22,153
Outpatient	21,688	21,317	22,356	20,765
Physician	10,074	9096	10,016	10,962
Home Health	1395	984	1464	1598
Skilled Nursing	1458	1174	1487	1633
Hospice	55	52	51	66

Source: HCFA ESRD Program Management and Medical Information System and National Claims History.

considerably greater than the $52,000 per person-year average cost for all dialysis patients.[13] This reflects the increased morbidity associated with vascular procedure creation and maintenance. Average expenditures were much greater for patients receiving a graft ($75,611 per person-year) or a catheter ($86,927 per person-year) than for persons receiving a fistula ($68,002 per person-year). Dialysis and erythropoeitin costs are largely fixed and there were no significant differences for outpatient services. Most of the differences were explained by higher costs for hospitalization and physician care. Second year costs following access placement ($54,206 per person-year) more nearly approximate average costs for all dialysis patients. As expected, outpatient costs remained fairly unchanged, while inpatient costs decreased by over $10,000 per person-year, and in the case of catheter patients, decreased by almost $20,000 per person-year. While expenditures decreased for all types of placements, there still remained a cost advantage to fistulae. As shown in table 14-5, there are many differences between the patients who receive the 3 types of vascular access. In order to control for these differences, a multivariate analysis was performed on the expenditure levels. The dependent variable was calculated as total Medicare expenditures per day of Medicare eligibility. Variables included in the model were age, sex, race, cause of renal failure, and type of access. In addition, 3 other variables were added to the model. Because there is usually some excess morbidity associated with the initiation of dialysis, a variable was added to indicate incident patients. Hospitalization for the initial procedure also adds greatly to the costs of the procedure but does not reflect on the success of the procedure itself. So a variable was added to control for the place of service for the

Table 14-7. Multivariate analysis of medicare expenditures following vascular access procedures.

Variable	Parameter Estimate	Annualized ($)	*P* value
Intercept	104.89	38,286	0.0001
0 to 24	1.36	496	0.7073
25 to 34	4.74	1731	0.330
35 to 44	5.19	1895	0.0032
45 to 54	Comparison	–	–
55 to 64	0.88	322	0.5736
65 to 74	2.42	883	0.0662
75 to 84	0.34	124	0.8154
85 and over	-3.52	-1286	0.1778
Female	Comparison	–	–
Male	-6.49	-2,369	0.0001
White	Comparison	–	–
Asian	-1.70	-621	0.5831
African American	7.27	2654	0.0001
Native American	-7.37	-2689	0.506
Other Race	8.32	3036	0.1589
Glomerulonephritis	Comparison	–	–
Diabetes	17.28	6307	0.0001
Secondary GN	8.21	2996	0.0022
Interstitial nephritis	3.44	1254	0.1089
Hereditary diseases	-3.98	-1452	0.0987
Neoplasms	14.97	5465	0.0001
Other diseases	34.23	12,495	0.0001
Unknown	3.16	1,153	0.1655
Missing	32.95	12,027	0.0001
Incident	21.63	7895	0.0001
Death	123.67	N/A	0.0001
Hospitalization	34.09	12,442	0.0001
Fistula	Comparison	–	–
Graft	12.23	4464	0.0001
Catheter	24.73	9026	0.0001

N/A is not applicable. *Source:* HCFA ESRD Program Management and Medical Information System and National Claims History.

original access placement. Finally, a crude measure of severity was added to the model. As it is highly unlikely that the access type itself would cause excess mortality, a bivariate indicator of death during the observation period was added to approximate severity of some patients.

The results of the multivariate analysis are shown in table 14-7. In addition to daily parameter estimates, estimates of annual expenditures are also shown. There were no consistent age effects although persons 25 to 34 years of age and 35 to 44 years of age had statistically higher expenditure levels than persons in the 45 to 54 years of age group ($P<.05$). Expenditures were higher for males ($P<0.0001$), African-Americans ($P<0.0001$), and persons whose renal failure was attributed to diabetes ($P<0.0001$), secondary glomerulonephritis ($P<0.003$), and neoplasms ($P<0.0001$). Higher expenditures were also associated with incident patients ($P<0.0001$) and with patients whose initial placement was in an inpatient facility ($P<0.0001$). Finally, compared with fistula recipients, persons who received a graft had $4464 in predicted additional annualized expenditures and catheter recipients had $9026 greater annualized expenditure levels.

Conclusions

The importance of vascular access as a source of both morbidity and costs for dialysis patients has received more attention in recent years. The publication of the DOQI guidelines has highlighted the low level of fistula placement in the United States compared to other countries. This study shows that there is evidence that the dialysis community is working to reverse the long-term trend to increased use of artificial grafts. Medicare billing data show that the number of fistula placements in 1999 represent almost a doubling of the number of these procedures since 1993. In addition, the placement of artificial grafts declined from 1997 to 1999. Although this shift in treatment patterns cannot be directly attributed to DOQI guidelines, given the congruence of this trend with DOQI, it is likely that dialysis professionals are working toward this end.[14]

Another trend shown by these data is the movement of vascular procedures from the inpatient setting to outpatient settings. Although there are no guidelines recommending a reduction in inpatient procedures, the shift has welcome economic benefits. Previous work has shown that, in 1994, hospitalizations for vascular procedures accounted for about one fourth of all hospital costs for dialysis patients.[3] By 1998, the shift in vascular procedures had decreased hospitalization costs by almost $500 per dialysis patient, a 12% decrease.

Finally, these data provide the strongest evidence yet of the economic advantages of fistula placement compared with either graft or catheter access types. Controlling for basic demographic and cause of renal failure variables, fistulae appear to have an annual savings to Medicare of $4 500 over grafts and $9 000 over catheter placement. However, this last finding needs to be regarded with considerable caution. It is almost certain that there is a great deal of patient selection when it comes to access placement, particularly with respect to catheters. It is not possible, using administrative data such as Medicare billing, to discern the intent of catheter placement. People who receive catheters probably fall into 1 of 2 categories. First, catheters are often used as a bridge therapy, often while a fistula is maturing. A catheter that is replaced by a functioning fistula within a few weeks or months cannot be considered a failed therapy. In fact, in this case, it probably makes more sense to consider the catheter cost as part of the total cost of the fistula, than as a separate procedure. The second group of catheter recipients not evident in the billing data are patients whose declining health makes a catheter the only available option. Controlling for patient selection effects would probably attenuate the apparent cost advantage to fistula placement.

Work on the cost-effectiveness of different access procedures can be enhanced by linking the Medicare expenditure data with clinically based data sets or trials. In this manner, selection effects can be mitigated and more accurate assessments of cost advantages and disadvantages can be obtained.

References

1. U.S. Renal Data System, USRDS 1997 Annual Data Report. National Institute of Health, National Institute of Diabetes and Digestive and Kidney Diseases, Bethesda, MD, April 1997.
2. Feldman HI, Held PJ, Hutchinson JT, Stoiber E, Hartigan MF, Berlin JA. Hemodialysis vascular access morbidity in the United States. Kidney Int 1993; 43:1091-96.
3. Eggers, PW. Medicare expenditures for vascular access in the ESRD program [syllabus]. The Sixth Biannual Symposium on Dialysis Access. Miami, FL; 1998.
4. Schwab SJ. Vascular access for hemodialysis. Kidney Int 1999; 55:2078-90.
5. Pastan S, Bailey J. Dialysis Therapy. N Engl J Med 1998; 338:1428-37.
6. Hakim R, Himmelfarb J. Hemodialysis access failure: A call to action. Kidney Int 1998; 54:1029-40.
7. Rocco MV, Bleyer AJ, Burkart JM. Utilization of inpatient and outpatient resources for the management of hemodialysis access complications. Am J Kidney Dis 1996; 28:250-56.
8. Hirth RA, Turrenne MN, Woods JD, et al. Predictor of type of vascular access in hemodialysis patients. JAMA 1996; 276:1303-08.
9. NKF-DOQI Clinical Practice Guidelines for Vascular Access. New York, National Kidney Foundation, 1997.
10. Wish J, Roberts J, Besarab A, Owen WF Jr. The cost of implementing the dialysis outcomes quality initiative clinical practice guidelines. Adv Ren Replace Ther 1999; 6:67-74.
11. Becker BN, Breiterman-White R, Nylander W, et al. Care pathway reduces hospitalizations and cost for hemodialysis vascular access surgery. Am J Kidney Dis 1997; 30:525-31.
12. Helgerson SD, McClellan WM, Frederick PR, Beaver SK, Frankenfield DL, McMullan M. Improvement in adequacy of delivered dialysis for adult in-center hemodialysis patients in the United States, 1993 to 1995. Am J Kidney Dis 1997; 29:851-61.
13. U.S. Renal Data System, USRDS 1999 Annual Data Report. National Institute of Health, National Institute of Diabetes and Digestive and Kidney Diseases, Bethesda, MD, April 1999.
14. Ascher E, Gade P, Hingoram A, et al. Changes in the practice of angioaccess surgery: Impact of dialysis outcome and quality initiative recommendations Vasc Surg 2000; 31:84-92.

DISCUSSION

Panelists:

Steven J. Schwab, M.D.
Timothy L. Pruett, M.D.
Mark H. Deierhoi, M.D.
Paul W. Eggers, Ph.D.

Discussant: I have a couple of questions for Dr. Schwab. What is the best blood flow that we can set on the pump for the catheters, granted that the high flow is associated with higher recirculation and this probably will give us a less clearance? The second question is what should be approached with somebody with persistent bacteremia regarding the catheter placement? Do you do "in and out" catheters in your setting or do you put temporary catheters for a week and then you replace it like over time?

Dr. Schwab: In regard to the first question, we believe that cuffed silicon catheters placed in the right atrium, in our studies and other studies, do not tend to re-circulate. So we see very little re-circulation because of the high volume of blood flowing past them. Their flow is principally limited by inflow. As the lumens get bigger the catheters will flow faster. It is just a matter of dynamics. What we routinely do is we set an upper negative arterial pressure that we recommend to our dialysis nurses they do not go beyond. We set that at minus 300. So we tend to run our arterial catheters at minus 300 and accept whatever blood flow we are getting, knowing that there is an enormous difference to what the pump says and what we are really getting probably by a 25% decrement. For those patients who have an active bacteremia and do not clear their blood stream, we do not replace a cuff tunnel catheter until we have cleared the blood stream. So that if someone is persistently bacteremic, our inclination is to get all of the artificial tissue out, treat them with antibiotics until we are at least not actively growing bacteria prior to replacing a cuff tunnel catheter.

SECTION V

15

BASILIC VEIN TRANSPOSITION INCREASES THE RATE OF AUTOGENOUS FISTULA CREATION

Richard L. McCann, M.D.

The National Kidney Foundation-Dialysis Outcomes Quality Initiative (NKF-DOQI) guidelines advocate that 50% of all new dialysis patients be provided with a native arteriovenous (AV) fistula for vascular access.[1] Construction of native AV fistulae is preferred over the use of synthetic graft fistulae or tunneled cuffed catheters because of their presumed better long-term patency rate, lower incidence of infection, and decreased requirement for revision. Fistulae constructed entirely from autogenous materials are potentially both medically and economically advantageous. In the United States the goal of 50% native fistula creation has not often been met.[2] Reasons for this include late referral of patients when requirement for initiation of dialysis is imminent, poor quality of subcutaneous superficial veins in the upper extremity (due to patient disease and prior utilization of these veins for intravenous therapy), and inadequate training or indifference on the part of vascular access surgeons.

Polytetrafluoroethylene (PTFE) grafts have been the dominant access used in the United States, but there has been a resurgence of interest in the use of native vessels for fistula creation. This has occurred as physicians have recognized the importance of an optimal surgical strategy, and that native fistulae, which require fewer revisions and replacements, may be more reliable and more economical than PTFE grafts. Since this increased interest has not been accompanied by referral of patients with more intact and usable superficial upper extremity veins, the use of other available veins has expanded. Dagher[3,4] described a technique of basilic vein transposition from the native subfascial location to a superficial subdermal position in the upper arm and anastomosis to the brachial artery forming a native AV fistula intended for dialysis access. The basilic vein is usually large, and its deep position makes it less vulnerable to damage from prior venipuncture and/or intravenous therapy, and thus, it is more likely available, even in patients who have required frequent venous access.

This report describes our early experience with this strategy in an effort to maximize the number of patients with totally autogenous fistulae for dialysis access.

Patient Selection

This study included 156 patients referred for vascular access surgery from July 1998 to December 1999 for creation of upper extremity dialysis access. The algorithm used for selection of a specific access procedure for each patient followed DOQI guidelines. A primary fistula at the wrist was considered first, followed by a brachial artery cephalic vein fistula at the elbow, and if neither of these sites appeared propitious on clinical examination, a basilic vein transposition was considered. An upper arm PTFE shunt was employed only if an autogenous fistula did not appear feasible.

Surgical Technique

Patients determined not to be candidates for radiocephalic (Cimino) or brachiocephalic fistulae were considered for a basilic vein brachial artery fistula. Preliminary duplex scanning was helpful and was used selectively if there was concern that the basilic vein was not suitable. Patent veins larger than 4 mm were preferred for use. Procedures were performed using general anesthesia, or axillary or scalene block. The basilic vein courses from the ulnar side of the forearm, across the antecubital space, and routes inferior to the brachial artery in the arm. The vein pierces the deep fascia in the upper part of the arm and joins with the venae comitantes to form the brachial vein. During this course, the basilic vein is intimately associated with the median cutaneous nerve of the forearm, then the median nerve higher in the arm. In order to ensure careful vein dissection, adequate control of all branches, and prevention of injury to adjacent neurovascular structures, we prefer a continuous, rather than serial interrupted, skin incisions. At the level of the antecubital fossa the vein splits into the basilic vein proper and the median antecubital vein. The latter is often the larger branch and may be selected in preference to the basilic vein in the forearm.

After a branch is selected, it is carefully dissected into the mid-forearm to provide adequate length. After complete dissection and mobilization, the vein is gently hydrostatically dilated to ensure adequate control of all side branches, which are either ligated or secured with clips. The distended vein is then placed on the skin in a curved arch, over the biceps muscle in its proposed final location. This path is outlined on the skin with a sterile marker. Using this mark as a guide, a sheathed tunneler is passed in the subdermal plane and the vein is passed through the sheath in a distended state. The sheathed tunneler is necessary to avoid potential dislodgment of any clips that secure the side branches, which may be caught and avulsed by local tissue if passed without the protection of a sheath. Great care must be taken to avoid any twisting of the graft. After passage of the graft through the tunnel, the anastomosis is made to the brachial artery in end-to-side fashion, usually using a side branch of the vein to improve the spatulation of the anastomosis.

After release of the clamps, flow is qualitatively evaluated by examining the magnitude of the thrill. The potential for vascular steal is estimated by palpating the pulse distally and by listening to the distal arterial flow with a sterile doppler. Additionally, a sterile pulse oximeter probe is placed on a finger. The presence of a pulsatile pulse oximeter tracing (with little change in waveform induced by clamping and unclamping of the fistula) is good evidence that adequate distal circulation is present. In cases of significant vascular steal, the pulse oximeter signal at the finger will be markedly attenuated or unobtainable. If there is inadequate distal circulation, an immediate jump graft is placed across the anastomosis by using another vein graft, either harvested from the ipsilateral arm or using the saphenous vein. This graft bridges the site of the AV anastomosis. The interval between the distal anastomosis and the AV fistula is then ligated to prevent reverse flow in the brachial artery (distal revascularization-interval ligation or DRIL procedure).[5]

Four to 6 weeks must be allowed for edema to subside and for the tunnel to seal before puncture is allowed. Dialysis technicians must be reminded that this upper arm graft is to be treated as a fistula rather than a PTFE graft in order to minimize the risk of double wall puncture and potential serious bleeding into the underlying muscle.

Results

During the study period, conventional native AV fistulae were created in 35 patients (24 wrist, 11 elbow). Basilic vein transposition fistulae were placed in 56 patients, and 65 required upper extremity PTFE grafts. Patients requiring leg grafts and chest wall grafts were not included. Thus the rate of native fistula creation in upper extremity access was 58%, meeting the DOQI requirement of an autogenous fistula rate greater than 50%. This compares favorably to the rate prior to the initiation of the basilic vein transposition (BVT) procedure in our program of 33%.

The group receiving BVT was comprised of 22 females and 34 males, with an average age of 55 years (range 22 to 89 years of age). Reflecting our dialysis population, 60% of the patients were African American and 54% had diabetes mellitus as the principle cause of their renal insufficiency. In many of the patients, basilic vein transposition was a secondary access procedure. Thirty-six percent of this population had 1 or more previous ipsilateral accesses created and 41% had a contralateral access as well. General anesthesia was selected for the majority (54%) of patients. Axillary or scalene block was used in 41% and local infiltration with sedation in 2 patients. Because of the extensive nature of the dissection, local anesthesia is usually not well tolerated and anesthetic volumes required approached toxic levels.

Clinical outcome parameters for the 3 groups are shown in table 15-1. During the study period 6 of 65 PTFE grafts were lost due to infection, compared with no infections in the patients receiving native fistulae. In patients with BVT, no wound or late infections were observed and no patients had nerve or vascular injury. Initial patency for BVT was 95%. Of the fistulae that were lost early, 1 was due to injudicious use of a small vein (<3 mm) and 2 grafts required ligation when hand ischemia persisted despite a DRIL procedure. The 1 year patency curve by lifetable analysis for BVT compared to conventional AV fistulae and primary and secondary patency of PTFE grafts is shown in figure 15-1. Seventy-seven percent patency of BVT, 65% patency of conventional AV fistulae, and 69% secondary patency of PTFE grafts compares favorably with values published in the literature.[6]

Table 15-1.

	BVT	AVF	PTFE
N			
Infection %	0	0	9
Steal %	7	3	11
1Yr Patency %	77	65	69*

*Secondary Patency

In the BVT group, 1 fistula was preserved with a late percutaneous transluminal angioplasty (PTA), but PTA in another resulted in thrombosis and loss of the access. Four additional fistulae were lost late: 3 due to small veins and 1 due to dehydration in the setting of chemotherapy for malignancy.

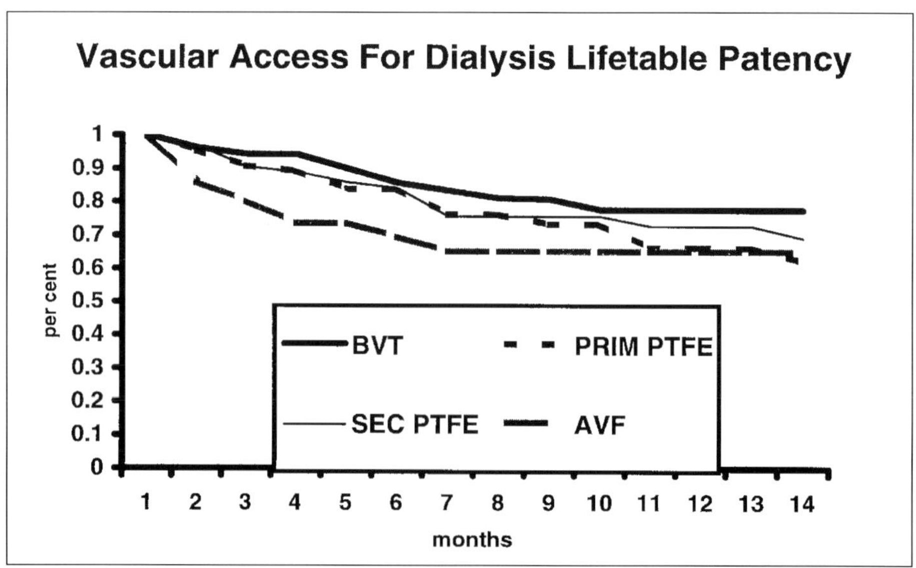

Figure 15-1.

Reimbursement Issues

Because BVT has become increasingly popular, it has been assigned its own Common Procedural Terminology (CPT) code (36819). Interestingly, despite the extensive dissection of the basilic vein that is required, it has been assigned smaller Relative Value Unit (RVU) than simple insertion of a PTFE graft. In our experience, BVT procedures require more than twice the operative time that is required for a PTFE graft insertion, and because of the extensive dissection of the neurovascular structures in the arm, the liability for serious complication is considerably higher. Despite this, the Medicare allowable reimbursement for basilic vein transposition is nearly identical with that for a PTFE shunt insertion. For comparison, the Medicare allowable reimbursements and the relative value units assigned to various access procedures are shown in table 15-2.

Table 15-2.

	CPT	MCA	RVU
BVT	36819	750	22.20
AVF	36821	558	17.09
PTFE	36830	747	23.57
SVG	36825	688	22.57
Fog Thrombectomy	36831	368	11.67

Conclusions

We conclude from this early experience that the use of basilic vein transposition is a good secondary access if superficial veins are not available for construction of a conventional AV fistula. This type of access has an early patency rate that compares favorably with both conventional AV fistula and PTFE graft patency. It enjoys relative freedom from infection and can be used in patients even when prior access has occurred in the extremity. It does have a relatively high rate of vascular steal occurrence and construction of this type of fistula is technically demanding. It requires an experienced access surgeon to avoid potential neurovascular compromise, which may result from the extensive dissection of the upper extremity that is required. The procedure has now been assigned its own CPT code, a fact that reflects its increase in popularity.

Our results confirm that the initial and short-term patency rates of the various access strategies are similar. Our data also suggest that native fistulae are potentially superior to synthetic grafts because of decreased requirement for revisions and thrombectomies. There may also be some theoretical advantage to the basilic vein fistula that does not have a venous anastomosis, as it is the graft-to-vein anastomosis where the majority of intimal hyperplasia occurs in PTFE grafts and that limits their longevity. Further long-term studies will be required to determine the durability and long-term utility of this access strategy.

References

1. Schwab S, Besarab A, Beathard G, et al. NKF-DOQI clinical practice guidelines for vascular access. New York: National Kidney Foundation; 1997:69.
2. Hirth RA, Turenne MN, Woods JD, et al. Predictors of type of vascular access in hemodialysis patients. JAMA 1996; 276:1303-08.
3. Dagher F, Gelber R, Ramos E, Sadler J. The use of basilic vein and brachial artery as a A-V fistula for long-term hemodialysis. J Surg Res 1976; 20:373-76.
4. Dagher FJ. The upper arm AV hemoaccess: Long term follow-up. J Cardiovasc Surg (Torino) 1986; 27:447-49.
5. Berman SS, Gentile AT, Glickman MH, et al. Distal revascularization-interval ligation for limb salvage and maintenance of dialysis access in ischemic steal syndrome. J Vasc Surg 1997; 26:393-402.
6. Burger H. Long-term outcome of different forms of vascular access. Conlon P, Nicholson M, and Schwab S, eds. Hemodialysis vascular access. Oxford UK: Oxford University Press; 2000.

DISCUSSION

Panelists:

Mitchell L Henry, M.D.
Richard L. McCann, M.D.

Dr. Henry: I would start off by saying that there are long-term studies available. They are not randomized prospective trials but there have been some 10-year patency data out there. This is in response to a comment made this morning that are in the very high 70% to 80% 10-year patency rates for people who are very experienced in doing this procedure. So I think there is some evidence that it has a very good long-term patency. I have a question for you in terms of the complications of the procedure. Have you, or anybody else in the audience, seen significant arm edema following this procedure?

Dr. McCann: We have only seen that in instances of central vein stenosis. If you get persistent edema, I would urge you to get a shuntogram to investigate it because that is a very high likelihood.

Dr. Henry: Just 1 other technical thing. I noticed in one of your slides that you make your tunnel curved. When I have tried to do that in some cases I have found that I did not really have enough vein to make a nice curve. What I started doing subsequent to that is making a straight tunnel from the brachial artery up the arm and then making my incision curved. I can make my tunnel straight and then you get more vein to use for access.

Discussant: I may have missed it but what was your incidence or steal in your patients? If you do have ischemic complications, how can you treat this in these patients?

Dr. McCann: Steal is relatively common and occurs in 9% of the basilic vein transpositions. It is obvious immediately. We find the pulse oximeter on the field to be very helpful and when you lose the pulse oximeter signal by opening the graft we proceed directly with a re-vascularization.

Discussant: Roughly a quarter, if I understood your statistics correctly, of these failed. What happens to the ipsilateral extremity? What options are there after you have done this operation for establishment of further access using this extremity?

Dr. McCann: You can still place a PTFE graft in the same extremity. You just have to go a little high in the axillary.

Discussant: Have you had any problems with aneurysms in this regimen?

Dr. McCann: We have not had that problem at this early juncture.

Dr. Henry: I think that it is very important as to how you handle that vein during the time of surgery. For instance, if you are used to dilating it up under pressure, that is something that can lead to stenoses. The cardiac surgeons have learned long ago to treat the vein very carefully at the time that you operate on it.

Discussant: This is a good access and it can be accessed very quickly and can last a long time and it is a good secondary access. Do you think we need to make any changes in our practice of jumping the forearm loop graft and it fails? Because if you do a jump graft of the upper arm, then you potentially lose this deep vein.

Dr. McCann: Yes, and in fact, in my practice I do very few forearm loop grafts because I think that if the vein is adequate at the anticubital level that it should either be used as a primary fistula or as a basilic vein transposition.

Discussant: I think I would agree with that. I think it depends on what the long-term patency really is. If we can be convinced that the long-term patency of the basilic vein transposition is really very good, and much different than the PTFE, then it is probably better to go directly to that rather than have all sorts of different operative procedures, costs, and pain to the patient than a loop PTFE. But it depends on what that long-term patency really is.

Discussant: We have been following a procedure protocol of trying to get the forearm brachial cephalic or upperarm brachial cephalic as the primary access. If it is not possible to have a forearm loop graft, or a straight, whatever is the surgeon's preferences. But once it has failed we try to do local revisions for that and try to prolong the graft as soon as possible but we do not jump into the upperarm. The secondary access is when we try to do upperarm basilic vein transposition. The other 35 to 40% of patients who tend to get a good long-term outcome from the forearm loop graft are the ones we do not want to exclude.

Discussant: There is another logic to that approach also. Even if they get a year out of their PTFE, their basilic vein will be hypertrophied by that time and is a better vein for the basilic vein transposition. So I think you could go either way. We just need more data.

16

FURTHER DEFINING THE TRANSPOSED BRACHIOBASILIC FISTULA

Gary W. Barone, M.D., Meredith L. Lightfoot, M.D., Mary Jo Shaver, M.D., and Beverley L. Ketel, M.D.

Since its first description in 1966, the Brescia-Cimino arteriovenous (AV) fistula has been the gold standard against which all types of hemoaccess for chronic hemodialysis have been compared.[1] This hemoaccess fistula is associated with both a high long-term patency rate and an overall low number of complications. Unfortunately, this type of fistula can only be constructed in a minority of hemodialysis patients.[2] A large percentage of patients are not candidates, usually due to the lack of a suitable superficial vein. Viable alternatives for the majority of hemodialysis patients have been either an AV bridge graft, usually of expanded polytetrafluoroethylene (PTFE), or an alternative endogenous fistula.[2-9]

Dagher and collegues[5] in 1976 are credited with first describing the transposed brachiobasilic fistula (TBF) as an alternative endogenous hemoaccess to the Brescia-Cimino fistula. Since then, many series have reported their results.[6-9] With the recent introduction of DOQI Clinical Practice Guidelines for Vascular Access, there is both an emphasis on using alternative endogenous fistulae instead of PTFE grafts and an increased interest in monitoring the specific long-term outcomes of the different types of hemoaccess.[10]

Our goal is to precisely define the role of the TBF. Should a TBF be an option for every hemodialysis patient? Where should the TBF be placed in the hemoaccess regimen? We started by investigating if potential previous vein maturation causes a secondary (after a previous forearm access) brachiobasilic fistula (SBF) to behave differently from a primary (no previous hemoaccess) brachiobasilic fistula (PBF).

The TBF's placement in the hemoaccess regimen could be affected by a difference between the SBF and the PBF.

Materials and Methods

Between October 1998 and February 2000, 186 new hemodialysis accesses (67 native AV fistula and 119 AV PTFE grafts) were created, either at the University of Arkansas Medical Center or at the John L. McClellan Veteran Affairs Hospital. Of the native fistulae, 26 of these were TBF, in 26 patients. These fistulae were followed prospectively. We used the transposed basilic vein technique, as described by Dagher et al.[5], Matsuura et al.[8], and Coburn et al.[7], rather than the translocated basilic vein technique as recommended by Humphries et al.[6]

In an attempt to reduce patient morbidity, we used a slightly modified technique that employs 2 separate skin incisions with a skin bridge, rather than the standard continuous upper arm incision.[6,8] All vein side branches were ligated or suture ligated with silk. In our experience, vessel clips have a tendency to drag and dislodge during tunneling. Heparin flush solution was used to gently dilate the mobilized basilic vein in an effort to assess the overall quality of the vein. The vein was then marked and tunneled superficially subcutaneously as described by Rivers et al.[9] Depending on the length of the vein, we anastomosed it to the above elbow brachial artery (using the same vein-harvesting incision) or to the below elbow brachial artery (new incision required). The below elbow brachial artery offers the advantage of tunneling with a resultant straight line arterial anastomosis, similar to a native upper arm cephalic vein fistula. A significant disadvantage of the below elbow technique is that it may interfere with the future placement of a forearm hemoaccess.

A PBF was defined as a fistula in a patient with no previous hemoaccess graft or fistula in the treated arm. A SBF was defined as a fistula in a patient who had a previous hemoaccess in the same arm. The diameter of the basilic vein was determined after the fistula was completed and blood was flowing. For convenience, basilic vein measurements were obtained at the level of the axilla. The diameter of the basilic vein was measured by flattening the vein against a metal ruler.

As with other types of native AV dialysis fistula, maturation time for a TBF can be very subjective. At 4 weeks postoperatively, we started to assess whether a TBF was sufficiently mature to allow cannulation (based on vein size and thickness). However, we considered a TBF matured only when it could be repeatedly cannulated and used regularly for hemodialysis without complication. The surgical literature suggests that by allowing TBF adequate maturation time, early fistula complications can be prevented, and it recommends a 6 to 8 week maturation period.[8,9] TBF that were not at least 4 weeks old were not included in our calculations.

Primary patency was defined as the time from surgical placement to the time that any surgical or radiological intervention was required, secondary to thrombosis, stenosis, or aneurysmal formation of TBF. Any patients who died, were transplanted, or stopped dialysis before TBF maturation were not included in calculations.

Results

Of the 26 TBF, 13 were PBF, with a mean follow-up of 10.2 ± 2 months (range 2 to 17 months), and 12 were SBF, with a mean follow-up of 9.7 ± 3 months (range 6 to 12 months). One patient died prior to maturation of a PBF and was not considered in the calculations. Both groups (table 16-1) were similar, and the majority of patients were hypertensive black males with diabetes mellitus. This patient profile is common in our institution's male veteran patient population.

Initial basilic vein size at the time of surgery was 10 ± 1 mm for the PBF and 13 ± 1 mm for the SBF, which is statistically significantly different ($P<0.05$). As of May 2000, the primary patency of PBF was 8 (62%) of 13, with 3 salvaged through combined lytic and surgical therapy. The primary patency of the SBF was 10 (83%) of 12, with 2 lost to thrombosis and none successfully salvaged. The overall primary patency of our group of TBF was 18 (72%) of 25, with no significant differences between PBF and SBF. Figures 16-1 and 16-2 demonstrate typical venous stenosis, which appeared to involve the distal half of the vein close to the arterial anastomosis. The time to fistula maturation for PBF was 15 ± 5 weeks compared with 10 ± 2 weeks for SBF, a statistically significant difference ($P<0.05$). The maturation rate for our TBF, as seen in figure 16-3, demonstrates that by 8 weeks, only approximately 40% of PBF and 60% of SBF were consistently usable. To date, 3 total TBF have failed to mature after 7 months.

Table 16-1. Patient demographics.

	PBF	SBF
Number of patients	13	12
Male	92%	83%
Black	62%	91%
Mean age, years (range)	53 (40-80)	50 (25-74)
Renal failure		
Hypertension	92%	100%
Diabetes mellitus	62%	66%
Mean follow-up (months)	10.2	9.7

(PBF: Primary brachiobasilic fistula; SBF: Secondary brachiobasilic fistula)

Discussion

The creation and maintenance of hemoaccess sites continues to be a significant source of morbidity for patients requiring chronic hemodialysis.[10] A well-functioning Brescia-Cimino AV fistula is the desired hemodialysis fistula type.[1] These hemoaccess fistulae can last a lifetime for a renal failure patient, if properly used. Unfortunately, the majority of patients are not considered candidates for fistulae

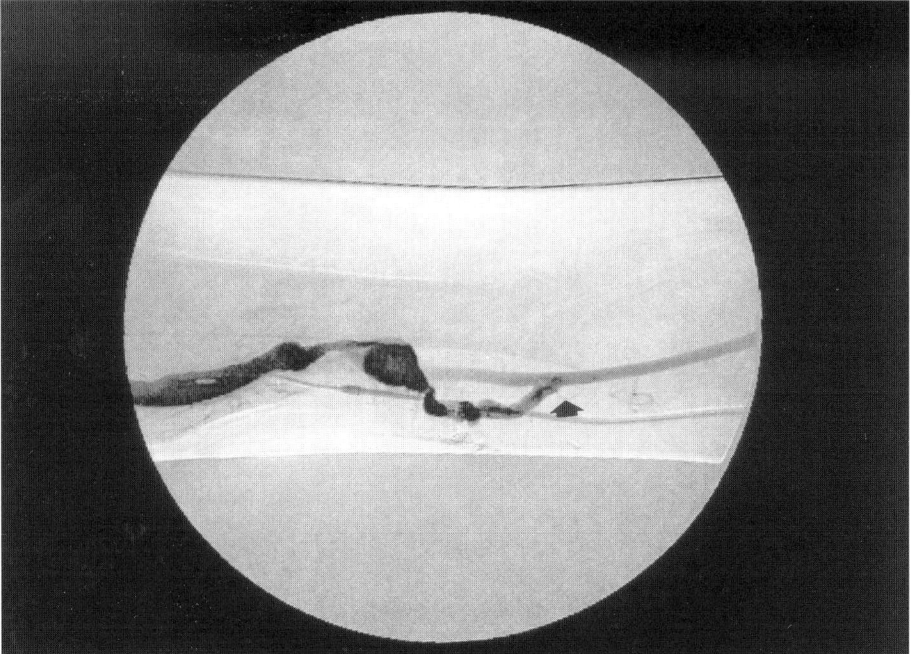

Figure 16-1. Venous stenosis and small pseudoaneurysm formation; arteriovenous anastomosis (arrow) and patient's hand to right.

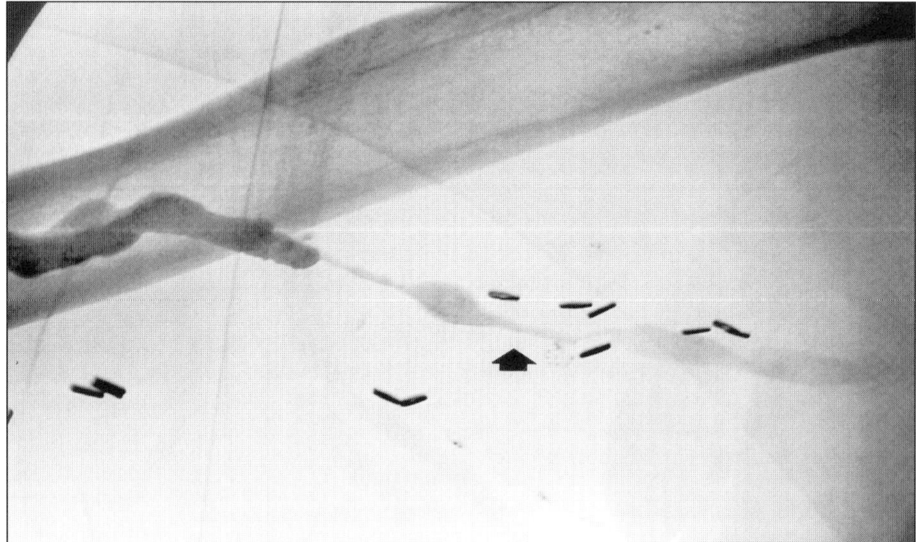

Figure 16-2. Venous stenosis in area of needle sites (arrow); patient's hand to left.

because of underlying arterial vasculopathy and/or the lack of suitable superficial veins. Prior to our use of TBF, our endogenous fistula rate was approximately 20%, which is similar to the 15% reported by Bell et al.[11] This is probably related to the large end-stage renal failure population of our older diabetic patients.

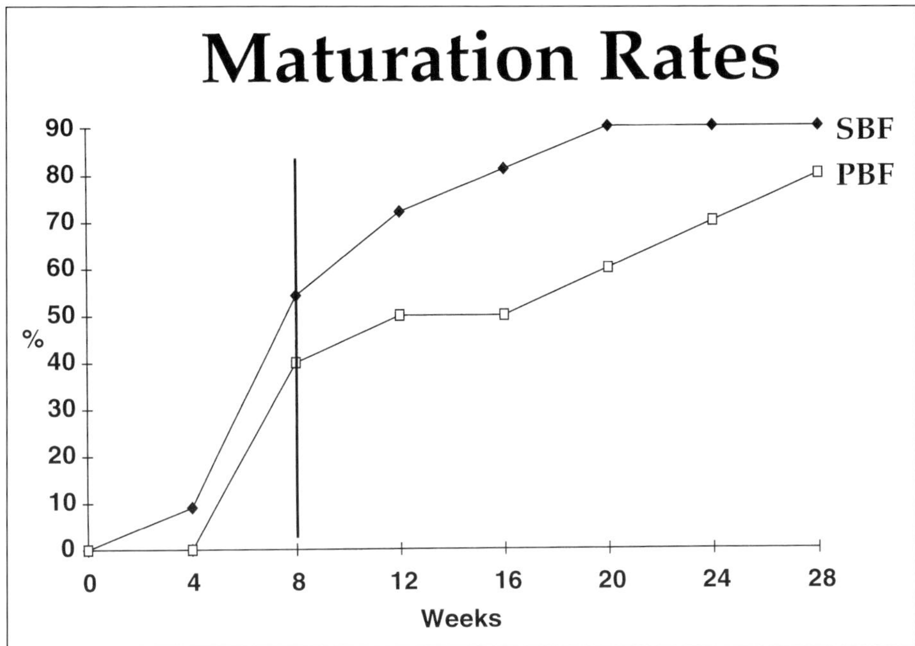

Figure 16-3. Maturation rate (weeks): SBF (Secondary brachiobasilic fistula), PBF (Primary brachiobasilic fistula).

Since expanded PTFE was introduced as an alternative prosthetic material for creating AV bridge grafts in 1976, PTFE has proven to be easy to handle, resistant to infection, and tolerant of repeated punctures.[3,12] A significant disadvantage of PTFE is that a majority of the grafts will thrombose within 2 years (versus our mean patency survival time of approximately 13 months).[13] PTFE graft thrombosis is typically associated with venous outflow obstruction due to focal anastomotic or extensive segmental venous neointimal hyperplasia. The use of alternative endogenous fistulae continues to be reported,[2,4-9] and there are several recent excellent reviews on the upper arm brachiobasilic fistula.[6-9]

Our study of TBF is limited by a relatively small number of patients and a short follow-up. However, the primary patency was 18 (72%) of 25 for our TBF group at about 1 year, similar to Matsuura et al.[8], which reported a rate of 25 (80%) of 30. Certainly, this may change as more TBF are performed with longer follow-ups. We could not identify any other series on TBF that specifically compared PBF versus SBF. The vein size for a SBF is larger than a PBF. This is probably due to previous arterialization of the upper arm outflow veins after previous forearm access.

Our results showed better early patency and earlier maturation for SBF. Again, confirmation of these results requires additional studies with more patients and longer follow-ups. Studies recommend between 6 and 8 weeks for the maturation of TBF.[6,9] Our mean maturation time of 15 weeks for the PBF and 10 weeks for SBF was longer than the maturation times previously reported. This may reflect our requirement that a TBF mature before attempts at consistent hemodialysis cannulation are initiated. It is important to note that this long apparent maturation time may place patients requiring immediate hemodialysis at an increased risk of infection and central vein injuries from required central venous catheters.

PBF may also preclude the future use of the treated arm for hemoaccess. Chronic hemodialysis continues as the only viable alternative for many of these patients. A hemodialysis patient has only 4 primary hemoaccess graft sites, 2 forearms and 2 upper arms. With many patients expected to survive 5 to 10 years or more on hemodialysis, conservation of these hemoaccess sites is extremely important. Matsuura et al.[8], Rivers et al.[9], and Coburn et al.[7] claim that a PTFE AV graft can easily and successfully be placed in the upper arm if the upper arm TBF should fail, but no studies have addressed the status of the forearm. If a PBF is anastomosed in the antecubital fossa below the elbow, the future use of the forearm as an access site may be compromised. For this reason, we no longer routinely recommend anastomosing TBF to this arterial site.

Finally, where can TBF be placed in an access regimen, and are there significant differences between PBF and SBF? As mentioned above, if TBF should be used primarily, then it would be best to avoid anastomosing below elbow antecubital fossa. Our early data suggested that SBF may have advantages over PBF. Figure 16-4 is one conceivable hemoaccess regimen. Bender et al.[2] also suggested that the antecubital fossa superficial cephalic vein offers excellent long-term patency and should be used before a forearm graft. We have no experience with the use of alternative endogenous forearm fistulae, and only after reviewing patients with longer follow-up periods will we be able to answer these questions.

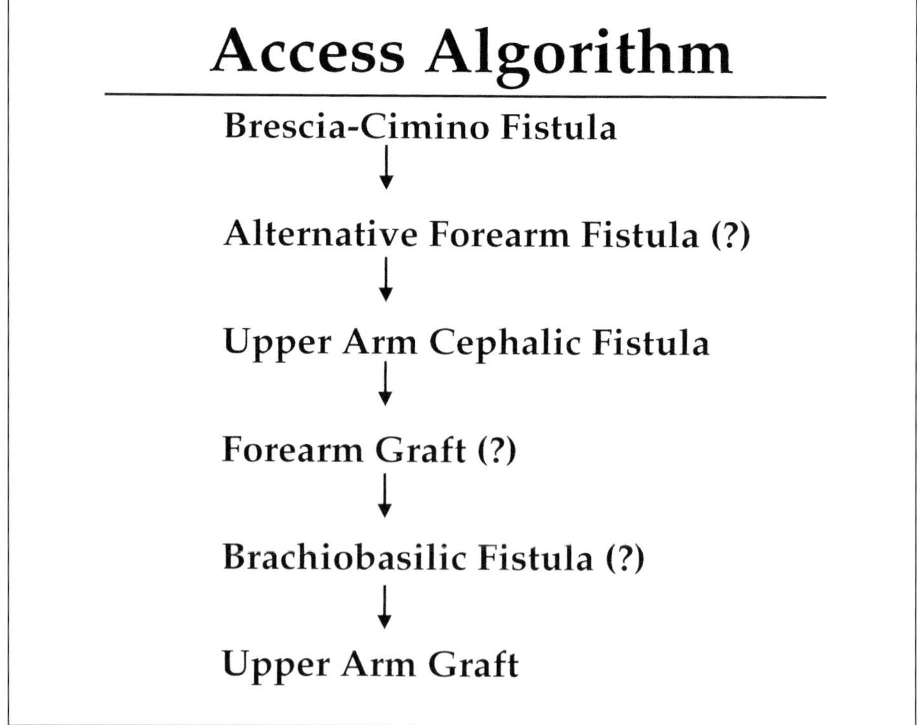

Figure 16-4. Access regimen.

References

1. Brescia MJ, Cimino JE, Appel K, Hurwich BJ. Chronic hemodialysis using venipuncture and a surgically created arteriovenous fistula. N Engl J Med 1966; 9:1089-92.
2. Bender MH, Bruyninckx CM, Gerlag PG. The brachiocephalic elbow fistula: A useful alternative angioaccess for permanent hemodialysis. J Vasc Surg 1994; 20:808-13.
3. Raju S. PTFE grafts for hemodialysis access: Techniques for insertion and management of complications. Ann Surg 1987; 206:666-73.
4. Silva MB, Hobson RW, Pappas PJ, et al. Vein transposition in the forearm for autogenous hemodialysis access. J Vasc Surgery 1997; 26:981-86.
5. Dagher F, Gelber R, Ramos E, Sadler J. The use of the basilic vein and brachial artery as an AV fistula for long-term hemodialysis. J Surg Res 1976; 20:373-76.
6. Humphries AL, Colborn GL,Wynn JJ. Elevated basilic vein arteriovenous fistula. Am J Surg 1999; 177:489-91.
7. Coburn MC, Carney WI. Comparison of basilic vein and polytetrafluoroethylene for brachial arteriovenous fistula. J Vasc Surg 1994; 20:896-02.
8. Matsuura JH, Rosenthal D, Clark M, et al. Transposed basilic vein versus polytrafluorethylene for brachial-axillary arteriovenous fistulas. Am J Surg 1998; 176:219-221.
9. Rivers SP, Scher LA, Sheehan E, Lynn R, Veith FJ. Basilic vein transposition: An underused autologous alternative to prosthetic dialysis angioaccess. J Vasc Surg 1993; 18:391-96.
10. Schwab S, Besarab A, Beathard G, et al. NKF-DOQI clinical practice guidelines for vascular access. New York: National Kidney Foundation 1997:15-78.
11. Bell DD, Rosental JJ. Arteriovenous graft life in chronic hemodialysis. J Vasc Surg 1989; 9:277-85.
12. Hines LH, Turner GR, King WS, McDaniel CE, Dodd DJ. 4-7 mm tapered expanded PTFE access grafts: Techniques of construction of preservation of graft life. In: Henry ML, Ferguson RM, eds. Vascular access for hemodialysis-III. Chicago: W.L. Gore & Associates and Precept Press, 1993;175-85.
13. Palder SB, Kirkman RL, Whittemore AD, Hakim KM, Lazarus JM, Tilney NL. Vascular access for hemodialysis: Patency rates and results of revision. Ann Surg 1985; 202:235-39.

DISCUSSION

Panelist:

Merideth L. Lightfoot, M.D.

Speaker: Thank you, that was a very nice presentation. Are there any questions?

Discussant: I was a little troubled by one thing. I think I heard you say that your patient population was elderly, yet the mean age was 52 and made me feel a little uncomfortable!

Discussant: I have done a couple of these basilic fistulas but I had the opportunity of having a permacath in. The basilic vein approach I used was actually to do your anastomosis first, let it mature for up to 2 or 3 weeks, and then transpose it just under the skin. If you look at secondary patency rates, they are better.

Dr. Lightfoot: I think that is very interesting and something definitely worth considering.

Discussant: Was there a vein size below which you would not perform a basilic vein transposition?

Dr. Lightfoot: Four millimeters is the number that is most often quoted in the literature.

Discussant: It looks like you are advocating creating a forearm loop graft first so as to help the basilic vein arterialize, which in theory I think is good. On the other hand, it seems to me once you have a graft in place then you get in this frame of mind to just try to keep the graft going. The next thing you know a year or 2 years have passed and the patient has had a number of procedures trying to keep that graft going. So, for that reason, I would just question that approach.

Dr. Lightfoot: I think that is certainly true and that is something that everyone would have to be mindful of. At our center it may be useful because there are 2 surgeons involved and they will see all the patients. So it would be very appropriate for us. But that is definitely a good point.

17

AN INNOVATIVE TWO-STAGE CONSTRUCTION TECHNIQUE OF TRANSPOSED BRACHIO-BASILIC ARTERIOVENOUS FISTULA

Joon H. Hong, M.D., Nabil Sumrani, M.D., Dale Distant, M.D., and Bruce Sommer, M.D.

An efficient and dependable vascular access is essential for the longevity of patients on long-term hemodialysis therapy. The autogenous arteriovenous fistula (AVF) continues to be the access of choice because it provides the best long-term performance with superior patency and a low complication rate.[1] In the United States, however, the frequency of AVF construction is low, and prosthetic arteriovenous grafts (AVGs) are placed in the majority of patients. This predominant use of AVGs results in increased vascular access morbidity and health care costs.[2]

Recently, an upper arm AVF, created between the brachial artery and a superficially transposed basilic vein (known as a brachio-basillic arteriovenous fistula [BB AVF]), has become popular in patients for whom the AVF cannot be created or maintained in the forearm.[3,4] The basilic vein, however, must be of optimal length and luminal size for successful construction of a transposed BB AVF. Patients with a previously functioning arteriovenous access in the forearm are ideal candidates for this procedure as a secondary access, while most new patients requiring an initial vascular access do not have adequate vessels for the construction of a transposed BB AVF.

We have developed an innovative approach for patients with suboptimal vessels for BB AVF by creating a preliminary distal AVF followed by the construction of a transposed BB AVF in the second stage.

Methods

Between January 1998 and December 1999, preliminary distal AVFs were created in a total of 37 patients with end-stage renal disease (ESRD) who required new vascular accesses for hemodialysis therapy. These patients were selected because they did not have adequate vessels for the creation of either a radio-cephalic AVF in the forearm or a one-stage transposition BB AVF in the upper arm. Of these patients, 24 were men and 13 were women. The patients ranged from 18 to 78 years of age and the mean was 51 years of age.

Surgical technique. In the first stage, an *in situ* AVF was created between the distal brachial artery and the basilic vein in the medial aspect of the antecubital fossa. If an adequately sized median cubital vein joined the basilic vein, it was anastomosed to the proximal radial artery instead. The vena comitans of the brachial artery was utilized when the basilic vein was not suitable. An anastomosis of length 7 to 10 mm was usually performed in a side-to-side fashion. The distal vein to the anastomosis was divided between ligatures, as were any immediate side branches, in order to ensure maximal blood flow into the main stream of the proximal vein.

After a preconditioning period of at least 1 month, the second stage of the procedure was performed. The interval between the 2 stages was extended to a maximum period of 3 months whenever the clinical situation allowed. The need to initiate dialysis therapy, the lack of dependable temporary access, and poor maturation without further improvement or the adequate maturation of the preliminary AVF were the deciding variables in the timing of the second stage procedure.

In the second stage, the *in situ* AVF was closed off by ligating the proximal vein close to the fistula. The entire length of previously arterialized basilic vein was dissected and mobilized from the antecubital area to the apex of the axilla through 2 or 3 separate incisions along the medial aspect of the upper arm. The brachial vein was also fully mobilized beyond the basilic vein junction toward the chest wall in the axilla. The mobilized vein was then flushed with heparinized saline solution using a 14 F catheter and any leak, kink, or stenosis was repaired. A superficial subcutaneous tunnel was created along the anterior aspect of the upper arm in a loop fashion utilizing a tunneling device and making a counter incision. The vein was transposed through the tunnel to the anterior aspect of the upper arm and the distal end of the vein was brought to the medial aspect of the midportion of the upper arm.

An oblique end-to-side anastomosis was performed between the spatulated distal end of the vein and the brachial artery in an antegrade fashion, as described previously.[4] If the length of the mobilized vein was not long enough for the transposition, a segment of a prosthetic graft was extended to the vein. An AVG fistula was placed when the vein was not large enough to accommodate a 14 F catheter freely. Upon completion of the access construction, the blood flow rate of the transposed BB AVF was measured intra-operatively using an electromagnetic blood flowmeter, CLINIFLOW II (Carolina Medical Electronics Inc, King, NC). Excessive flow rates, above 2 liters/min, were reduced by banding the inflow at the anastomosis.

Results

Of the 37 patients, the preliminary distal AVF remained patent in 35 patients and thrombosed in 2 patients during the preconditioning period.

In patients with patent distal AVFs, transposed BB AVFs were successfully constructed in 32 patients. Also, a hybrid access of a prosthetic graft extension to the mobilized basilic vein was constructed in 2 patients because of the short length of the vein, and an AVG fistula was constructed in 1 patient because of the poor maturation of the vein. In the 2 patients with thrombosed distal AVFs, a transposed BB AVF was created in 1 patient and an AVG fistula in the other.

The mean blood flow rates of the distal AVF were 438 ± 210 mL/min during the first stage and 555 ± 424 mL/min during the second stage. The flow rate was 1,105 ± 427 mL/min after completion of the transposed BB AVF.

In the follow-up analysis, 33 accesses were functioning at the time of this writing, 26 of which were without complication. Four required surgical revisions to control excessive inflow, and 2 required surgical revisions to control thrombectomy. Percutaneous angioplasty was required in 3 patients for the dilation of the venous outflow stenosis. Three accesses failed beyond salvage due to subclavian vein thrombosis in 2 patients, and poor arterial inflow resulting in diffuse stricture of the transposed vein in 1 patient. One patient died of an HIV-related disease.

Discussion

The 2-stage construction technique of the transposed BB AVF described here allowed for the creation of an autogenous AVF in most of our patients. Because of suboptimal vessels, the only other option for these patients would have been a prosthetic graft access. Of the 37 patients selected for a new access creation, a preconditioning approach allowed transposed BB AVF creations in 33 patients (89.2%), hybrid access in 2 patients (5.4%) and AVGs in 2 patients (5.4%). Hybrid access is comprised of a minor prosthetic graft for the delivery of blood flow from the artery and mostly of a transposed vein, which is used for repeated needle puncture for dialysis therapy. In comparison to AVGs, the resilient nature of the vein against repeated needle punctures helps to reduce the incidence of intimal hyperplasia, luminal narrowing, and the subsequent thrombosis of the access.

Vessels that are dilated from the preconditioning approach not only simplify needle puncturing, but also have and allow a high blood flow rate for efficient dialysis therapy, due to the creation of a large anastomosis. Many of the access flow rates were excessive (over 2 liters/min). For these patients, especially the elderly ones, banding of the inflow was required to avoid high-output cardiac failure. Our personal experience, however, tells us that once the vein is transposed from its original location, it rarely dilates, even with arterializations. This may explain some of the discrepancies among the transposed BB AVF patency rates within the published data.[3-6] We emphasize the need for adequate vein dilation before transposition.

In this report, we observed a reduced incidence of distal ischemia caused by steal syndrome, presumably because of enhanced arterial collateral circulation associated with fistula preconditioning. Arm edema was also observed less frequently in these patients, since the proximal veins were already dilated to accommodate a further increase in the blood flow with the transposition. Also, patients seemed to better tolerate increased cardiac output following the 2-stage procedure with the stepwise increment of cardiac preload from the AVF. Even if a preliminary fistula fails to lead to the creation of a transposed BB AVF, these observed merits suggest that AVGs constructed following the distal AVF fare better than the AVGs placed without preconditioning.

We cannot ascertain from the data presented in this report whether the hemodynamic parameters measured at the time of access construction can predict the fate of the access in the future. The mean blood flow rates of the brachial artery and the basilic vein prior to creation of distal AVF were about 100 mL/min and 45 mL/min, respectively. It is noteworthy that the flow increased approximately 5-fold through the brachial artery and 10-fold through the basilic vein after fistula creation. The access flow rate only moderately increased (by 20%) during the preconditioning period, probably because of the retrograde nature of the flow through the side-to-side anastomosis of the distal fistula. However, the flow was increased by almost 100% with the creation of the transposed BB AVF despite the similar size (7 to 10 mm) of the anastomosis. This may be partly explained by the large vessel size, but more significantly by the antegrade nature of the flow through the oblique end-to-side anastomosis.

Conclusions

The 2-stage construction technique of the transposed BB AVF provides a satisfactory autogenous AVF in the majority of patients with suboptimal vessels. A desirably high blood flow rate, low morbidity rate, and a superior patency rate of the access are additional merits provided by this technique. We prefer the two-stage transposition BB AVF to AVGs in patients for whom no forearm AVF can be created.

References

1. Mehta, S. Statistical summary of clinical results of vascular access procedures for hemodialysis. In: Sommer BG, Henry ML, eds. Vascular access for hemodialysis-II. Chicago: W.L. Gore & Associates and Precept Press, 1991; 145-57.
2. Held PJ, Port FK, Webb RL, et al. Excerpts from United States Renal Data System 1995 Annual Data Report. Am J Kidney Dis 1995; 26 (suppl 2):140-56.
3. Dagher FJ, Gelber R, Reed W. Basilic vein to brachial artery, arteriovenous fistula for long-term hemodialysis: A five-year follow-up. Proc Clin Dial Transplant Forum 1980; 10:126-29.

4. Hong JH, Sumrani N, Distant DA, Sommer BG. A modified basilic vein transposition arteriovenous fistula. In Henry ML, ed. Vascular access for hemodialysis-VI. Chicago: W.L. Gore & Associates and Precept Press, 1999; 231-39.
5. Cantelmo NL, Logerfo FW, Menzonian JO. Brachiobasilic and brachiocephalic fistulas as secondary angioaccess routes. Surg Gynecol Obstet 1982; 155:545-48.
6. Rivers SP, Scher LA, Sheehan E, Lynn, R, Veith F. Basilic vein transposition: An underused autologous alternative to prosthetic dialysis angioaccess. J Vasc Surg 1993; 18:391-97.

DISCUSSION

Panelist:
Joon H. Hong, M.D.

Discussant: I just want to make sure I understand this. You would use this 2-stage procedure in every patient that you wanted to create an access or did you select patients who perhaps had small basilic veins by venography?

Dr. Hong: Our philosophy is to try to create a native vessel fistula in any patient coming for dialysis for this procedure. If we are able to create a native fistula in the forearm that is our first choice. If we cannot make an AV fistula in the forearm, then we move on to the 2-stage procedure, if a patient consents. Some of the patients do not like to have 2 operations, then we have no choice but to put in a graft.

Discussant: It would seem to me that there are many patients who wouldn't really need the 2-stage procedures. Some would, as you pointed out, but are you not subjecting a high percentage of patients to an additional operation?

Dr. Hong: About 20% of basilic vein transposition fistula are a primary fistula. That means without a pre-condition stage, we are able to create it especially in those patients who had intravenous drug usage. The superficial veins are gone but in some this basilic vein is preserved very well. Those are the good candidates for the primary transposition fistula.

Discussant: Do you get venography in on the patients beforehand?

Dr. Hong: We depend on physical examinations.

Discussant: I think it is fair to say that we are not clear why some of these brachial basilic fistulas do not mature, even though the vein is significantly dilated at 5 mm or more in diameter. Some of them develop stenotic disease when they are done as a first stage procedure, as a 1-stage procedure. I, in fact, used to do that as 1-stage procedures but now I have moved to the idea of the 2-stage procedure. I rarely get the stenotic problems. You can do the first stage with a local anesthetic. It does not take a long time and then a few weeks later, transpose it.

Dr. Hong: Once the vein is transposed, they are ready to dilate. So you have to have a good vein to begin with, otherwise you prematurely do the transposition and the failure rate is high. If you look at the published papers, some of them have a 10-year patency rate of 80%. It depends on how you select the patients or I think that you have to have some experience with choosing this patient.

18

VIDEO-ASSISTED BASILIC VEIN TRANSPOSITION FOR HEMODIALYSIS VASCULAR ACCESS

Jan H.M. Tordoir, M.D., Ph.D., Ruben Dammers, M.S., and Maurits de Brauw, M.D., Ph.D.

A well-functioning vascular access site remains the lifeline for patients with end-stage renal disease (ESRD), who are treated with chronic intermittent hemodialysis. Vascular access through the creation of Brescia-Cimino (BC) radio-cephalic arteriovenous fistulae (AVF) at the wrist has been the first method of choice during the past decades. When initially successful, BC AVF have a low incidence of complications and high patency rates.

Nevertheless, an increasing number of elderly patients either will lack suitable vessels for BC AVF construction or have developed irreversible thrombosis of such fistulae. The implantation of prosthetic bridge-grafts in the upper extremity position using polytetrafluoroethylene (PTFE) prostheses is usually the second choice for vascular access. Such grafts have proven to be valuable, but thrombosis and infection rates are high, and patency rates are low for PTFE, compared with BC AVF.[1-3]

There has been a renewed interest in the use of elbow and upper arm AVF, anastomosing the brachial artery to the cephalic vein or the transposed basilic vein.[4-9] Reported patency rates of brachio-basilic vein AVF range from 70% to 86% after 2 years of follow-up.[7,10] The incidences of thrombotic occlusion and infection are relatively low, compared with prosthetic AVF.

The conventional surgical technique of basilic vein transposition consists of dissection and mobilization of the basilic vein at the medial side of the upper arm. After dissection, the basilic vein is transposed to a subcutaneous tunnel on the anterior surface of the arm and anastomosed to the brachial artery.[10,11] The large incision needed for this operation, with the excessive vein dissection, may result in postoperative wound infection, skin necrosis, lymphatic leakage, or nerve injury. In peripheral arterial bypass surgery and coronary artery revascularization, less invasive techniques for harvesting of the saphenous vein have been shown to be technically feasible and were associated with fewer wound complications.[12-14]

In this report, we outline our first experience with a minimally invasive, video-assisted method for basilic vein dissection and transposition for the creation of brachio-basilic vein AV fistulae.

Patients and Methods

Patients. In a total of 14 patients, brachio-basilic vein AVF were created because of previously failed vascular accesses (mean number 3.3; range 1 to 7). The patients' characteristics are outlined in table 18-1. All patients underwent preoperative assessment of upper extremity arteries and veins by means of duplex ultrasound investigation. The diameters and patency of the brachial, radial, and ulnar arteries were determined. Also, cephalic and basilic vein diameter and continuity in the forearm and upper arm were assessed. AV fistula volume flows were measured 2 months postoperatively by means of duplex ultrasound.

Table 18-1. Patient characteristics.

No. of patients		14
Female/male		8/6
Mean age (years)		52 (range=26 to 74)
Mean no. of previous accesses		3.3 (range=1 to 7)
Comorbidities	Diabetes	6 (43%)
	Cardiac	5 (36%)
	Hypertension	6 (43%)

Operative technique. Video-assisted vein dissection was carried out with the use of a video monitor situated at the superior end of the patient. A reusable hook, with a channel suitable for introduction of a 5-mm 30° view endoscope (Storz Medical, Kreuzlingen, Switzerland) was used. A transverse incision is made at the medial site just above the elbow, and the basilic vein was localized and a few centimeters were dissected. Then the hook was introduced along the vein, and a blunt dissection was performed, with continuous visualization of the vein. Standard endoscopic scissors and dissection clamps were used to facilitate the dissection.

The median cutaneous nerve was identified and eventually freed from the basilic vein. The side branches were carefully dissected and clipped with a disposable, 5-mm clip instrument (Auto Suture Europe SA, Elancourt Cedex, France). Then a small longitudinal incision was made in the axilla, and the basilic vein was removed after complete circumferential dissection and transection at the elbow level. The proximal part of the vein remained attached to the deep vein. Subsequently, the anterior surface of the vein was marked to avoid rotation during tunneling, and the quality and diameter of the vein were tested by injecting saline. A subcutaneous tunnel was created anterior in the upper arm, and the vein was brought through the tunnel and anastomosed, in an end-to-side fashion, to the brachial artery with a running 7-0 polypropylene (Prolene®) suture. Completion angiography was performed to determine technical problems. Needle puncturing for hemodialysis was permitted after 4 to 6 weeks postoperatively.

Results

The mean total operation time was 146 minutes (range 110 to 240 minutes). The mean time for the endoscopic vein dissection was 42 minutes, with a range of 30 to 90 minutes. A mean of 4.6 side branches per patient (range 2 to 7 side branches per patient) were clipped with endoscopic instruments. No conversions to an open technique or specific complications of the video-assisted dissection were observed. One patient developed early postoperative thrombosis, necessitating surgical revision. There were no postoperative wound complications or infections. One patient developed a hematoma in the subcutaneous tunnel, necessitating surgical exploration, with salvage of the access.

The mean hospitalization time was 3 days (range 2 to 4 days). The median follow-up was 13.4 months (range 6 to 18 months). There were 3 late elective interventions after 6, 9, and 13 months in 2 patients, because of a decreased bloodflow through the AV fistula, as measured with Transonic flowmetry. These patients were successfully treated with percutaneous transluminal angioplasty of a significant venous outflow stenosis at the level of the axilla. The primary, assisted-primary, and secondary patency rates after 12 months of follow-up were 78%, 93%, and 100%, respectively. All AVF were patent at the time of the latest follow-up and were satisfactory for use as hemodialysis vascular access treatment.

The mean AV fistula volume flow after 6 weeks postoperatively, was 1250 cc/min (range 500 to 1805 cc/min), as measured by duplex scanning.

Discussion

Patients requiring long-term hemodialysis treatment need adequately functioning vascular accesses. The radiocephalic fistula at the wrist has been the vascular access of first choice during the past 3 decades. Unfortunately, superficial veins in the forearm suitable for the creation of an AV fistula are unavailable and an increasing number of patients require the implantation of prosthetic graft material (usually PTFE prosthesis). These prosthetic bridge-grafts, however, have a high incidence of thrombotic and infectious complications, necessitating a great number of surgical and interventional revisions.

The basilic vein in the upper arm is relatively large and has been called the hidden vein because it is not visible through simple inspection and palpation.

Therefore, it can escape the damage inflicted by repeated iatrogenic venipunctures or intravenous lines. The use of the native basilic vein offers certain advantages over the prosthetic PTFE graft: (1) a high flow through the large vein is possible; (2) only 1 anastomosis is required, and the distal venous anastomosis, usually the site for stenoses in PTFE graft AV fistulas, is avoided; and (3) the risk of infection is low and does not mandate removal of the native vein AVF.

Today, a basilic vein transposition for vascular access is usually necessary because of the failure of previous BC AVF or forearm prosthetic bridge-grafts. If there is no suitable cephalic vein in the upper arm, a sufficient basilic vein may often be detected by duplex scanning and used as an access site. In patients with active infections or a high risk of infection, as documented in 2 study patients (HIV-positive and immunosuppressive treatment), the avoidance of implantation of foreign-body materials, such as prosthetic grafts, is essential. A native brachio-basilic vein AVF may be a good solution for such patients.

The patency rates of transposed basilic vein AV fistulae, as reported from the literature, range from 70% to 90% after 1 year, 70% to 86% after 2 years, and 50% to 60% after 3 years of follow-up, and are likely to be superior to PTFE grafts.[6,7,10] Also, the incidence of thrombotic occlusion (18% versus 80% in the first postoperative year), infection (3% versus 16%) and aneurysm formation (3% versus 6%) seem to be significantly lower when compared with prosthetic grafts.[7-9]

The technique for creation of brachio-basilic AVF was initially described by Dagher et al.[10] in 1974. Presently, many physicians have adopted and used this same operative method. Usually, large incisions are needed to dissect the basilic vein from the elbow up to the axilla. The risk of cutaneous nerve damage, hematoma, wound complications, and postoperative pain is not insignificant. Also, lymphoedema, due to the extensive dissection, may occur. This edema may hamper successful needling of the AVF. Using the conventional operation, an incidence of 2% to 5% of postoperative wound infections and lymphatic problems has been reported.[15] No data on cutaneous nerve damage and persistent edema have been reported in the literature.

Video-assisted basilic vein transposition demonstrated several advantages compared with open basilic vein dissection. It avoided a large wound with all the risks of wound complications. A perfect, continuous visualization of the vein was possible with a good sight on structures, such as the median cutaneous nerve and basilic vein side branches, which facilitated adequate dissection. The most important advantage of this minimally invasive technique was that patients had little or no pain after the operation.

In conclusion, video-assisted basilic vein transposition is a valuable surgical technique for the creation of a secondary vascular access in patients receiving hemodialysis treatment. Prospective studies are needed to prove the value of this new technique for the prevention of wound complications and postoperative pain sensation.

References

1. Kherlakian GM, Roedersheimer LR, Arbaugh JJ, Newmark KJ, King LR. Comparison of autogenous fistula versus expanded polytetrafluoroethylene graft fistula for angioaccess in hemodialysis. Am J Surg 1986; 152:238-43.

2. Tordoir JHM, Herman JM, Kwan TS, Diderich PM. Long-term follow-up of the polytetrafluoroethylene (PTFE) prosthesis as an arteriovenous fistula for haemodialysis. Eur J Vasc Surg 1988; 2:3-7.
3. Ascher E, Gade P, Hingorani A, et al. Changes in the practice of angioaccess surgery: Impact of dialysis outcome and quality initiative recommendations. J Vasc Surg 2000; 31:84-92.
4. Hibberd AD. Brachiobasilic fistula with autogenous basilic vein: Surgical technique and pilot study. Aust NZ J Surg 1991; 61:631-35.
5. Hatjibaloglou A, Grekas D, Saratzis N, et al. Transposed basilic vein-brachial arteriovenous fistula: An alternative vascular access for hemodialysis. Artif Organs 1992; 16:623-25.
6. Rivers SP, Scher LA, Sheehan E, Lynn R, Veith FJ. Basilic vein transposition: An underused autologous alternative to prosthetic dialysis angioaccess. J Vasc Surg 1993; 18:391-97.
7. Coburn MC, Carney WI Jr. Comparison of basilic vein and polytetrafluoroethylene for brachial arteriovenous fistula. J Vasc Surg 1994; 20:896-904.
8. Stonebridge PA, Edington D, Jenkins AM. Brachial/basilic vein transposition for vascular access. J R Coll Surg Edinb 1995; 40:219-20.
9. Butterworth PC, Doughman TM, Wheatley TJ, Nicholson ML. Arteriovenous fistula using transposed basilic vein. Br J Surg 1998; 85:653-54.
10. Dagher F, Gelber R, Ramos E, Sadler J. The use of the basilic vein and brachial artery as an AV fistula for long term hemodialysis. J Surg Res 1976; 20:373-76.
11. LoGerfo FW, Menzoian JO, Kumaki DJ, Idelson A. Transposed basilic vein-brachial arteriovenous fistula. A reliable secondary access procedure. Arch Surg 1978; 113:1008-10.
12. Folliguet TA, Le Bret E, Moneta A, Musumeci S, Laborde F. Endoscopic saphenous vein harvesting versus open technique. A prospective study. Eur J Cardiothorac Surg 1998; 13:662-66.
13. Allen KB, Griffith GL, Heimansohn DA, et al. Endoscopic versus traditional saphenous vein harvesting: A prospective randomized trial. Ann Thorac Surg 1998; 66:26-31.
14. Robbins MR, Hutchinson SA, Helmer SD. Endoscopic saphenous vein harvest in infrainguinal bypass surgery. Am J Surg 1998; 176:586-90.
15. Humphries AL Jr, Colborn GL, Wynn JJ. Elevated basilic vein arteriovenous fistula. Am J Surg 1999; 177:489-91.

DISCUSSION

Panelists:
Jan H. M. Tordoir, M.D.
Allan Lumsden, M.D.

Discussant: That is a very interesting approach I must say. I have just 1 question. I guess it is not really in the main part of your presentation, which I think is spectacular. But you said that the secondary patency is 100%, and the primary patency is 80%, which means you rescued some of the grafts that presumably thrombosed. How do you rescue a basilic vein transposition that thromboses?

Dr. Tordoir: Many of you have a surveillance program with flow measurements in these patients and if you see the flow go down in this brachial basilic transposition access, we do angiography and do usually an elective PTA. Therefore you can raise your patency rates.

Discussant: So they were not completely thrombosed. They just had poor flow.

Dr. Tordoir: Correct.

Discussant: Did you ever consider to ligate the side branches after elevation of the vein?

Dr. Tordoir: To make the separation easier, we usually clip the side branches, then take out the vein, and then we perform a suture ligation of the side branches of the vein itself.

Discussant: I just wanted to put this into perspective a little bit because video-assisted harvest has been around for 5 or 6 years; in fact, our group published the first 2 reports about endoscopic vein harvest. It is not something we do a lot of now. We do not do a lot of it now because this is a very difficult procedure to perform. I do not know of anyone who has done deep venous dissection, which is essentially what you are doing with an endoscopic vein harvest. One of the reasons for that is that these veins are different from the superficial veins. You are dissecting an extremely challenging vessel to take out with an endoscope because it is extremely thin and it has numerous side branches. So I am surprised about your vein harvest time, even it is a relatively short segment that you are dissecting. It is not actually more than 40 minutes. One of the complications is nerve injury. Those are superficial cutaneous nerve injuries you are talking about. My concern is that you are going to change that to ulnar nerve and median nerve injuries. How do you get the experience and do you think this is something that can be generalized? My concern is half the audience is now going to go and try to do endoscopic vein harvest of a basilic vein and I think that will be catastrophic, quite frankly.

Dr. Tordoir: I certainly agree that this is a very difficult procedure and you have to have a lot of experience. I am not doing this by myself alone. There also is an endoscopic surgeon involved. We perform these operations with 2 surgeons. There is certainly a risk to damage the basilic vein because it is very thin. You have to be very careful. One patient did have a temporary sensation loss due to a small nerve injury and that was completely restored after 2 months. Of course the long-term results are as good for forearm fistulas. But we can declot physiologically the transposed fistulas.

Discussant: What is your time limit for that?

Dr. Tordoir: It is 2 weeks, but the older the thrombosis, the more difficult is removal of the thrombosis because it becomes hard.

Discussant: You mentioned that there was a lot of time in the dissection of the tissues into the basilic vein. Why was it so much time to dissect? Was it because you were looking for the basilic vein or was it removing the tissues away from the basilic vein?

Dr. Tordoir: Usually it is not very difficult to find the basilic vein but it is difficult to dissect the structures from the basilic vein. There are a lot of patients with the nerve circulating around the vein and it is very difficult to free the vein from the nerve. That took a lot of time.

Dr. Lumsden: These catheters have been made for veins that actually emit infrared radiation. Then, to the endoscope, you can build an infrared detector. So when you put a catheter inside the vein and you view the arm for example with the infrared camera, you can see these lights flashing up and down the vein. It is also very helpful at the time you are actually doing the dissection. You will see it is like a runway of flashing lights up the length of the vein and it does help you do the dissection.

19

EFFECTS OF ARTERIAL AND VENOUS ANASTOMOTIC DESIGN ON HEMODYNAMICS IN ARTERIOVENOUS PROSTHETIC GRAFTS

Ulf Krueger, Ph.D., Michael Heise M.D., Almut Huhle, Kerstin Krys, Juergen Zanow, M.D., and Hans Scholz, M.D.

Prosthetic graft material, such as expanded polytetrafluoroethylene (ePTFE), is increasingly used for arteriovenous access if in situ autologous vein is not suitable for fistula construction. Relatively high blood flow rates are required in an arteriovenous graft to perform adequate hemodialysis and prevent thrombosis. High flow rates are maintained by low graft resistance and outflow into the compliant venous system. High flow rate, however, leads to flow disturbances that are severe enough to produce perivascular vibrations.[1] Palpation of a thrill in the distal graft is often recommended as proof for a well-constructed bridge graft.[2,3] Anastomotic intimal hyperplasia at the venous anastomosis has been widely accepted as the main reason for graft stenosis and consecutive occlusion. We observed the occurrence of occlusion in the arterial side-to-end anastomosis in selected cases.

Despite extensive investigation, the specific etiology of intimal hyperplasia has not been clearly understood. Numerous studies suggest that hemodynamic phenomena, such as disturbances of flow patterns, flow separation, oscillation, and abnormal wall shear stress may induce this process.[1,4-17] The creation of an arteriovenous access sometimes leads to forearm or hand ischemia, accompanied by dialysis access-associated steal syndrome. Ischemia has been managed with surgical reduction of graft flow, however, the delicate balance between essential graft flow and an adequate limb perfusion pressure is difficult to achieve.

This study investigated the effect of arterial and venous anastomotic design on hemodynamics. An arterial anastomosis had a narrowly shaped segment between the artery and the graft. Flow patterns and the effect of segment length on flow reduction was investigated in a flow circuit. Computational fluid dynamics (CFD) characterized local hemodynamics and wall shear stresses in conventional venous end-to-side anastomosis and a patch form anastomosis, such as Venaflo™ (Impra, Tempe, AZ). The main differences in size and geometry comprised not only the enlarged anastomotic room but also the curved design of vein floor (figure 19-1). Three-dimensional flow simulations were performed and were used to further examine the results of previous 2-dimensional studies.[18]

Materials and Methods

Arterial anastomosis flow visualization. An in vitro study was performed to investigate the effect of a narrow segment (diameters between 4 and 5 mm) at the arterial end of a graft. A series of 48 anastomotic models with differing diameters (artery 2, 3, 4, and 5 mm; graft 5, 6, 7, and 8 mm) and segment lengths (10 and 20 mm) were constructed. Hand-made wax models were used to create a silicone rubber model into which a special molten metal alloy (HEK Medizintechnik,

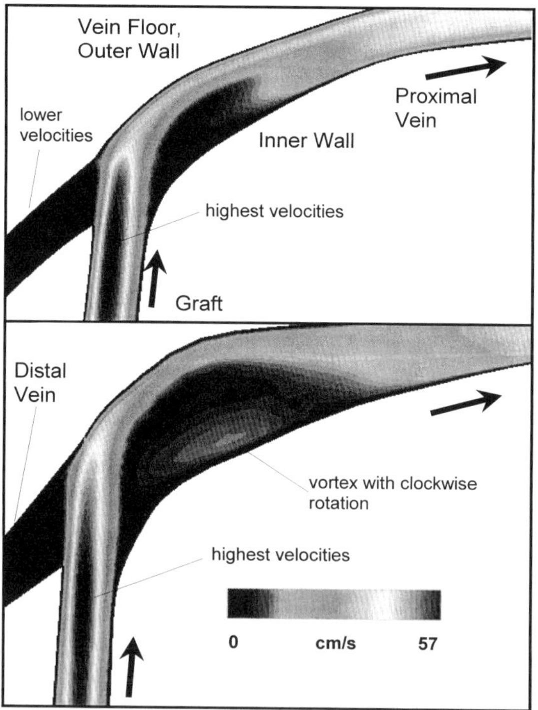

Figure 19-1. Velocity distribution at the beginning of the diastolic period in the symmetric plane. (Conventional venous end-to-side anastomosis, upper panel; patch form anastomoses, lower panel). Fluid enters at the inlet boundary and is split into distal and proximal outflows (systolic). The arrows indicate the flow direction. The color scale is associated with the velocity magnitude.

Luebeck, Germany) with a melting point of 48°C was injected to produce a male cast. The metal cast was polished and then embedded in Sylgard 184 clear silicone rubber (Dow Corning Corp, Midland, MI). The metal was melted out after curing in a water bath, leaving the transparent anastomotic models used in the flow experiments.[19]

Models were investigated in the circulating model described previously.[18] Briefly, the circulating model was based on the connection of 2 pressure-controlled reservoirs at systolic and diastolic pressure by a proportional magnetic valve. A function generator supplied control voltage for the proportional magnetic valve. In superposition with an air-reservoir (Windkessel), the result was a nearly physiological pressure curve at the outlet of the circulating model. The circulating fluid was an aqueous glycerol solution with the dynamic viscosity η = 3.6 mPas. A thermostat with heat exchanger maintained a constant fluid temperature of 25°C. The flow was visualized over a range of Reynolds (Re) numbers from 130 to 950 Re with direct dye injection. An MV1 digital video camera (Canon Inc, Tokyo, Japan) was set up on a tripod at a fixed distance to point vertically down at the model. Video images were viewed frame by frame using Panasonic DV Studio software (Matsushita Electric Industrial Co Ltd, Osaka, Japan).

Arterial anastomosis flow measurement. In addition, the influence of the length of narrow segment on graft flow was investigated, which is depicted in figure 19-2. An example for a straight graft in upper arm position is shown. To simulate the different anastomotic regions, the flow rates were reduced by small tubes with variable length and diameter. The flow in every basic combination of artery and graft diameters with segment length zero was measured under different pressure conditions (mean pressure 80, 100, and 120 mm Hg). Subsequently, flow measurements were performed in the models with segment lengths of 10 mm and 20 mm. At the time of the measurement, it was essential to keep a constant pressure amplitude. Because the fluid viscosity strongly depended on the temperature (ascertained regression equation $\eta = 6.459 - 0.114 * T$, with T = temperature in °C), the fluid temperature was measured. Small deviations of 25°C temperature led to calculation of current viscosity, using a flow normalization of 25°C.

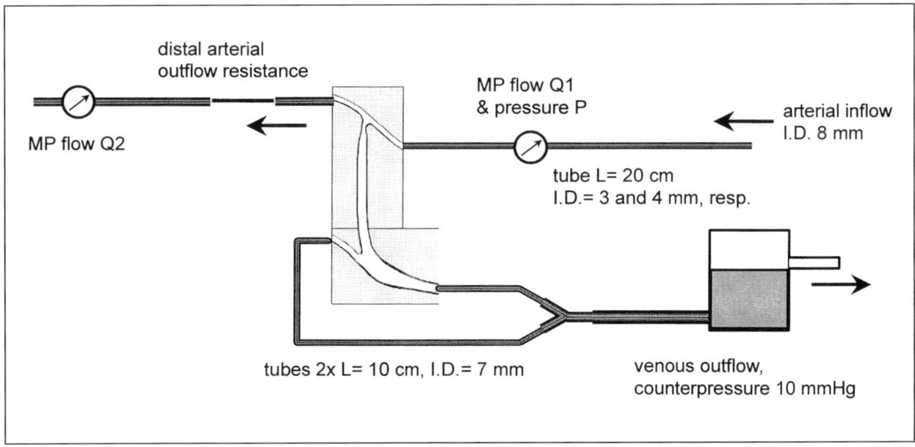

Figure 19-2. Diagram of the narrow segment. MP-measuremnet point, L = length, ID = inner diameter.

Venous anastomosis. Two different forms, conventional and Venaflo™ patch forms, were analyzed with Computational Fluid Dynamics (CFD) using a finite volume-based algorithm. Flow simulations were carried out 3-dimensionally and extended the results of our previous 2-dimensional studies.[18] Geometry and size of anastomotic forms were both defined on a scale of 1:1 according to an idealized image of conventional venous graft anastomosis and patch form anastomosis for upper arm grafts. The diameters of the graft and distal veins were 6 mm; the proximal vein diameter was set to 7 mm.

The anastomoses were divided for computational analysis into controlled volume meshes, with the obtained numerical solutions for the velocities and pressures. The number of grid cells governed the accuracy of CFD solution. Larger numbers of cells were correlated with longer calculation times. Fluid simulations were limited by memory capacity and performance of computing hardware. One compromise was to increase the cell numbers in areas where large flow variations occured (in the immediate vicinity of junction) and to use a coarser grid in the region with relatively little change (the graft inlet and the distal and proximal vein outlet). Because of its idealized geometry, the anastomotic flow is symmetric about a plane that passes through the axes of the graft and vein, with no flow across the symmetric boundary. Normal vectors of velocities are set to zero at this boundary, and for the calculation, only half the model was needed.

The number of control volumes of the conventional anastomosis and patch form anastomosis amounted to 7260 and 9120, respectively. The no-slip condition (zero velocities) was assigned to all rigid walls. A non-Newtonian, pulsatile mass flow profile with flow rates of 1000 mL/min (systolic) and 500 mL/min (diastolic) was specified as the inlet boundary conditions[19] (ie, corresponding Re numbers amounted to 980 and 490 Re, respectively). The distal vein outlet was defined by an oscillating mass flow to simulate the acute case immediately after graft implantation.[20] The distal vein shows antegrade flow (flow toward hand) in systolic period (-100 mL/min) and retrograde flow (flow toward heart) in diastolic period (+70 mL/min) in agreement with the results of intraoperative measurements. The proximal outlet was selected remote from geometrical disturbances and was defined by the von Neumann condition that requires gradients of all variables (except pressure) to be zero in the flow direction. The wall shear stress was calculated by using the quadratic method.[21]

RESULTS

Arterial anastomosis flow visualization. The presentation of the results (figures 19-3 and 19-4) only describes 1 model with different segment lengths (straight graft upper arm, artery diameter 4 mm, graft diameter 7 mm, diameter of narrow segment 4 mm, segment length 0 mm and 10 mm). Figure 19-3 gives flow patterns in the arterial anastomosis without any narrow segment at an Re of 165. As the fluid from the proximal artery enters the anastomosis, the central stream remains nearly in a central position and flows up into the distal artery. The bottom and lateral stream parts bend into the graft, forming a large vortex with a clockwise rotation that reaches into the artery.

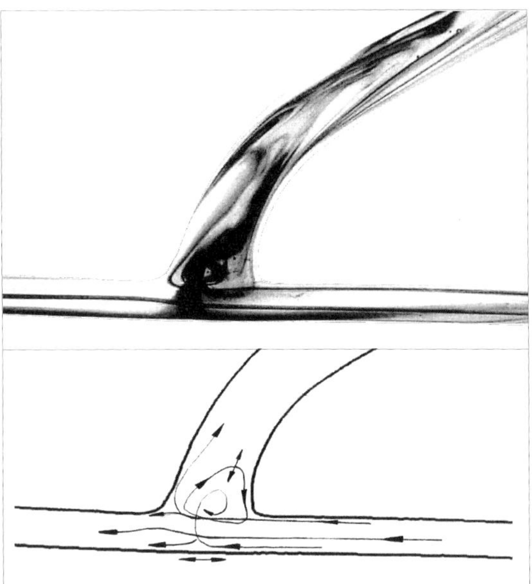

Figure 19-3. Flow visualization in an arterial anastomosis without narrow segment. The lower image is a diagrammatical representation of the same.

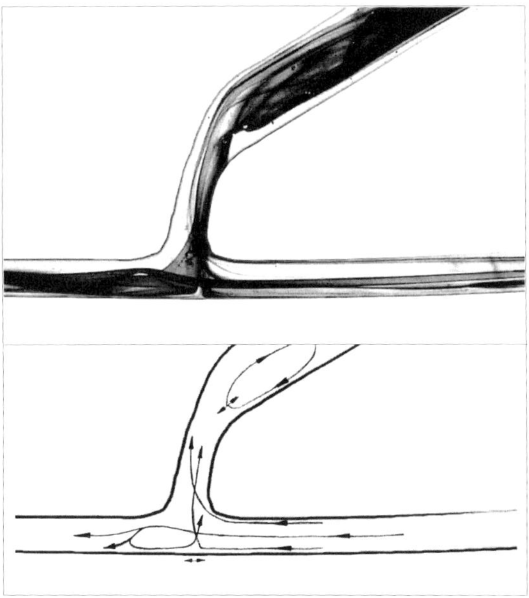

Figure 19-4. Flow visualization in an arterial anastomosis with a 4 mm segment, segment length 10 mm.

During the deceleration phase, the vortex becomes larger. The upper stream part impinges on the distal anastomotic angle, creating a stagnation point and splits into 2 parts with 1 stream moving in the direction of the distal artery and the other stream moving in the direction of the graft. Location of the stagnation point oscillates with the simulated cardiac cycle. The point moves into the graft in the systolic period and into the distal artery in the diastolic period. At an Re of 490, the overall flow pattern remains unchanged except for the central stream (not directly illustrated, but refer to figure 19-4 to get an impression of this feature). When the central stream enters the region below the distal anastomotic angle, it is edged out of the central position into the direction of the distal anastomotic angle and splits into 2 parts. One part moves into a distal direction and the other turns back and is skewed toward the graft. The point on the artery floor, where the bottom stream impinges on the retrograde flow part of the central stream (called impact point), oscillates in the axial direction.

In all models using a narrow segment, the oscillating anastomotic vortex disappeared. The main features of the flow patterns observed at diastolic beginning are given in figure 19-4 (Re=165, identical diameters compared with figure 19-3). The arterial central stream is pushed away from a central position and splits into 2 parts as described before. The distance of impact point oscillation is smaller compared with the anastomosis without a narrow segment. The graft inflow is composed by all stream parts and is presented nearly undisturbed. As the flow enters the well-rounded expansion of the graft, it separates from the vessel wall and a large vortex with clockwise rotation can be seen. No appreciable differences of flow patterns could be observed when the Reynolds number was increased to an Re of 490. Above an Re of 800, the flow is highly disturbed, and it becomes difficult to discern any organized structures in both of the models.

Arterial anastomosis flow measurement. The investigated models were separated into 3 groups:

- Models of group 1 (straight graft forearm) consisted of different combinations of 2- and 3-mm arteries, grafts with 5- and 6-mm and narrow segment diameters of 4 mm. Two tubes (first 20-cm length and inner diameter [ID] of 4 mm; second length 25 cm, ID 2 or 3 mm) restricted the inflow and the outflow was limited by a 5-mm tube (with a length of 25 cm).

- Models of group 2 (straight graft upper arm) were built from different combinations of 3- and 4-mm arteries, 6- and 7-mm grafts, and narrow segment diameter of 4 and 5 mm. A tube with a 20-cm length (ID 3 or 4 mm) restricted the inflow, and the outflow was limited by a 7-mm tube (length=10 cm).

- Models of group 3 (loop graft upper arm) were built from different combinations of 4 and 5-mm arteries, 6- and 7-mm grafts, and narrow segment diameters 4 and 5 mm. The inflow was restricted by a tube with a 10 cm length (ID 4 or 5 mm), and the outflow was limited by a 7 mm-tube (length=10 cm).

The results of flow measurements are summarized in table 19-1. The mean flow reduction in group 1 was 4.8% for a segment length of 10 mm and 6.5% for a segment length of 20 mm, compared with basic combination without narrow segment. In group 2, the flow reduction amounted to 5.9% for a 10-mm segment length and 10.4% for a 20-mm segment length. The highest flow reduction was in group 3: 8.5% for a 10-mm segment length and 13.2% for a 20-mm segment length. Differences of the mean values between group 1 and group 2 and between group 2 and group 3 were not significant ($P>0.05$), whereas the differences between group 1 and group 3 were significant ($P<0.05$).

Table 19-1. Effect of length of narrow segment on flow reduction in percent.

Type of graft	10 mm (%)	20 mm (%)
Straight graft forearm	4.8	6.5
Straight graft upper arm	5.9	10.4
Loop graft upper arm	8.5*	13.2**

*$P<0.01$, when compared with straight graft forearm.

**$P<0.05$, when compared with straight graft forearm.

An impressive result was observed following the removal of the tubes that were for flow restriction (model with an arterial diameter of 4 mm, a graft diameter of 7 mm, a segment length of 0 versus 20 mm): under identical hemodynamic conditions (mean pressure=120 mm Hg), a 17% reduction of mean flow from 880 mL/min to 730 mL/min was seen (figure 19-4). The dotted lines mark the calculated values of flow reduction for segment length from 30 mm to 70 mm (linear regression analysis). The solid line at 400 mL/min labels the limit of poor graft flow.

Venous anastomosis. Characteristic results of flow simulation in the venous anastomosis are presented in figures 19-1 and 19-6 through 19-8. The flow field was at the beginning of diastolic period, with the pressure distribution and shear stress on the vein floor at the systolic maximum velocity (figure 19-1). At the beginning of diastole, the distal outlet flow was nearly 0 demonstrating the reversal of flow direction. The maximum inlet velocity amounted to 57 cm/s. The color scale is associated with the magnitude of the velocity.

When the flow stream enters the host vein, the velocity profile becomes skewed toward the outer wall in both investigated models. The highest anastomotic velocities are seen at the outer wall, and the lowest velocities occur near the inner wall during the entire cardiac cycle. A point of stagnation is recognized at the vessel outer wall. At this point, the flow stream splits into 2 parts with the main stream moving in the direction of the proximal outlet branch and the other stream moving in the direction of the distal outlet branch (best seen at systolic maximum, which is not shown). The stagnation point oscillates with the simulated cardiac cycle. During the acceleration phase, the stagnation point moves distally. From minimum systole to the diastolic end, the stagnation point moves proximally. In the patch form (see lower panel of figure 19-1), the flow streamlines detached from the inner wall of host vein and created a separated region. As a result of flow separation from the wall, a backflow region was formed.

The characteristic 3-dimensional vortex exists over the whole simulated period. Both the intensity and the location of the vortex depend on the phase of the flow cycle. In contrast, the velocity distribution in the anastomotic region of the conventional form is highly disturbed (see upper panel of figure 19-1). In a cross-sectional view (not demonstrated), a secondary flow pattern was seen. The secondary flow was responsible for the intermittent increase of velocity in the center and near the inner wall of the proximal outflow branch. During the simulated cardiac cycle, the location of a recognizable beginning of velocity increase oscillates in a violent manner downstream in the systolic period and upstream in the diastolic period. The magnitude of the velocity near the outer wall was significantly higher than the velocities in the patch form. The computed results were compared with the experimental data of flow visualization and corresponded very well.[18]

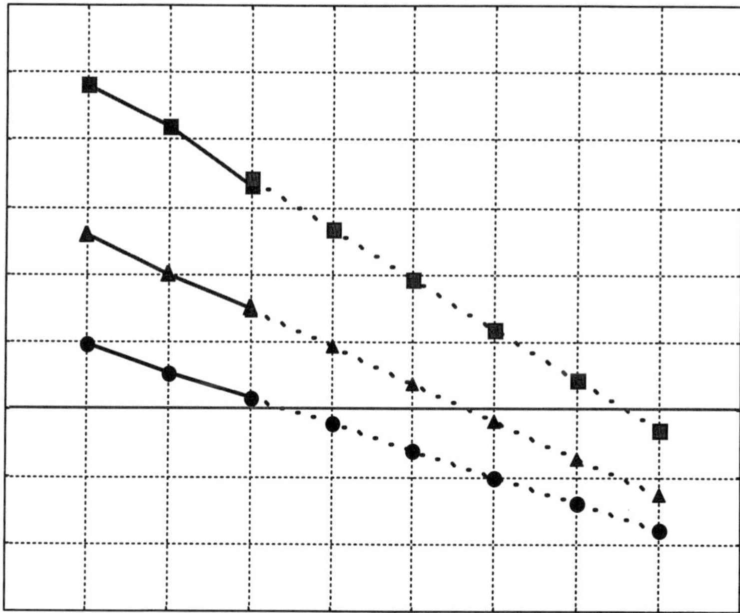

Figure 19-5. Example for flow reduction (arterial diameter 4 mm, graft diameter 7 mm, 4 mm segment). The dotted lines mark the calculated values of flow reduction for segment length from 30 mm to 70 mm (linear regression analysis). Note the horizontal solid line at 400 mL/min, which marks the limit of poor graft flow.

Static pressure. An important result of numerical simulation is presented in figures 19-6 and 19-7, which depict the relative static pressure distribution at the systolic maximum of simulated cardiac cycle (Re=980). Values of pressure were related to the proximal outlet pressure (reference pressure). The color scale was associated with the magnitude of the pressure.

Within the conventional anastomosis (figure 19-6), a high local pressure maximum on the floor of the host vein occurred directly opposite the midpoint of the graft lumen. Simultaneously, corresponding systolic velocities were very slow. This region is therefore defined as a stagnation point with a 3-dimensional extension, representing the conversion of all of the kinetic energy into a pressure rise. In contrast, the local pressure maximum was reduced in the patch form (figure 19-7; note the same scaling of pressure values in figure 19-6). The relative peak value amounted to 372 Pa (ie, 2.8 mm Hg) in the conventional form and 200 Pa (ie, 1.5 mm Hg) in the patch form.

Wall shear stress. The diagram in figure 19-8 depicts the wall shear stress distribution on the vein floor at the systolic peak flow (Re=980). For better guidance, the corresponding cut of the mesh was drawn in the bottom of figure 19-8 (only the grid of the patch form; the values of distance are identical to the conventional form).

The estimated peak shear stress was 59 dyn/cm^2 at the conventional anastomosis versus 44 dyn/cm^2 in the patch form. In the patch form, there was a general decrease in wall shear stress as compared with the conventional form. Shear stress is reduced up to 50% on the average. Although the depicted situation refers to the time of systolic maximum, these reductions in wall shear rates were observed during the entire

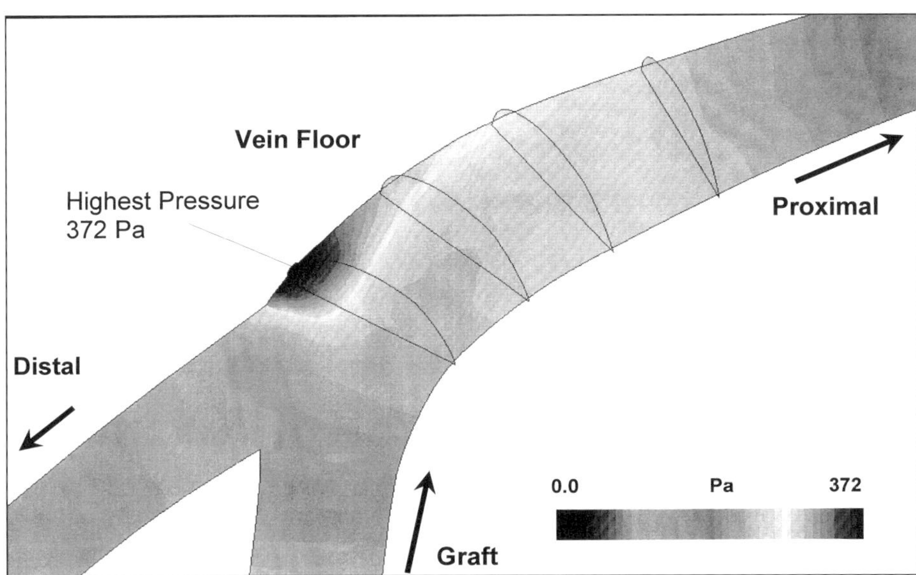

Figure 19-6. Conventional form: Static pressure distribution at peak flow in a 3-dimensional view. The color scale is associated with the magnitude of the pressure. Note the high local pressure maximum on the floor of host vein with 3-dimensional extension.

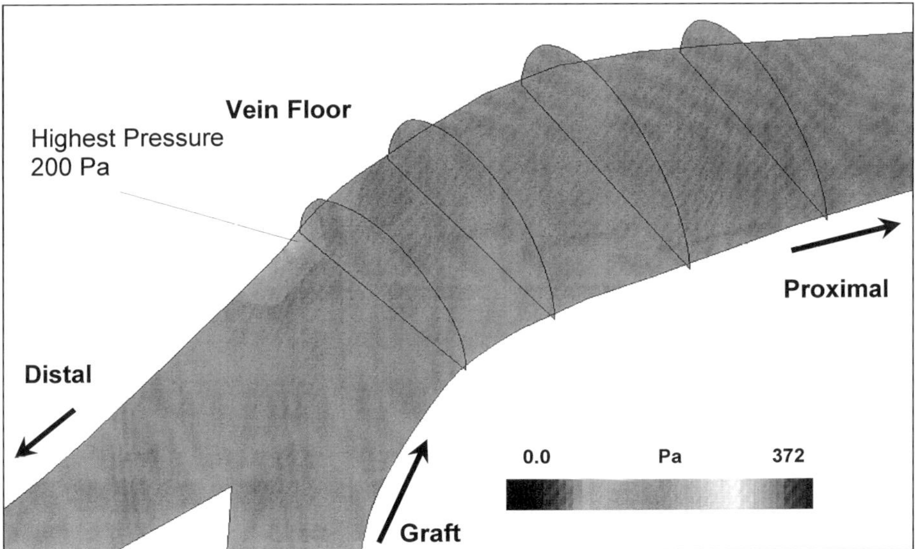

Figure 19-7. Patch form: Static pressure distribution at peak flow. The local pressure maximum is reduced in the patch form (identical scaling of pressure values in figure 19-6).

cardiac cycle. The ascertained small region of shear stress drop in the conventional form (in vicinity to distance 0) corresponded to the very slow velocities at the stagnation point (compare with figure 19-6).

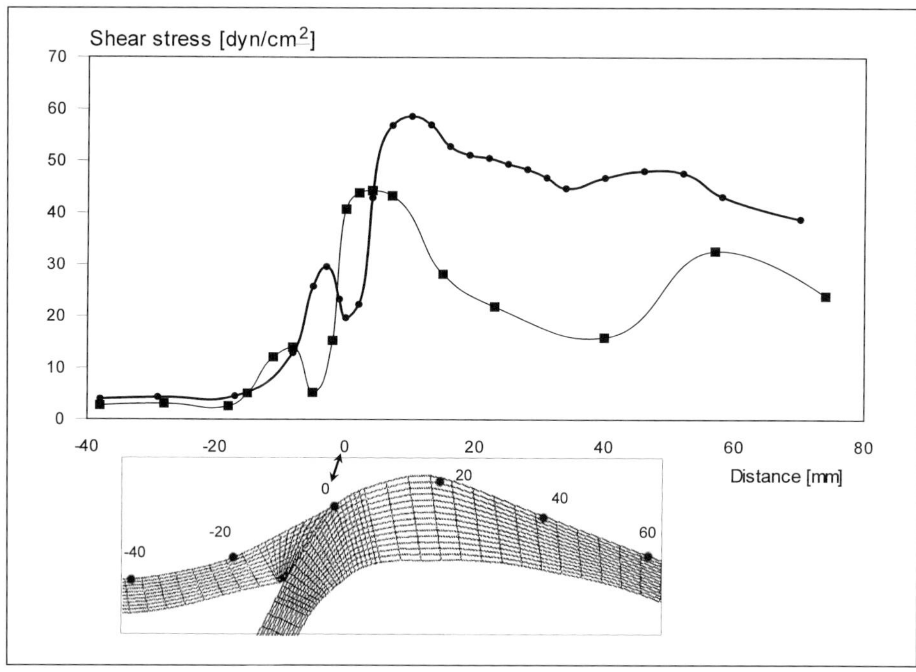

Figure 19-8. Wall shear stress distribution on vein floor (top). Conventional: ●, patch form: ■, time: peak flow. Note the general decrease in wall shear stress in the patch form. Corresponding cut of the mesh is depicted in the bottom.

Discussion

The findings of this study clearly demonstrated the potent influence of anastomotic geometry on hemodynamics.

When the graft was directly connected to the artery, a large vortex was observed in the graft inflow region. Using a narrow segment in the arterial anastomosis, the vortex disappeared and the graft inflow appeared highly stable. A large vortex existed in the region of the well-rounded expansion of the graft. This vortex persisted for the whole cardiac cycle without any changes in flow direction. The anastomosis with a narrow segment showed a lower shift of the bottom impact point. No essential differences of flow patterns were observed with regard to the length of the narrow segment.

Length influenced the graft flow quantity directly-the larger the segment length, the lower the graft flow. The value of flow reduction correlated to the anatomic region. The reason was the existence of smaller diameters and bigger length of inflow arteries and outflow veins in order of loop upper arm grafts, straight upper arm grafts, and straight forearm grafts. An additional narrow segment connected to small arteries in a series caused only a slight flow reduction, while the use of a narrow segment in the upper arm position led to a clear decrease of the graft flow lower than we originally expected. A limitation of this study was that the measurements were only included for segment lengths of 0, 10, and 20 mm. Although it may be incorrect to assume a linear course of flow reduction caused by segment length, the results of linear regression analysis (ie, figure 19-5) were helpful for assessing the use of longer segment length. In hypotonic patients (mean pressure=80 mm Hg), a segment length of 30 mm decreased the graft flow below 400 mL/min, which is widely accepted as a critical limit to perform adequate hemodialysis and prevent thrombosis. For the same reason, the segment length should be shorter than 45 mm in normotonic patients.

The 3-dimensional simulation of blood flow in venous anastomoses resulted in detailed results.[18] The velocity profile of the patch form anastomosis was better than for the conventional form. The enlarged anastomotic room led to durable flow separation from the inner wall. As a result of flow separation, a large 3-dimensional vortex existed during the whole simulated cardiac cycle that may lead to an improved washout effect and a more stable outflow. An added factor may be that the vortex avoided the contact between blood elements, especially platelets, in the vein wall, preventing activation. In contrast, the flow patterns of the conventional anastomosis were highly irregular. The time-dependent shift of center velocity increase caused by the secondary flow was the main feature in this model. The flow disturbance was strong enough to produce perivascular vibrations, which could be responsible for hyperplasia.

The fluid stagnation on the vein floor was a main finding of the CFD. It demonstrated the development of a high static pressure region at the systolic peak flow. It represented the conversion of all kinetic energy into a pressure rise. The related peak value amounted to 2.8 mm Hg in the conventional form and 1.5 mm Hg in the patch form. To assess the pressure rise, the consideration of venous anastomotic pressure was necessary. Intraoperative measurements of pressure course in arteriovenous grafts demonstrated that the arterial anastomotic pressure within the graft decreased to venous values along a distance of centimeters in the immediate vicinity of the arterial anastomoses. Subsequently, the mean pressure in the venous anastomosis amounted to typical venous pressure values. At a value of 10 mm Hg for the venous mean pressure, the wall strain would increase to about 130% due to the stagnation pressure in the conventional anastomosis. In the patch form, this pressure rise was distinctly reduced to 50% compared with the conventional form. The reason for this pressure decrease was the curved design of the vein floor. The central stream crashed against the vein floor in the conventional anastomosis, but became softly diverted toward the proximal vein outlet in the patch form. Thus, the surgical creation of a curved design of the vein floor was essential. For the same reason, it is highly recommended that clinicians avoid performing the Venaflo anastomosis such as a hooded anastomosis with straight vein floor.[22]

As noted by Zarins et al. the adaptive response of arteries to increased blood pressure results in increased intimal thickness.[23] A rise in intraluminal pressure will increase wall tensile stress (Laplace's Law) and stimulates an increase in wall thickness to reduce tensile stress to normal. In our study only a local pressure rise on the vein floor was seen, but no general increase in intraluminal or venous anastomotic pressure was observed. It was probably because the pressure rise led to an increase in local wall tensile stress with a subsequent stimulus of increased wall thickness. Regions with high wall shear stress and high pressure linked with biochemical reactions may play a role in the development of intimal hyperplasia.[13,15,17,24,25] Contrary to those findings, other authors have reported on the correlation between intimal hyperplasia and areas with low shear stress. [4,5,10,12,14,24,26] This type of hyperplasia can be regarded as an appropriate adaptive thickening of the arterial vessel wall, which may normalize shear stress.[24]

In assessment of these contrary findings, it is useful to compare the absolute values of wall shear stress. If anastomotic intimal thickness was a direct function of low wall shear stress in arteriovenous grafts the shear stress amounted to 2 or 5 dyn/cm^2.[14,26] In contrast, the shear stress values accompanied with intimal thickness in arteriovenous loop grafts was 34 to 130 dyn/cm^2 (calculated from presented hemodynamic data[1], for calculation viscosity was assumed to be 3.6 mPas). Therefore, comparison of low-shear versus high-shear hypothesis has to be performed with regard to the range of shear stress, which was obtained in different studies.[27]

It can be assumed that reduction in wall shear stress within the patch form may lead to delayed or less formation, even preventing the development of intimal hyperplasia and venous anastomotic stenoses. The decreased pressure stress on the floor of the host vein was the second positive effect of the bulb-like venous anastomosis. The large 3-dimensional vortex leads to an improved wash-out effect and a more stable outflow. Additionally, the graft flow reduction caused by using a narrow segment between the artery and the graft may augment the decrease of wall shear stress and pressure drop on the vein floor. The results of this study strongly support the use of the patch form.

References

1. Fillinger, MF, Reinitz, ER, Schwartz RA, et al. Graft geometry and venous intimal-medial hyperplasia in arteriovenous loop grafts. J Vasc Surg 1990; 11:556-56.
2. Richman P, Wilson SE. Bridge grafts for angioaccess. In: Ernst CB, Stanley JC eds. Current therapy in vascular surgery. Philadelphia and Toronto: B.C. Decker Inc, 1991: 927-32.
3. Sivanesan S, How TV, Black RA, Bakran A. Flow patterns in the radiocephalic arteriovenous fistula: An in vitro study. J Biomech 1999; 32:915-25.
4. Banerjee RK, Cho YI, Back LH. Numerical studies of three-dimensional arterial flows in reverse curvatory geometry: Part I - peak flow. J Biomech Eng 1993; 115:316-26.
5. Bassiouny HS, White S, Glagov S, Choi E, Giddens DP, Zarins CK. Anastomotic intimal hyperplasia: Mechanical injury or flow induced. J Vasc Surg 1992; 15:708-17.
6. Da Silva AF, Carpenter T, How TV, Harris, PL. Stable vortices within vein cuffs inhibit anastomotic myointimal hyperplasia? Eur J Vasc Endovasc Surg 1997; 14:157-63.
7. Fatemi RS, Rittgers SE. Derivation of shear rates from near-wall measurements under steady and pulsatile flow conditions. J Biomech Eng 1994; 116:361-68.

8. Friedman MH. A biologically plausible model of thickening of arterial intima under stress. Arteriosclerosis 1989; 9:511-22.
9. Heethaar RM. Atherosclerosis and blood flow. In: Strackee J, Westerhof N, eds. The physics of heart and circulation. Bristol and Philadelphia: Institute of Physics Publishing, 1993; 321-34.
10. Hughes PE, How TV. Effects of geometry and flow division on flow structures in models of the distal end-to-side anastomosis. J Biomechanics 1996; 29:866-72.
11. Keynton RS, Rittgers SE, Shu MCS. The effect of angle and flow rate upon hemodynamics in distal vascular graft anastomoses: An in vitro model study. J Biomech Eng 1991; 113:458-63.
12. Kim YH, Chandran KB, Bower TJ, Corson JD. Flow dynamics across end-to-end vascular bypass graft anastomoses. Ann Biomed Eng 1993; 21:311-20.
13. Ojha M, Cobbold RS, Johnston KW. Flow and shear stress patterns at proximal and distal ends of bypass grafts: Implications for the development of intimal hyperplasia. In: Callow AD and Ernst CB, eds. Vascular surgery-theory and practice. Stamford, CT: Prentice-Hall International Inc, Appleton & Lange, 1995; 1231-36.
14. Salam TA, Lumdsden AB, Suggs WD, Ku DN. Low shear stress promotes intimal hyperplasia thickening. J Vasc Investigation 1996; 2:12-22.
15. Sottiurai VS. Biogenesis and etiology of distal anastomotic hyperplasia. Int Angiol 1990; 9:59-69.
16. Staalsen NH, Ulrich M, Winther J, Pedersen EM, How T, Nygaard H. The anastomosis angle does change the flow fields at vascular end-to-side anastomoses in vivo. J Vasc Surg 1995; 21:460-71.
17. Steinmann DA, Vinh B, Ethier CR, Ojha M, Cobbold RC, Johnston KW. A numerical simulation of flow in a two-dimensional end-to-side anastomosis model. J Biomech Eng 1993; 115:112-18.
18. Krueger U, Scholz H. Comparison of two different arteriovenous anastomotic forms by in vitro investigation. In: Henry ML, ed. Vascular access for hemodialysis-VI. Chicago: W.L. Gore & Associates and Precept Press, 1999; 335-45.
19. Krueger U. Hämodynamische optimierung von Gefäflprothesen. Verlag Dr. Köster: Berlin, 1998: 40-64 (German).
20. Gordon IL. Physiology of the Arteriovenous Fistula. In: Wilson SE ed. Vascular access- principles and practice. St. Louis, MO: Mosby Year Book Inc, 1996; 29-41.
21. Lou Z, Yang WJ, Stein PD. Errors in the estimation of arterial wall shear rates that result from curve fitting of velocity profiles. J Biomech Eng 1993; 26:383-90.
22. Escobar FS, Schwartz SA, Aboulijoud M, et al. A preliminary study comparing a new "hooded" vs. conventional ePTFE graft in hemodialysis patients. In: Henry ML, ed. Vascular access for hemodialysis-VI. Chicago: W.L. Gore & Associates and Precept Press, 1999:205-11.
23. Zarins CK, Bassionuny HS, Glagov S. Intimal hyperplasia. In: Haimovici H ed. Haimovici's vascular surgery. Cambridge, MA: Blackwell Science, 1996; 678-87.

24. Fillinger MF, Kerns DB, Bruch D, Reinitz ER, Schwartz RA. Does the end-to-end venous anastomosis offer a functional advantage over the end-to-side venous anastomosis in high-output arteriovenous grafts? J Vasc Surg 1990; 12:676-90.
25. Hofstra L, Bergmans DC, Leunissen KM, et al. Anastomotic Intimal Hyperplasia in Prosthetic arteriovenous fistulas for hemodialysis is associated with initial high flow velocity and not with mismatch in elastic properties. J Am Soc Nephrol 1995; 6:1625-33.
26. Zhuang YJ, Singh TM, Zarins CK, Masuda H. Sequential increases and decreases in blood flow stimulates progressive intimal thickening. Eur J Vasc Endovasc Surg 1998; 16:301-10.
27. Hofstra L, Bergmans DC, Leunissen KM, Hoeks AP, Kitslaar PJ, Tordoir JH. Prosthetic arteriovenous fistulas and venous anastomotic stenosis: Influence of a high flow velocity on the development of intimal hyperplasia. Blood Purif 1996; 14:345-49.

DISCUSSION

Panelist:
Dr. Krueger

Discussant: We heard this morning that the Venaflo graft had not shown any real differences in overall patency rates with the non-Venaflo. Is there any insight that you can give us based on your studies as to why that might be the case?

Dr. Krueger: We believe the use of the Venaflo is not a simple thing because there are many points you have to be aware of with the geometrics of the Venaflo. I think it is a very important point. Many surgeons don't know about this.

20

ISCHEMIC MONOMELIC NEUROPATHY AS A COMPLICATION OF FOREARM PTFE LOOP GRAFTS IN UREMIC DIABETIC PATIENTS

John Raheb, D.O., Robert Esterl, M.D., Robert Reuter, M.D., William Washburn, M.D., Jim Lowe, M.D., Greg Moorman, M.D., Francisco Cigarroa, M.D., and Glenn Halff, M.D.

Ischemic monomelic neuropathy (IMN) is a rare but devastating complication after placement of polytetrafluoroethylene (PTFE) grafts for chronic hemodialysis.[1] The pathophysiology of IMN remains obscure, although alteration in blood flow to the vasa nervosum appears to be the major factor.[2] The hallmark of IMN is the acute and often irreversible dysfunction of the radial, median, and ulnar nerve without tissue necrosis in the affected upper extremity.[1,2] This article describes a single-center, retrospective study of the incidence, diagnosis, and treatment of IMN after forearm PTFE loop grafts for hemodialysis.

Material and Methods

Two hundred and seventy-three patients with chronic renal failure underwent forearm PTFE loop grafts at the University of Texas Health Science Center at San Antonio, Texas between August 1992 and October 1999. All grafts were 4- to 7-mm PTFE grafts that originated at the brachial artery and drained into the cephalic, median cubital, or basilic vein. All PTFE grafts were performed by surgical residents under the supervision of 3 faculty surgeons.

Results

Twelve (4.4%) of 273 patients developed IMN after placement of the PTFE loop graft. All 12 patients were women (mean age 60 years, range 32 to 73 years) with diabetes mellitus as the cause of renal failure. In addition to diabetes mellitus, comorbid factors for vascular disease included hypertension (10 patients), cardiac disease (6 patients), smoking (3 patients), peripheral vascular disease (2 patients), and cerebrovascular accident (2 patients).

Symptoms of IMN included pain (12 patients), paresthesia (12 patients), poor wrist flexion (12 patients), poor wrist extension (12 patients), and poor movement of intrinsic hand musculature (12 patients), edema (8 patients), and coolness of the digits (4 patients). Symptoms of IMN were present within 24 hours in all 12 patients. Physical examination revealed a palpable radial pulse in 8 patients and a dopplerable radial pulse in 4 patients. No patient developed skin or muscular necrosis in the digits, wrist, or forearm.

Diagnosis of IMN was established greater than 24 hours after development of symptoms in all 12 patients. Diagnosis of IMN was made on clinical grounds alone (8 patients) or with adjuncts of noninvasive arterial studies (4 patients) and nerve conduction studies, or electromyelographs (EMG, 4 patients). All 4 patients who underwent noninvasive studies had improvement in radial artery blood flow when the graft was temporarily occluded.

Treatment of IMN included banding only (5 patients), banding followed by radiographic or surgical occlusion (2 patients), or observation only (5 patients). Patients who underwent observation only had very limited sites for future vascular access. Banding occurred with a mode 5 days (mean 22 days, range 4 to 111 days) after placement of the forearm PTFE graft. All patients underwent aggressive physical therapy immediately upon diagnosis of IMN.

A 7-year follow-up revealed a wide spectrum of recovery, where patients demonstrated complete recovery (1 patient), partial recovery (10 patients), or no recovery (1 patient) of sensorimotor function. The patient with complete recovery underwent banding 111 days after placement of the PTFE graft, and this patient required 9 months of aggressive physical therapy for complete recovery. The patient with no recovery underwent surgical occlusion of the PTFE graft. All 5 patients with observation and aggressive physical therapy had partial recovery. Three patients with partial recovery have expired from cardiovascular disease.

Discussion

IMN is a rare but serious complication of forearm PTFE (and bovine) grafts for chronic hemodialysis. The pathophysiology of IMN is unclear, but acute alteration of arterial blood flow to the vasa nervosum appears to be the primary cause.[2] The hallmark of IMN is acute, profound, and often irreversible sensorimotor dysfunction of the radial, median, and ulnar nerves without tissue necrosis in the affected extremity.[1,2] Severe neurologic dysfunction out of proportion with the mild ischemia in the affected extremity is the rule that clearly differentiates IMN from vascular steal syndrome.[1] Therefore, IMN is characterized by acute ischemia, which can induce global sensorimotor dysfunction, but which is too brief and insufficient to cause skin or muscle ischemia.[2]

Descriptions of IMN after forearm PTFE grafts are limited in the literature; in fact, only 5 articles describe a total of 18 patients who developed IMN after creation of forearm PTFE or bovine grafts (see table 20-1).[1-5] Our experience suggests that IMN may be a more frequent occurrence than the literature reports.

Table 20-1. Ischemic monomelic neuropathy in the literature.

Author	Age	Gender	Disease (associated illness)	Op	Sensory Dys	Motor Dys	NCS	NAS	A	Rx	Outcome
Bolton 1979	58	N/A		LFA	X	X	X			0	SI
	50	N/A		LFA	X					0	CI
Wilbourn 1983	58	Female		LFA	X	X	X			L	SI
	Three other patients not characterized										
Wytrzes 1987	34	Female	DM	LFA	X	X	X			B	SI
	76	Female	DM	LFA	X	X	X			B	SI
	72	Male	DM	RFA	X	X	X			L	SI
Riggs 1988	63	Female	DM (AKA, HTN)	LFA	X	X				R	NI*
	64	Female	DM (bruit, HTN)	LFA	X	X				R	NI*
	63	Male	DM (CVA HTN)	LFA	X	X	X			R	NI*
	64	Male	DM (CABG, HTN)	LFA	X	X	X			0	NI*
Hye 1994	64	Male	DM (PVD, HTN, CVA)	LFA	X	X	X	X	X	a	NI
	62	Male	DM (PVD)	LFA	X	X	X	X		0	NI
	51	Female	DM	LFA	X	X				L	SI
	64	Male	DM (PVD)	LFA RFA	X X	X X	X X	 X	 X	0 L	SI NI
	56	Female	DM	LFA	X	X	X			E	NI

Abbreviations: O-none; a-angioplasty; A-arterial angiogram; AKA-above knee amputation; B-banding; CABG-coronary artery bypass graft; CI-complete improvement; CVA-cerebral vascular accident; DM-diabetes mellitus; dys-dysfunction; E-embolectomy; HTN-hypertension; L-ligation; LFA-left forearm loop; N/A-not available; NAS-noninvasive arterial study; NCS-nerve conduction study; NI-no improvement; Op-operation; PVD-peripheral vascular disease; R-removal; RFA-right forearm loop; Rx-prescribed treatment; SI-slight improvement; *-except in causalgia

The population at risk for IMN appears to be elderly uremic diabetics with comorbid vascular disease.[4] At-risk patients undergo forearm PTFE loop grafts, which originate at the distal brachial artery and terminate at an antecubital vein. IMN has also been described after a patient developed thrombosis of a functional forearm PFTE loop graft.[1] IMN has not been described in patients who have forearm straight PTFE grafts or wrist Brescia-Cimino fistulae.[1]

The most common symptoms of IMN are pain, numbness, and paresthesia in the wrist and hand.[1] Another common symptom is weakness of the wrist and hand.[1] These symptoms often occur immediately after creation of the forearm PTFE loop graft. Physical examination reveals radial, median, and ulnar sensorimotor dysfunction with a proximal (better) to distal (worse) gradient.[2] Often the sensory deficits are more prominent than the motor deficits, because the forearm muscles that supply the hand are often spared relative to the intrinsic hand musculature.[2] Complete paralysis of the intrinsic hand musculature is common with less severe, but still disabling, weakness of wrist flexion and extension.[1] No patients develop sensorimotor defects proximal to the arterial anastomosis of the PTFE loop graft.

EMG studies confirm the sensorimotor deficits described on physical examination. The EMG findings are consistent with axonal degeneration of sensory and motor nerves in the distal affected extremity.[2] In EMG studies, the sensorimotor amplitudes deteriorate in a proximal (better) to distal (worse) fashion.[2] Therefore, the sensorimotor amplitudes are nearly normal in the proximal forearm, but the sensorimotor amplitudes are low or unobtainable in the hand, and sensory amplitudes in particular are usually more severely affected.[2] The sensorimotor latencies and conduction velocities, if obtainable, are often normal or nearly normal.[2] Because there is progressive, instead of discrete, deterioration in sensorimotor amplitudes, ischemia that produces infarction of a major nerve trunk is not a likely cause of IMN.[2]

Although physical examination of the hand often demonstrates an element of decreased perfusion, tissue necrosis is absent.[1] Noninvasive arterial studies usually demonstrate mild ischemia. Digital pressure indices are often not consistent with a threatened limb.[1] Digital pressure indices may improve slightly with temporary manual occlusion of the forearm PTFE graft. Most patients exhibit palpable or dopplerable radial pulses after creation of the forearm PTFE loop graft. Angiography is often unnecessary in the diagnosis of IMN, but an angiogram may define a proximal or anastomotic lesion, which is amenable to angioplasty or surgical correction.[1]

Although most symptoms of IMN occur immediately after graft placement, delay in diagnosis is common.[1] Initial symptoms are often attributable to local or block anesthesia, neuropathy from position on the operating table, edema which interferes with hand motion or surgical trauma.[1]

Treatment options for IMN include observation, banding, surgical or radiographic ligation, and removal of the graft. Observation as a treatment should occur only when the patient has very limited vascular access sites. Whenever possible, patients with IMN require immediate intervention, with the understanding that most patients have a residual neuropathy.[1] All patients require aggressive physical and occupational therapy. The response to therapy is clearly unpredictable. A rare patient who has only sensory deficits may develop complete recovery with observation only.[5] Other patients with prompt ligation or removal of the PTFE graft may demonstrate limited or no recovery of sensorimotor function.

In our series, the population at risk for IMN appeared to be elderly diabetic women with comorbid factors for vascular disease. All patients developed severe dysfunction of the radial, median, and ulnar nerves without tissue necrosis after placement of forearm PTFE loop grafts. All patients had palpable or dopplerable radial pulses after placement of the PTFE grafts. There was a delay in diagnosis greater than 24 hours in all patients. Treatment options included observation, banding and ligation of the forearm PFTE grafts, and recovery was unpredictable. Banding or ligation of the PTFE graft rarely resulted in complete recovery from IMN. Complete recovery from IMN may take several months. Prompt diagnosis and treatment of IMN may not change outcome, but IMN must be differentiated from other correctable etiologies when patients complain of weakness, pain, and paresthesia after placement of forearm PTFE grafts. If noninvasive arterial studies suggest an element of vascular steal, we recommend at a minimum banding of the PTFE graft, because differentiation of vascular steal from IMN is exceedingly difficult immediately after graft placement. We currently perform complete vascular examinations, noninvasive arterial studies, and nerve conduction studies on all elderly women with diabetes, both pre- and postoperatively, in an attempt to identify patients at risk for IMN. Further research is needed to elucidate the pathophysiology of this debilitating complication after forearm PTFE graft placement.

References

1. Hye RJ, Wolf YG. Ischemic monomelic neuropathy: An under-recognized complication of hemodialysis grafts. Ann Vasc Surg 1994; 8:587-82.
2. Wilbourn AJ, Furlan AJ, Hulley W, Ruschhaupt W. Ischemic monomelic ischemia. Neurology 1983; 33:447-51.
3. Wytrzes L, Markley HG, Fisher M, Alfred HJ. Brachial neuropathy after brachial artery-antecubital vein shunts for chronic hemodialysis. Neurology 1987; 37:1398-1400.
4. Riggs JE, Moss AH, Labosky DA, Liput JH, Morgan JJ, Gutmann L. Upper extremity ischemic monomelic neuropathy: A complication of vascular access procedures in uremic diabetic patients. Neurology 1989; 39:997-98.
5. Bolton CF, Driedger AA, Lindsay RM. Ischemic neuropathy in uraemic patients caused by bovine arteriovenous shunt. J Neurosurg Psychiatry 1979; 42:810-14.

DISCUSSION

Panelists:
John Raheb, D.O.
Miltos Lazarides, M.D.
Ali Bakran, M.D.

Discussant: I am scheduled to testify in defense of a surgeon who was performing an abdominal procedure, not an access procedure, in a diabetic elderly patient who developed something that sounds a lot like this from presumably an issue of positioning of the arm. In your review of the literature, did you find cases that were similar to this that were not access type issues?

Dr. Raheb: There were patients who had intravascular procedures done in the lower extremity that had similar type symptoms. Presumably a similar type of damage to the nerve but I do not think any were associated with just operative positioning.

Discussant: I guess I have to review my neurology a little bit, but is this pathology consistent with any kind of brachial plexus stretch injury?

Dr. Raheb: The real hallmark of this is that it starts right at the anastomosis and goes distal, so the march of the decreased amplitude is almost linear down and distal from the anastomosis. These forearm PTFE grafts are distal to the brachial plexus. I do not think you would see these specific changes.

Discussant: In your review of the literature, were any of the cases that were listed following fistula placements instead of graft placements?

Dr. Raheb: The ones that were listed were really following PTFE and all loop grafts. I did not find any that were associated with AV fistulas. There may have been some incidental reports but not that I recall.

Discussant: Do you have any strict criteria for deciding which ones to observe? You mentioned difficulty with access sites but any specific criteria to help one decide?

Dr. Raheb: You need to use judgement on the patient who already has a disabled hand, or 1 upper extremity who has very limited access. Perhaps trying to putting them at risk for the other extremity to become disabled is something you have to consider, especially in the elderly patient or a disabled patient who might not tolerate more procedures. So it is a difficult problem, especially when you see that despite operative intervention, their deficits persist. So the answer is there is strict criteria.

Dr. Bakran: I think this is not necessarily to do with PTFE grafts quite frankly, it deals with steal syndrome with a proximal vessel. It is the brachial artery, whether you use a PTFE or whether you use a brachial basilic or even brachial cephalic. You can get the same syndrome. It is a question of steal. Even though you can feel the radial artery. If you actually do the pressures at the wrist. I think you will find that it is reduced and can be considerably reduced even in those patients who can feel a weak radial artery pulse. So, I think it is severe steal syndrome that you are describing. To get reversal of this, you have to do it very quickly. You have to reverse your fistula very quickly indeed.

Dr. Raheb: I think that it does not have anything to do with PTFE. I think it is an ischemic event, but a steal syndrome I would expect to be more reversible and not necessarily have the associated EMG changes.

Discussant: Yes, but what I am saying to you is that clearly some patients' veins are more sensitive than others. If you measure the pressure in all those patients at the wrist with Doppler pressure, you will find there is a considerable change.

Dr. Raheb: It seems to be out of proportion to the amount of ischemia; however, it is such a severe disability. That is true.

Dr. Lazarides: I agree with Dr. Bakran. Some of your cases were steal cases and there was a Doppler signal, that is not enough. So if you have to confirm severe steal, why you choose the banding technique instead of the so-called ligation-bypass technique, which has better results in the literature?

Dr. Raheb: The fact is that none of these patients, very few of these patients, got better even with increased arterial inflow, decreasing what you would think would be vascular steal. I think that this is a problem of nerve damage from ischemia, even a transient ischemia, in the operating room during the technique or postoperatively. But it is not an ongoing ischemia because I would expect that to be more reversible. The problem is there is not much to do to fix that except physical therapy and time. However, since it is difficult to discern from vascular steal, I think it is appropriate to make interventions to try to decrease the amount of steal.

Discussant: I think what we are hearing is that the diabetic may be irreversible at a very early point and no matter what you do after that, it may not be a fixable problem.

21

DIAGNOSIS AND DIFFERENTIATED TREATMENT OF ISCHEMIA IN PATIENTS WITH ARTERIOVENOUS VASCULAR ACCESS

Jurgen Zanow, M.D., Michael Petzold, M.D., Karen Petzold, M.D., Ulf Kruger, M.D., and Hans Scholz, M.D.

Ischemic changes may occur in about 4% of patients after creation of arteriovenous (AV) angioaccess for hemodialysis.[1,2] The pathophysiology of access-related ischemia (ARI) is not fully known. The main pathological mechanism is the fall of peripheral arterial perfusion pressure below the level necessary for full tissue vitality. This critical pressure varies individually. The drop of arterial pressure results from the low peripheral resistance and high outflow in the connected vein. A reversed flow in the distal artery may occur with retrograde supply to the AV fistula with a side-to-end anastomosis, resulting in decreased perfusion pressure in the tissue distal to the fistula, but this so-called steal syndrome is not essential for ARI.[1,3]

Preferential risk factors for the development of ARI include the following:

- Microangiopathy (diabetes mellitus),
- Macroangiopathy (stenoses of inflow or outflow arteries),
- Persistent hypotonia.

Symptoms of ARI differ with clinical progression. We use the following classification to distinguish clinical stage:

Degree I:	Dialysis induced pain, coldness, numbness
Degree II:	Pain on exertion and debility of muscles, coldness of fingers and cyanosis, temporary paresthesia
Degree III:	Rest pain, muscular atrophy, persistent sensory lost, beginning trophic changes of cutis
Degree IV:	Ischemic ulcers, gangrene.

Patients and Methods

Patients. A retrospective review was conducted of the medical records of 188 patients who underwent surgical treatment for ARI during a 12-year period. One hundred nineteen patients (63.3%) were referred from 28 other hospitals.

Treatment of ARI. Patients who could tolerate the symptoms were asked to wait for 3-5 weeks. If symptoms did not reverse or markedly improve after this time, a recovery could not be expected. Surgical correction was also indicated when symptoms were intolerable. The measurement of flow was used as a parameter to choose one of the following as the optimal procedure:

1. When the flow was much higher than the minimal required flow volume for optimal hemodialysis and for avoiding thrombosis, flow was reduced by narrowing the vessel close to the AV anastomosis (figure 21-1).
2. When the flow was within the range of the required flow volume, the AV anastomosis was closed, and blood was supplied to the fistula by a graft from a more proximal artery (central feeding, figure 21-2).
3. Only in cases of extreme stenosis of the brachial or axillary artery was the AV access abandoned and a central angioaccess created at the subclavian or femoral site.

Operative procedure. ARI was treated either by flow reduction by plication or by central feeding. All operations were performed under local anesthesia. Flow reduction was effected either by simple plication, by interposition of narrow segment of a polytetrafluoroethylene (PTFE) graft, or by plication and banding (figure 21-1). Plication was performed by a continuous, narrowing suture resulting in progressive, spindle-like stenosis near the AV anastomosis, with more than 1.5-2.5 cm under permanent flow control.

Central feeding (figure 21-2) was performed in patients with a preoperative venous flow insufficient for proper hemodialysis and prevention of thrombosis. Either a 4-6 mm PTFE graft or a stepped 7 mm graft was used. The latter was used only to extend the distance to the puncture of the fistula vein. Otherwise, the graft served only as a feeder and was not cannulated to use the advantages of the fistula vein. A suitable fistula vein and proximal artery were required to achieve good results. The preceded maturation of the fistula vein makes this technique easier.

Results

The mean age of the 188 patients was 63.7 ± 13.1 years (range 24 to 88 years). There were 83 male (44%) and 105 female (56%) patients. The mean length of end-stage renal disease (ESRD) was 4.8 ± 3.9 years. Diabetes was diagnosed in 92 patients (48.9%). Sixty-two patients (32.9%) had signs or symptoms of chronic obstructive arterial disease. Iatrogenic arterial stenosis was observed in 42 patients (22.3%).

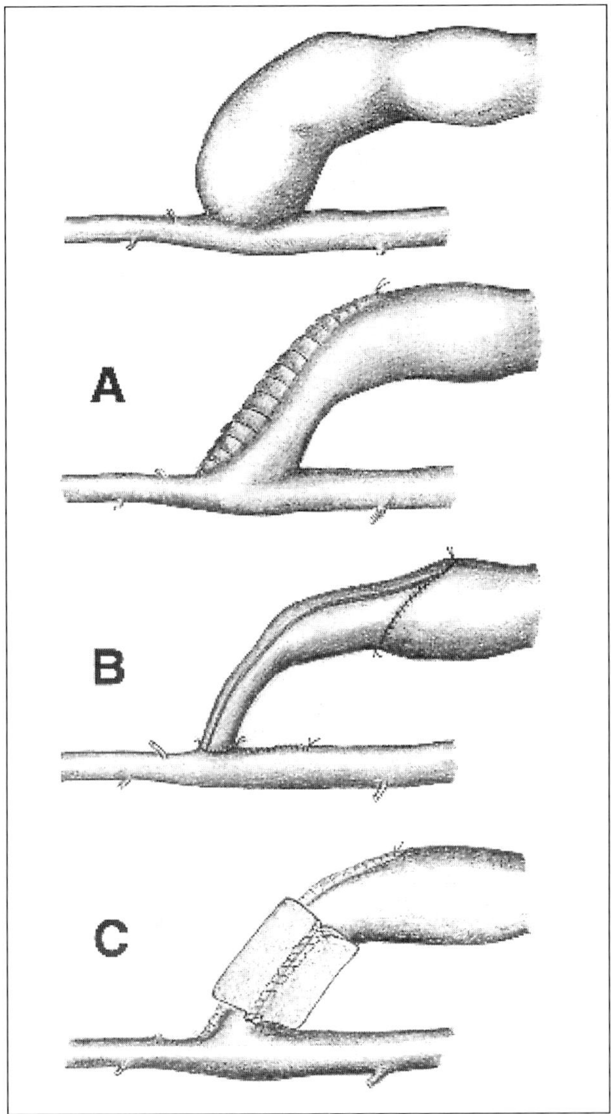

Figure 21-1. Flow reduction of AV fistula by plication (A), use of tapered graft (B), or plication, and additional banding (C).

Forty-one patients (21.8%) had disease classed as degree I; 32 (17.0%) as degree II; 56 (29.8%) as degree III; and 59 (31.4%) as degree IV. Patients with fourth degree disease showed finger necroses and reasonably severe destruction of several fingers and a hand. Forty-two patients (71.2%) with degree IV ischemia had been referred from other hospitals.

The kind of AV access associated with ARI is shown in table 21-1. Data were analyzed according to whether patients were referred from other hospitals or were originally treated in our institution. The observed incidence of steal syndrome could be estimated for patients in our own institution only.

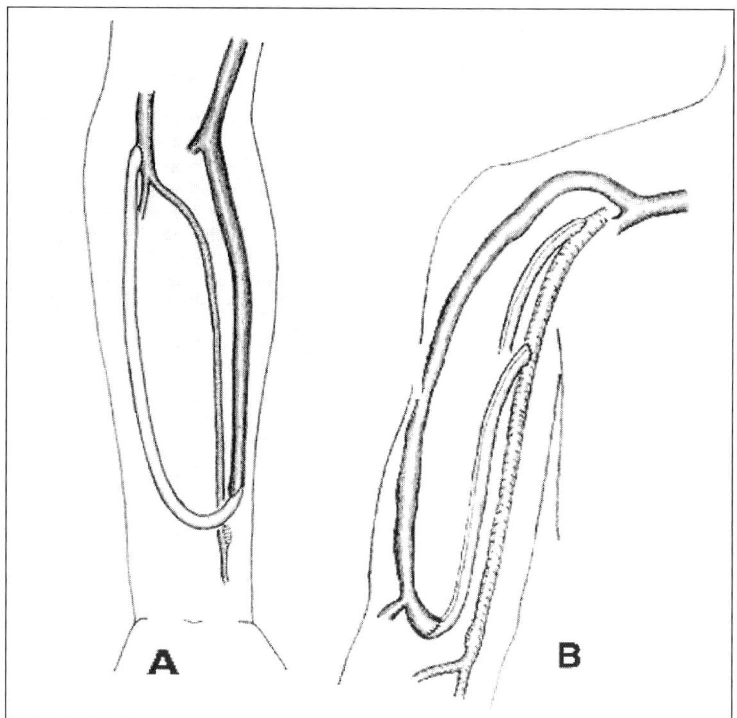

Figure 21-2. Central feeding of cephalic vein at forearm (A) and upper arm (B).

Table 21-1. Patients treated for ARI and incidence of ARI related to vascular access performed in our institution.

AV access	Number of patients with ARI (n)			Performed accesses (n)	Incidence of ARI (%)
	Total	Referred patients	Own patients	Own patients	Own patients
Snuffbox fistula	0	0	0	59	0.0
Wrist fistula	13	8	5	1999	0.3
Radio-cephalic	12	8	4	1885	0.2
Ulno-basilic	1	0	1	104	1.1
Elbow fistula	113	79	34	1870	1.8
Brachio-cephalic	46	34	12	1345	0.9
Brachio-basilic	23	14	9	274	3.7
Brachio-cephalo-basilic	44	31	13	251	5.2
PTFE shunts	62	42	20	925	2.2
Forearm straight	2	2	0	2	0.0
Forearm loop	5	4	1	12	8.8
Upper arm straight	42	28	14	564	2.5
Upper arm loop	12	7	5	213	2.3
Subclavian loop	2	1	1	132	0.8

Time of ischemic onset was defined as the time between the creation of AV access and the date of surgical reconstruction to correct steal syndrome. These data are presented in table 21-2.

Table 21-2. Ischemic onset time of ARI.

Ischemic onset time	Native fistula	PTFE shunt
Acute (<30 days)	37 (29.4%)	23 (37.1%)
Subacute (30-365 days)	30 (23.8%)	27 (43.6%)
Chronic (>1 year)	59 (46.8%)	12 (19.3%)

In accordance with treatment guidelines for surgical reconstruction of ARI, flow reduction was performed in 121 patients (64.3%). Elimination of AV anastomosis and arterial supply of the fistula vein from a more central artery was affected in 56 cases (29.8%). In 11 patients (5.8%), the AV access was abandoned because of unsuitable characteristics of the vessel, and a new access was created (table 21-3).

Table 21-3. Surgical treatment of ARI.

AV access	Flow reduction	Central feeding	Abandonment
Wrist fistula			
Radio-cephalic	3	7	2
Ulno-basilic	0	1	0
Elbow fistula			
Brachio-cephalic	29	15	2
Brachio-basilic	17	5	1
Brachio-cephalo-basilic	32	10	2
PTFE shunts			
Forearm straight	1	2	0
Forearm loop	7	0	2
Upper arm straight	21	16	1
Upper arm loop	9	0	1
Subclavian loop	2	0	0
Total	121	56	11

A concomitant existing stenosis of the subclavian or axillary artery was treated by percutaneous angioplasty in 3 cases. A complete improvement after reconstruction was seen in 127 patients (74.7%) 2 weeks postoperatively. In 43 patients (24.3%), ischemic symptoms partially improved with mild coldness of fingers during dialysis. Complete improvement was experienced by 85 (70.3%) of 121 patients with flow reduction and 49 (87.5%) of 56 patients with central feeding. The primary method of flow reduction was insufficient in 2 patients. In 1 patient, a further flow reduction lead to a sufficient improvement of symptoms; in another patient, a conversion of the straight upper arm access into a looped 1 resulted in complete improvement.

A thrombosis of the access after surgical flow reduction was seen in 3 patients during the early postoperative period: 2 had brachiocephalic fistula and 1 had a straight upper arm PTFE shunt. In all cases, after thrombectomy and reduction of the created stenosis, the access remained patent with ischemic symptoms absent or mild. Late thrombosis of the access was observed during the first year in 4 additional cases after flow reduction and in 3 cases after central feeding. Six patients died during the first postoperative year.

In 7 patients who had flow reduction (4.1%), a dilatation of the narrowed segment of the fistula vein developed during the first year, and the symptoms of ischemia reappeared. In all these patients, surgical flow reduction was repeated, with plication and additional banding with a PTFE stripe; this second procedure provided good results. Partial amputation of 1 or more fingers was necessary in 13 patients, and in 7 patients, full amputation of 1 or more fingers was required (33.9% of the 59 patients with degree IV).

Discussion

Access-related ischemia is an infrequent but disturbing and often debilitating complication after creation of AV access. The pathophysiology of ARI is not entirely clear. The oft-cited steal phenomena is not essential for ARI. The reversal of flow is a normal sign of created side-to-side or side-to-end AV anastomosis, but cannot be observed by duplex scan in a number of patients with ARI, as ARI may also develop after AV access is created with end-to-end anastomosis.

Different surgical techniques to correct ARI are described:

- Distal ligation of cephalic vein below an end-to-side AV-anastomosis
- Ligation of distal radial artery, end-to-end anastomosis
- Ligation of proximal artery
- Plication, banding
- Distal arterial feeding
- Distal revascularization interval ligation (DRIL)
- Ligation of fistula

The main problem with various surgical techniques to correct steal is subsequent thrombosis of the fistula or persistence of distal ischemia. A measurement of flow by duplex scan and assessment of the artery and fistula vein provide essential information for decisions regarding surgical correction.

The favored techniques in this series were flow reduction by plication and central feeding. The results of flow reduction prove its efficiency. A stenosis to close the AV anastomosis increases the resistance in the segment where there is a relatively high pressure. That reduces the risk of thrombosis and the development of fistula aneurysm as an artificial stenosis distant to the anastomosis. The subsequent flow reduction and ensuing drop of distal arterial pressure can be measured. A stenosis of more than 60% is necessary to achieve significant flow reduction. Flow control can be achieved by intraoperative duplex control most safely.[4] An experienced surgeon can manage this problem relatively safely by palpating finger, by comparing actual with preoperative estimated flow and by controlling the pressure of distal arteries. A postoperative duplex scan is mandatory. The problems of recurrent dilatation of stenotic segments and recurrent appearance of steal symptoms (which we have observed in 7 patients during the first postoperative year) can be prevented by additional banding with an adequate PTFE strip. The advantage of plication to banding alone is seen in the better adjustment of desired flow reduction.

The main advantage of the technique of central feeding in treating ARI is the diminished drop of pressure when access is supplied by a large artery (figure 21-3).

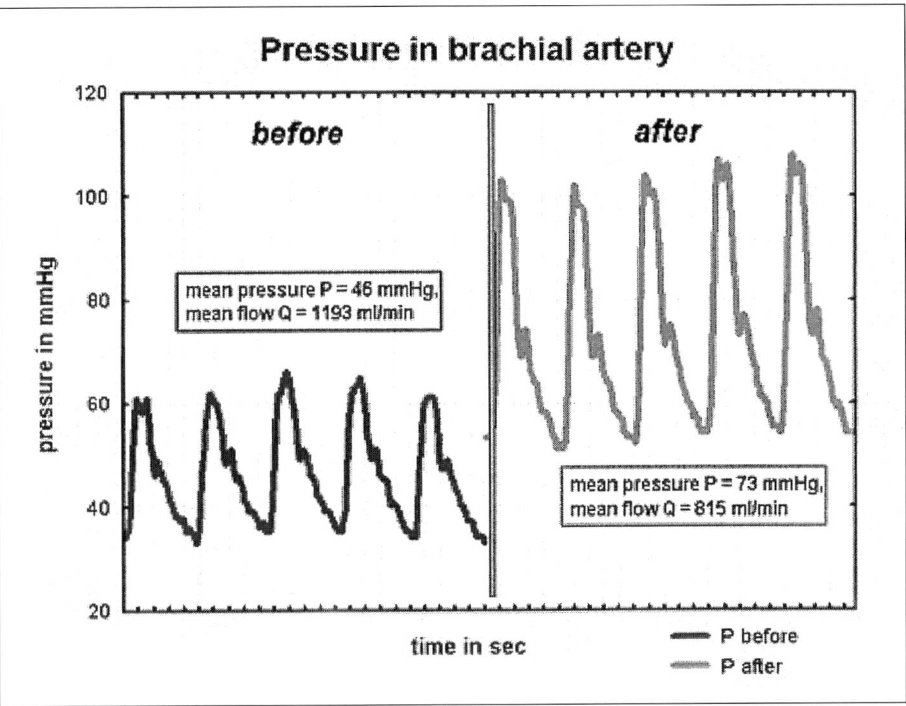

Figure 21-3. Arterial pressure of brachial artery before and after central feeding of cephalic vein at upper arm.

The achieved rate of complete steal improvement of 88% and a patency of more than 90% after 1 year is encouraging and at least comparable to results with the DRIL procedure.[5-7] In our opinion, the DRIL procedure represents an extensive method yielding a dubious prognosis at the wrist and forearm level.

A ligation of the fistula as the ultimate treatment of steal can be avoided in most cases. The prognosis of the fistula vein and possible treatment alternatives should be considered before performing such reconstruction.

Preventing steal syndrome is better than treating it. Besides the preoperative diagnosis and definition of optimal access, several points of intraoperative technique offer preventive effects:

- Creation of side-to-end AV anastomosis. A retrograde venous flow of side-to-side anastomosis results (in rare cases) in an improvement of the fistula only, but more commonly in problems such as steal syndrome and venous hypertension.

- Selective venous arterialization. Especially at the elbow level, a flow into the selected vein brings a faster maturation, whereas a diffuse arterialization results in high flows and other problems, without effective improvement of fistula function.
- Use of stepped or tapered grafts for bridging. We use stepped PTFE grafts (4-7 mm) with a short (5-20 mm) portion of the narrow segment only to prevent excessive flow and improve flow characteristics in the anastomotic area.

References

1. Duncan H, Ferguson L, Faris I. Incidence of the radial steal syndrome in patients with Brescia fistula for hemodialysis: Its clinical significance. J Vasc Surg 1986; 4:144-47.
2. Morsy AH, Kulbaski M, Chen C, Isiklar H, Lumsden AB. Incidence and characteristics of patients with hand ischemia after a hemodialysis access procedure. J Surg Res 1998; 74:8-10.
3. Valji K, Hye RJ, Roberts AC, Oglevie SB, Ziegler T, Bookstein JJ. Hand ischemia in patients with hemodialysis access grafts: Angiographic diagnosis and treatment. Radiology 1995; 196:697-701.
4. Shemesh D, Mabjeesh NJ, Abramowitz HB. Management of dialysis access-associated steal syndrome: Use of intraoperative duplex ultrasound scanning for optimal flow reduction. J Vasc Surg 1999; 30:193-95.
5. Berman SS, Gentile AT, Glickman MH, et al. Distal revascularization-interval ligation for limb salvage and maintenance of dialysis access in ischemic steal syndrome. J Vasc Surg 1997; 26:393-402.
6. Haimov M, Schanzer H, Skladani M. Pathogenesis and management of upper-extremity ischemia following angioaccess surgery. Blood Purif 1996; 14:350-54.
7. Schanzer H, Schwartz M, Harrington E, Haimov M. Treatment of ischemia due to "steal" by arteriovenous fistula with distal artery ligation and revascularization. J Vasc Surg 1988; 7:770-73.

DISCUSSION

Panelist:
Jurgen Zanow, M.D.

Discussant: How do you decide how long to make your interposition graft?

Dr. Zanow: The narrowed segment, from our experience, is less than 20 millimeters.

Discussant: We have tried to devise an easy way to intraoperatively decide if somebody was at high risk for a steal. What we just started doing was to do a 10 digit pulse oximetry in the operating room both before and after we placed a graft. Indeed, those people that we found developed a steal had a marked reduction either in the absolute pulse oximeter number or in the amplitude of the pulse wave in the fingers. Since I started measuring that, I found a decrease in either the pulse oximetry O2 saturation or the signal strength, I have then defunctionalized the graft at that point. Since I have started doing that, I have had a much decreased incidence of steal in those patients. I presented it as an easy way for anybody to do that intraoperatively.

Discussant: What would you define a marked reduction?

Discussant: In the pulse oximetry machines that we have in the operating room, you can see signals strength and it will measure it as either strong or it will go on different scales downward. If I see a significant change in that, and I do not have a specific definition of that, but it is pretty dramatic sometimes.

Dr. Hong: The steal syndrome is one of the main problems the surgeons are facing every day. If you change the geometry of the anastomosis between the artery and the graft so that the antegrade blood flow goes smoothly into the graft, the incidence of steal syndrome is much reduced. In your situations you try to band the inflow while you keep the same geometry which is in favor of ischemia. If you could move this graft proximally and make it antegrade flow, I think then it would help the flow graft flow intake and it could also reduce the incidence of steal.

SECTION VI

22

LONG-TERM RESULTS OF PROCOL® BIOPROSTHETIC VASCULAR GRAFTS

Pierre Bourquelot, M.D.

There are a rapidly increasing number of patients with end-stage renal disease (ESRD) who are at extremely high risk because of complications associated with vascular access. In most instances, these individuals have experienced numerous failed autologous and prosthetic access sites with septic and hemodynamic complications.

For these patients, each subsequent procedure is generally more complex and susceptible to complications that threaten conduit accessibility or patency; it is therefore important to attempt to maximize the utility of each intervention. Midterm results were previously reported for ProCol® Vascular Bioprosthesis utilized for vascular access in patients with previously failed access and significant circulatory complications associated with the remaining vasculature.[1] This study reports the long-term results for this patient cohort.

Patients

All of the patients (n=70) in this study presented with 1 or more previously failed fistula or prosthetic shunt. In most instances (>75%), there was significant arterial or venous stenosis associated with the remaining vasculature. Due to the variability of patients' surviving vascular anatomy (including previously placed shunt remnants and significant venous thromboses) and presenting conditions (including stenotic venous stents, infected catheters, and previously placed infected prosthetic grafts), implant procedures varied. However, a 6-mm diameter bioprosthesis and a microsurgical graft implantation technique were used in all patients.

Results

The Kaplan-Meier cumulative patency (figure 22-1) was 87%, 79%, 52%, and 46% at 1, 2, 3, and 4.3 years, respectively, including patients censored because of death or transplantation. The mortality rate was 17% (n=12), and in all instances the bioprosthesis was patent at the time of death. The overall complication rate not including incidents of thromboses or recurring stenoses was 16% (n=11). Of these complications, there were 8 infections, 2 skin necroses at puncture sites, and 1

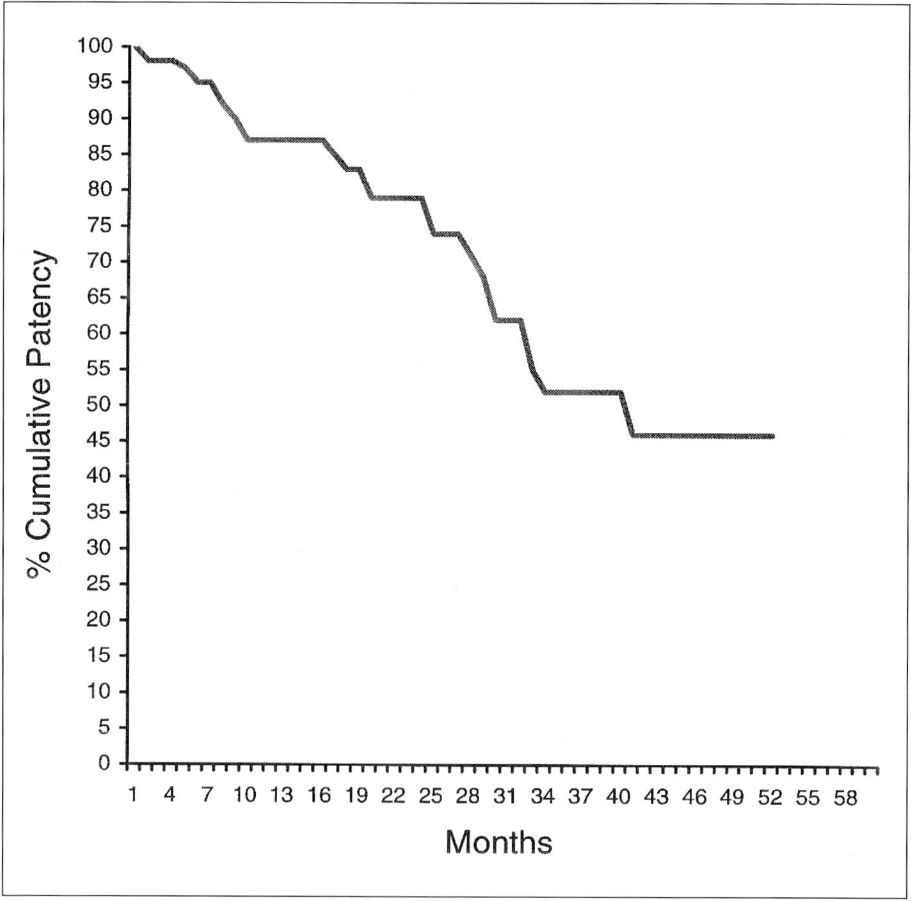

Figure 22-1. ProCol® cumulative patency.

ischemic event. During the study period, there were 30 procedures performed to remove thrombus (0.26 per patient year); midgraft thrombus was a rare event. Recurring outflow stenosis was observed in 8 cases. There were 2 surgical revisions and 1 graft was electively closed subsequent to transplantation. For the entire study period only 2 grafts were replaced, at 24 and 29 months, consequent to focal dilatation not associated with mural degeneration or false aneurysms commonly described for other biologic grafts. In the 4 years of this study, there have been no instances or evidence of graft-related inflammation, immunologic mediated events, or patterns of graft degeneration.

Though not directly examined in this study, the patency rate for the bioprosthesis appears to be significantly improved compared with those reported for polytetrafluoroethylene (PTFE) grafts. This rate suggests that bioprosthesis may be a desirable alternative, especially for patients with failed PTFE conduits. Trend analyses of bioprosthesis patency compared with our own series of PTFE grafts[2] (figure 22-2) suggested that bioprostheses may show almost twice the utility of PTFE grafts against this challenging condition.

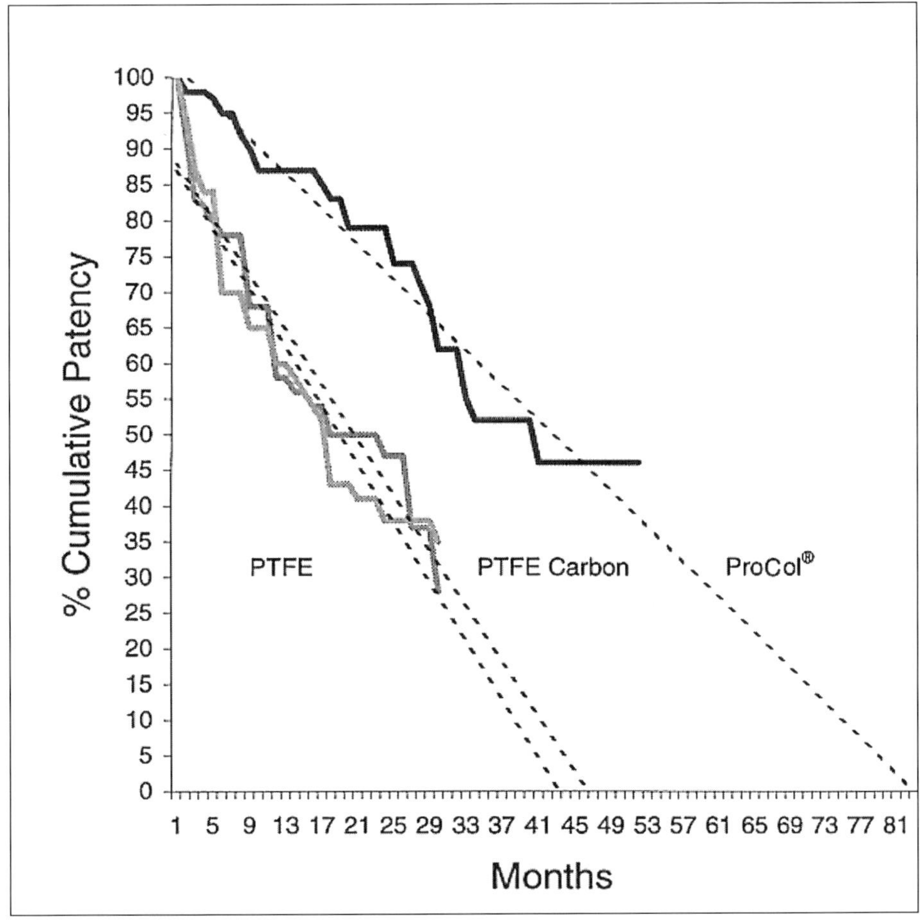

Figure 22-2. Trend analysis-ProCol (versus PTFE).

Discussion

These results indicate that the 6-mm ProCol® Bioprosthetic Vascular Graft can be successfully utilized for vascular access in a group of patients with difficult and complex vascular conditions.

References

1. Bourquelot P. ProCol Bioprosthetic Vascular Grafts for Dialysis Access. In: Henry ML, Ferguson RM, eds. Vascular access for hemodialysis-VI. Chicago: W.L. Gore & Associates and Precept Press, 1999:223-29.
2. Bourquelot P, Stolba J, Chèret P, Fournier F, Mouton A. Carbon-PTFE versus Standard-PTFE A-V bridge grafts for chronic hemodialysis. In: Henry ML, Ferguson RM, eds. Vascular access for hemodialysis-IV. Chicago: W.L. Gore & Associates and Precept Press, 1995:303-07.

DISCUSSION

Panelist:
Pierre Bourquelot, M.D.

Discussant: Dr. Bourquelot, could you just describe the ProCol® graft for those of us who are not terribly familiar with it?

Dr. Bourquelot: Yes, I am sorry that I do not have any slides about that. It is 6-millimeters. The branches of the vein have been ligated. There are valves inside the veins so you have to insert the graft in the correct direction. It is a very thin prosthesis and it is very easy to suture to distal arteries.

23

TAPERED AND STRAIGHT GRAFTS FOR HEMODIALYSIS ACCESS: A PROSPECTIVE, RANDOMIZED COMPARISON STUDY

Toshiyuki Hiranaka, M.D.

High-output failure and peripheral steal syndromes after placement of prosthetic arteriovenous (AV) grafts remain serious problems of vascular access. Rosental et al.[1] developed a tapered graft designed to prevent these complications. Some studies have suggested that the use of tapered grafts prevents high-flow problems, but no randomized clinical investigation has compared the complications of these grafts with those of nontapered grafts.

In an experimental study, Fillinger et al.[2] found no significant difference between 6-mm straight grafts and 4- to 7-mm tapered grafts in volumetric flow rates, although the tapered grafts had less venous intimal-medial hyperplasia. Shaffer[3], however, showed that the initial use of tapered grafts in patients with diabetes was associated with a significantly higher risk of thrombosis, compared with straight grafts, during the first year after implantation. No clinical studies have reported the effect of graft tapering on venous stenosis. We addressed several possible complications of prosthetic AV grafts in a prospective, randomized study comparing tapered and straight grafts with respect to early access flow, development of venous stenosis, and patency rates.

Materials and Methods

Between January and December 1999, 60 patients with end-stage renal failure requiring a prosthetic AV fistula were randomly assigned to undergo implantation of a 6-mm straight expanded polytetrafluoroethylene (ePTFE) graft (Carboflo graft, Impra, Tempe, AZ) or a 4- to 6-mm tapered ePTFE graft, either a Venaflo graft (Impra) or a Gore-Tex Stretch Vascular Graft (W.L. Gore & Associates, Flagstaff, AZ). Patients needing early graft cannulation were excluded from this randomization. The geometric configurations of the tapered graft types are shown in figure 23-1. Twenty patients were assigned to each of the 3 graft groups (table 23-1). Overall, 20 men and 40 women (mean age, 65 years; range, 40 to 87 years) were enrolled in the study. Twenty-six (43%) of the patients had diabetes and 30 (50%) had hypertension.

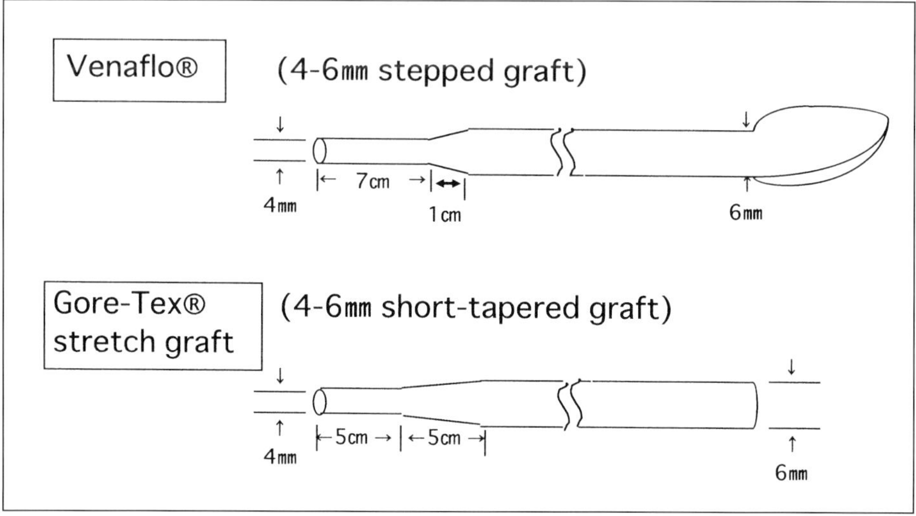

Figure 23-1. Geometric configurations of Venaflo and Gore-Tex tapered grafts.

Table 23-1. Characteristics of 60 patients in 3 graft groups

	Carboflo straight graft (n = 20)	Venaflo tapered graft (n = 20)	Gore-Tex tapered graft (n = 20)
Mean age (yr)	65.0	64.7	64.2
Sex: M/	5/1	5/1	10/10
Diabetic (n)	7	7	12
Hypertensive (n)	12	9	9

Fifty-five grafts (92% of the total) were placed in the forearm in a loop configuration; 5 grafts (8%) were placed in the upper arm (table 23-2). Carboflo and Venaflo grafts were anastomosed venous end first. Gore-Tex stretch grafts were anastomosed arterial end first. The venous ends of the Venaflo grafts were trimmed by 10 mm because the diameter of the veins that were anastomosed to the grafts was generally less than 6 mm.

Access flow was measured with a Crit Line Monitor (In-Line Diagnostics, Salt Lake City, UT) by using an optical dilution technique.[4,5] The mean time from graft

Table 23-2. Characteristics of grafts in the 3 graft groups

	Carboflo straight graft	Venaflo tapered graft	Gore-Tex tapered graft
Forearm loop (n)	15	13	18
Forearm/upper arm loop (n)	5	3	1
Upper arm curved (n)	0	4	1
Primary graft (n)	18	16	17
Graft in new site (n)	2	4	3
Mean follow-up (days)	276	283	205

implantation to flow measurement was 21 days (range, 14 to 60 days). Fistulography occurred 3 months after implantation.

Statistical methods used to compare results in the 3 graft groups included unpaired Student *t*-test (assessment of access flow), chi-square test (venous stenosis with >75% obstruction on fistulography), Kaplan-Meier evaluation (primary and secondary graft patency rates), and log-rank test (comparisons of graft patency rates).

Results

As measured in a total of 48 patients, mean (± SD) access flow rates were 1280 ± 490 mL/min for the Carboflo straight grafts (n=18), 1040 ± 340 mL/min for the Venaflo tapered grafts (n=16), and 1340 ± 370 mL/min for the Gore-Tex tapered grafts (n=14). Thus, the flow rate in the Venaflo grafts was generally lower than the rates for the other 2 graft types; however, the difference was not significant. The Gore-Tex and Carboflo grafts had flow rates that were stastically similar.

Postoperative fistulography of 41 patients showed venous stenosis in 8 (50%) of 16 patients in the Carboflo group, 8 (67%) of 12 in the Venaflo group, and 8 (62%) of 13 in the Gore-Tex group. Statistical analysis found no significant differences among the 3 groups in the occurrence of venous stenosis 3 months postoperatively.

One patient died during follow-up due to causes unrelated to graft implantation. Other complications treated during the follow-up period for the 3 graft groups are shown in table 23-3. Acute thrombosis occurred with 1 Venaflo graft and 3 Gore-Tex grafts. Early thrombosis (before postoperative fistulography was performed) occurred with 1 Carboflo graft, 3 Venaflo grafts, and 1 Gore-Tex graft. Late thrombosis occurred with 3 Carboflo grafts, 2 Venaflo grafts, and 3 Gore-Tex grafts.

Figures 23-2 and 23-3 show the primary and secondary patency rates, respectively, for the 3 graft groups. At 6 months, the primary patency rate was 63% for the Carboflo group, 60% for the Venaflo group, and 47% for the Gore-Tex group. At 12 months, the secondary patency rate was 95% for the Carboflo group, 83% for the Venaflo group, and 90% for the Gore-Tex group. There were no significant differences among the 3 groups in either primary or secondary patency rates.

Table 23-3. Number of complications in the 3 graft groups

	Carboflo straight graft	Venaflo tapered graft	Gore-Tex tapered graft
Acute thrombosis in less than 24 hours (n)	0	1	3
Early thrombosis in less than 3 months (n)	1	3	1
Late thrombosis in greater than 3 months (n)	3	2	3
Venous stenosis (n)	7	5	5
Steal syndrome (n)	2	0	0
Seroma (n)	1	2	0
Arterial stenosis (n)	0	1	1
Graft stenosis (n)	0	1	0

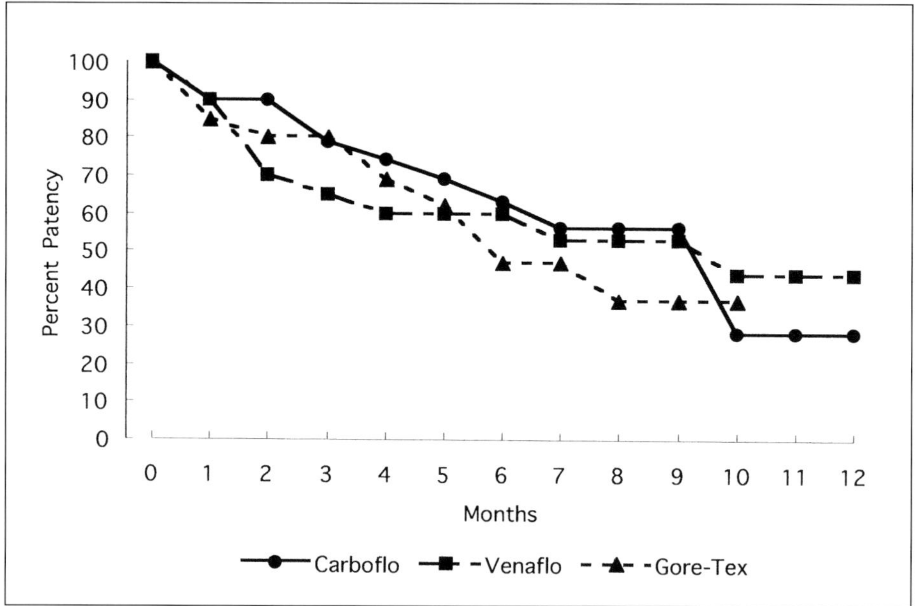

Figure 23-2. Central feeding of cephalic vein at forearm (A) and upper arm (B).

Discussion

Various modifications in the geometric configuration of prosthetic grafts have been made with the aim of improving their performance as vascular accesses for hemodialysis, but the clinical efficacy of these alterations is uncertain. Using computer modeling, Lei et al.[6] found that more uniform access flow and lower wall-stress gradients could be obtained with a larger anastomosis, smoother

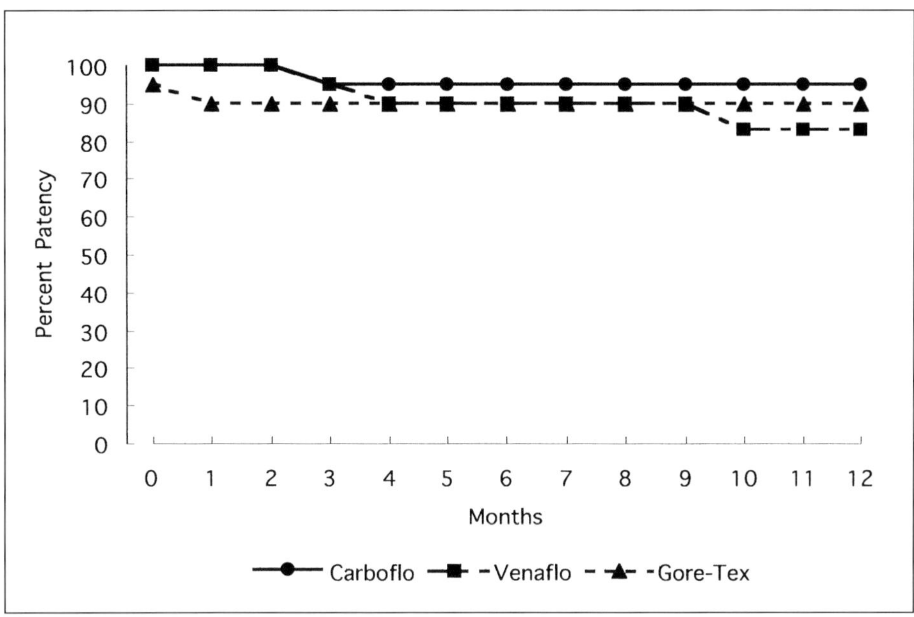

Figure 23-3. Secondary patency in the 3 graft groups

curves, and a 10-degree anastomosis angle. On the basis of this finding and the clinical studies of an AV patch prosthesis by Scholz et al.[7], a new, hooded, and tapered ePTFE graft (Venaflo) was developed.[8] In the prospective, randomized study reported here, however, flow rates with the 4- to 6-mm tapered Gore-Tex ePTFE grafts were similar to those with the 6-mm straight Carboflo ePTFE grafts. Moreover, flow rates with the Venoflo grafts, though lower than that of the other 2 prostheses, were not significantly different from the rates in either of the other 2 grafts. These results are consistent with the experimental findings of Fillinger et al.[2]

In our study, distal ischemia due to steal syndrome occurred in 2 patients with straight grafts and none with tapered grafts. The possible preventive effect of graft tapering on distal ischemia warrants further investigation. We found no difference between tapered and straight grafts in the occurrence of venous stenosis on fistulography 3 months postoperatively, a finding that suggests that neither tapering nor a venous-limb hood prevents venous stenosis in prosthetic AV fistulae. Additional studies are required to clarify the mechanisms of venous intimal hyperplasia and develop techniques to prevent venous stenosis in such fistulae.

Secondary patency rates at 12 months for the Carboflo, Venaflo, and Gore-Tex grafts were equally high. These favorable results may be due to our protocol for access monitoring. If the access flow rate decreased to 600 mL/min, we performed fistulography and treated venous stenosis with balloon angioplasty or surgical revision. Early detection and treatment of venous stenosis decreases the primary patency rate but improves the secondary patency rate.[9]

In conclusion, we found that the tapering of the arterial limb in prosthetic AV fistulae did not significantly improve access flow, decrease venous stenosis, or increase patency rates.

References

1. Rosental JJ, Bell DD, Gasper MR, Movius HJ, Lemire GG. Prevention of high flow problems of arteriovenous grafts. Development of a new tapered graft. Am J Surg 1980; 140:231-33.
2 Fillinger MF, Reinitz ER, Schwartz RA, et al. Graft geometry and venous-medial hyperplasia in arteriovenous loop grafts. J Vasc Surg 1990; 11:556-66.
3. Shaffer D. A prospective, randomized trial of 6 mm versus 4-7 mm PTFE grafts for hemodialysis access in diabetic patients. In: Henry ML, Ferguson RM, eds. Vascular access for hemodialysis-V. Chicago: W.L. Gore & Associates and Precept Press, 1997:91-94.
4. Krivitski NM. Theory and validation of access flow measurement by dilution technique during hemodialysis. Kidney Int 1995; 48:244-50.
5. Lindsay RM, Rothera C, Blake PG. A comparison of methods for the measurement of hemodialysis access recirculation: An update. ASAIO J 1998; 44:191-93.
6. Lei M, Archie JP, Kleinstreuer C. Computational design of a bypass graft that minimizes wall shear stress gradients in the region of the distal anastomosis. J Vasc Surg 1997; 25:637-46.
7. Scholz H, Zanow J, Petzold K, Kruger U, Settmacher U, Petzold M. Five year's experience with an arteriovenous patch prosthesis as access for hemodialysis. In: Henry ML, ed. Vascular access for hemodialysis-VI. Chicago: W.L. Gore & Associates and Precept Press, 1999: 241-53.
8. Escobar FS, Schwartz SA, Abouljoud M, et al. Comparison of a new 'hooded' graft with a conventional ePTFE graft: A preliminary study. In: Henry ML, ed. Vascular access for hemodialysis-VI. Chicago: W.L. Gore & Associates and Precept Press, 1999: 205-11.
9. Schwab SJ, Raymond JR, Saeed M, Newman GE, Dennis PA, Bollinger RR. Prevention of hemodialysis fistula thrombosis. Early detection of venous stenoses. Kidney Int 1989; 36:707-11.

DISCUSSION

Panelist:
Toshiyuki Hiranaka, M.D.

Discussant: I like the experimental design. It is a very important study that you have done. My sense of it was that the numbers were not as large as they need to be to have the power to show a real difference at 12 months. Do you plan to do more patients in this study or are these just the preliminary results?

Dr. Hiranaka: This study is ongoing. I intend to increase the number of patients.

Discussant: The other thing I thought was remarkable was at 3 months the rate of venous outflow stenosis was more than 75% of the luminal diameter, which occurred in more than 50% of cases. Dr. Hiranaka, I have no explanation for that but it was in each of the groups.

24

PROSPECTIVE RANDOMIZED TRIAL OF A SILASTIC BASED HEMODIALYSIS GRAFT

Earl S. Schuman, M.D., Marc Glickman, M.D., Mark Odland, M.D., Jill Linberg, M.D., and Kent Bodily, M.D.

Many different graft materials have been tried as conduits for hemodialysis access. However, polytetrafluoroethylene (PTFE) remains the model for comparison by providing an off-the-shelf graft that is durable, relatively nonthrombogenic, and resistant to infection. It also has a reasonable maturation time (2 to 3 weeks), and acceptable primary and secondary patency rates. Attempts have been made to improve this technique by developing a graft that can be used immediately, seals quickly after needle withdrawal, and maintains the other characteristics of PTFE.

Perma-Seal is a new conduit for dialysis access that is constructed of electronically spun silicone on a polyester yarn base. It can be used within 24 hours of implantation and has quick-sealing properties. A prospective, randomized, multicenter trial comparing Perma-Seal to PTFE was started in 1993. Our early experience was reported in 1996. At that time, there were 152 patients enrolled at 4 sites. The average follow-up was 6 months. There was no significant difference between the grafts for primary or secondary patency rates. Sealing times and early use after implantation were significantly better with the Perma-Seal graft.[1] The conclusion indicates that the theoretical benefit of a silicone elastomer graft was realized with decreased dependence on temporary access (due to immediate use of graft) and improved sealing times. There was no significant difference between the 2 grafts in primary and secondary patency rates and no difference in major complications. This paper presents the final data from the completed study.

Materials and Methods

This study started in July 1993 and was completed in March 1997. At conclusion, there were 250 patients at 6 sites. Data were collected at each site and sent to the sponsor for compilation and data analysis. Demographics and complication and patency rates were determined for each site as well as for each arm of the study. Gender and race were compared using the Fisher exact test. Student *t*-test was used to compare age and graft sealing times. Complication and patency rates were compared using the Kaplan-Meier life table with Breslow-Wilcoxon statistic.

The inner diameter of both Perma-Seal and PTFE grafts was 6 mm. While PTFE is 7.4 mm in outer diameter, Perma-Seal is 8.6 mm (figure 24-1). All patients were scheduled to receive antibiotics. However, at 1 site some patients were not given the ordered antibiotic and they had a higher infection rate. This failure was divided equally between both study arms.

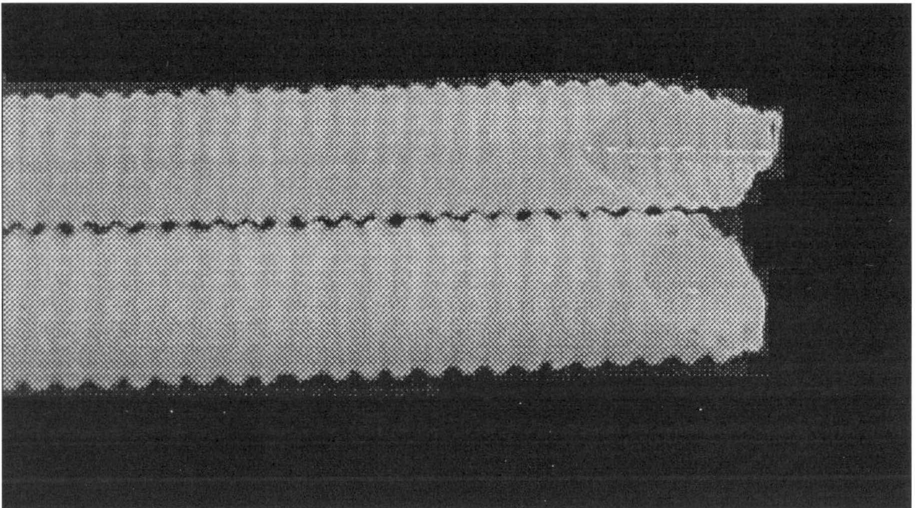

Figure 24-1. Thin wall (on top) and original version of Perma-Seal silastic grafts.

Results

There were 133 females (57%) and 117 males. The average age was 58 years (range, 21 to 84 years). Overall, there were 99 white patients (40%) and 138 black patients. In 2 cities, black patients were greater than 50%, while in 3 cities blacks comprised 20% of patients enrolled in this study. Average follow-up was 1.08 years. Forearm grafts were utilized in 78% of the study patients. Demographics are summarized in table 24-1.

As shown in table 24-2, the Perma-Seal graft had significantly more complications than PTFE. Primary and secondary patency rates were significantly lower with

Table 24-1. Demographics.

	PTFE	Perma-Seal	P value
Age	59.6	58.2	.429
Percent Male	23.1	24.4	.898
Percent Black	28.9	26.9	.352
Flow rate	412.7	405.7	.135
Venous resistance	213.3	204.3	.004

Perma-Seal. However, the Perma-Seal sealing time after dialysis needle withdrawal was significantly shorter than PTFE. This sealing characteristic allowed the Perma-Seal graft to be accessed earlier than PTFE. Fifty Perma-Seal grafts were accessed within 10 days of implantation, while all of the PTFE were accessed 10 days after implantation.

Table 24-2. Patency rates, sealing times, and times to first hemodialysis treatment.

	PTFE	Perma-Seal	*P* value
Cumulative primary patency at 6 months	60%	42%	.001
Cumulative primary patency at 1 year	40%	26%	.001
Cumulative secondary patency at 6 months	79%	64%	.001
Cumulative secondary patency at 1 year	73%	44%	.001
Sealing times	9.18 minutes	4.29 minutes	.001
Time to first hemodialysis	37 days after graft implant	29.5 days after implant	.001

Discussion

Two configurations of the Perma-Seal graft were used in this study. The first version had a much larger outer diameter (10 mm) with a 6-mm inner diameter. The second (current) version had an outer diameter of 8.6 mm while maintaining an inner diameter of 6 mm. Final data were pooled after evaluating each version separately and after finding no significant difference in any measured parameter.

Interestingly, significant differences were noted between the various study sites in race, complication rates, number of procedures performed, and primary and secondary patency rates. However, the differences between the study arms were consistent at each site, giving validity to the results. As an example, there were significantly more black patients at sites in the East and South than in the West.

The outcome of these individuals across study arms was not statistically different. Similarly, differences in patency rates between sites may reflect differing approaches to patient selection, graft maintenance techniques, or comorbidities. However, at each site PTFE patients had fewer complications and better patency rates than Perma-Seal patients did, and at each site Perma-Seal patients had earlier use and quicker sealing times than PTFE patients.[2]

The handling characteristics of Perma-Seal were markedly different than PTFE, with some differences noted between the 2 formulations of Perma-Seal. PTFE was more compliant, easier to suture, and more flexible around curves. Perma-Seal had less bleeding at the suture line upon completion of the anastamosis. The current version of Perma-Seal was much more compliant and flexible than the original version. Its smaller outer diameter made it more comfortable for, and appealing to, the patients.

Conclusion

Unlike the original report, this long-term study of Perma-Seal graft material shows it produced more complications and required more surgeries to maintain patency than PTFE. Primary and secondary patency rates were significantly shorter with Perma-Seal grafts. However, the goal of early use and quick sealing times with Perma-Seal was realized and was significantly better than PTFE.

In May 1998, the FDA gave the Perma-Seal graft limited-use approval. In those individuals who require immediate dialysis access and chronic access but who cannot tolerate a temporary hemodialysis catheter, the Perma-Seal graft is worthy of consideration. However, because of its superior long-term results, PTFE remains the material of choice in those patients who require chronic hemoaccess with synthetic graft material.

References

1. Glickman MH, Hurwitz RL, Fogle MA, et al. Early experience with the Perma-Seal graft for hemodialysis. In: Henry ML, ed. Vascular access for hemodialysis-V. Chicago: W.L. Gore & Associates and Precept Press, 1997: 112-17.
2. Possis Perma-Seal Clinical Study: FDA Final Report. Possis Medical, Inc. 1998.

DISCUSSION

Panelist:
Earl S. Schuman, M.D.

Discussant: Well, that is a very interesting paper. It makes a lot of sense to me. I am wondering if there are some logistical problems trying to extrapolate it to my own institution. I think our angiographers would have a problem with not knowing what was going to happen in their scheduling. They are busy and if you go on to an operative procedure, do you then have to involve anesthesia or do you do it under local anesthesia?

Dr. Schuman: We do it under local anesthesia, as these are all our patients. They are done in the operating room, with virtually all under sedation. The endovascular procedure is all done in that same setting.

Discussant: This is a totally logical approach. When you think about what it is you do surgically when you take a patient to the operating room, is that you make your best guess about why that graft failed. Statistically, it is usually the venous anastomosis so you go after that. Then you pass a balloon through the arterial anastomosis. If it squirts blood over the anesthesiologist, that is the finding of good inflow. If the catheter goes downstream and pulls back without too much resistance, that is the finding of patency downstream. The limitations are finding concurrent lesions. We know that most grafts that fail have more than 1 lesion. The surgeons miss that every time. We do a best guess type thing. Adding an angiogram allows you to pick up all these lesions and potentially address every lesion, and identify the lesion or lesions that made the graft fail. So why not go to the interventional suite and do all of this? Because there is only 1 tool and that tool is an angioplasty plus a stent. Stents have never been shown to add anything as far as I know with a venous anastomosis or a central venous stenosis. What the radiologist does is that he defines the problem much better than the surgeon does. But he has 1 arm tied behind his back because he only has 1 way of addressing that. What we are doing is combining both of these and I think what we need is to know what the right tool for the right lesion is. My bias is the lesion is at the venous anastomosis, but I do not know that. The reason surgery has done so badly, in my opinion, is because you miss all of the other lesions and it is not directed in terms of what you are doing. One of the things we are doing is to do an angiogram picking up those patients with only a venous structure at the anastomosis and then randomizing that lesion knowing that there is no contaminant problems elsewhere.

25

BRACHIAL ARTERY FLOW MEASUREMENT AS AN INDICATOR OF FOREARM NATIVE FISTULA MATURATION-EARLY EXPERIENCE

Surendra Shenoy, M.D., Ph.D., William D. Middleton, M.D., David W. Windus, M.D., Thomas Vesely, M.D., Nirmal K. Veeramachaneni, M.D., V. Ramachandran, M.D., Jeffrey A. Lowell, M.D., and Todd K. Howard, M.D.

Over 300,000 patients in the United States receive some form of dialysis, providing lifesaving renal replacement therapy for end-stage renal disease (ESRD). This poses a tremendous financial burden on the health care system. The estimated ESRD expenditure in the year 1996 was $15 billion.[1] The National Kidney Foundation-Dialysis Outcomes Quality Initiative (NFK-DOQI) published the first evidence-based clinical practice guidelines in 1997, with the objective of increasing the efficiency of patient care, and to positively impact patient outcomes and survival. The NFK-DOQI Vascular Access Work Group emphasized the placement of native arteriovenous (AV) fistulae as the first of 2 primary goals in achieving improvement of quality of life and overall outcomes in hemodialysis patients.[2] This has lead to an increased effort by the surgical community to create such AV fistulae.

Determination of fistula maturation, however, has always been based on subjective opinion. A native vein fistula is considered mature and suitable for use when the vein's diameter is sufficient to allow successful cannulation, but not sooner than 1 month and preferably 3 to 4 months after construction.[2] Assessment of fistula maturity is simple when patients develop large, superficial outflow veins that have a good thrill on clinical exam. Unfortunately, a large number of patients present with equivocal physical examination findings leading to a clinical dilemma. Attempts to use nonmature fistulae result in either low flows with inadequate dialysis or infiltration of blood. Patients with clinically nonmature but patent fistulae often continue to receive catheter dialysis while awaiting fistula maturation indefinitely and are thus exposed to catheter dialysis associated problems.[3,4] There are also patients who present for permanent access placement after initiation of catheter dialysis. The general perception that native vein fistulae take a long time to mature prompts many surgeons to create synthetic graft AV fistulae despite having clinical findings conducive for creation of native vein fistulae. Hence, an objective method to assess fistula maturation and to predict their successful use is necessary.

Hypotheses

We hypothesize that the flow in the main feeding artery to the extremity, bearing the AV fistula, reflects fistula flow. Thus, measuring brachial artery flow in the upper extremity predicts maturation of the forearm native vein fistulae.

Methods

We studied 53 patients with native vein radiocephalic primary fistulae created between July 1998 through July 1999. Suitability of the patient for creation of native vein fistulae was determined by clinical examination of the cephalic vein and radial artery. An elbow tourniquet and percussion of the vein for a 1 to 2 minute period was used to distend veins. A vein that was over 2.5 to 3 mm in size and was continuous from wrist to elbow was considered suitable. In addition, an artery with a reasonably palpable pulse was considered suitable for fistula creation. Duplex Doppler ultrasonic scanning was used to evaluate arterial flow measurements. Fistula flow was determined by measuring flows in the brachial artery at the level of the elbow at 1, 2, and 3 months. Flow measurements were discontinued after fistulae were used successfully for 6 consecutive dialysis treatments. Fistulae that were not suitable for use after 6 months were considered failures. Death, successful renal transplant, perioperative thrombosis, and noninitiation of dialysis were considered exclusion criteria.

Results

Fifty-three patients underwent creation of a native vein radiocephalic primary fistula. Twelve patients were excluded from this flow study (table 25-1). Of the 41 patients included in the study, 30 (73%) fistulae were successfully used for dialysis and 11 (27%) fistulae failed to mature.

Mean age and sex were similar between the fistulae that matured and those that failed. The age range was 19 to 84 years of age, with a mean of 56 years of age, in fistulae that matured and 25 to 81 years (mean 52 years of age) in fistulae that failed. Six of 8 patients who had arterial calcifications noted during the surgical procedure failed to mature (P=0.006). There were also significantly more patients with diabetes in the failure group.

Table 25-1. Exclusions from the study.

Death	1
Transplant	1
Technical failure	3
Working fistulae on dialysis	7
Total patients excluded	12

Table 25-2 summarizes duplex Doppler flow measurements. The mean blood flow of 795 mL/min (standard deviation [SD]=243 mL) at first measurement (mean=27 days, n=26) for fistulae that successfully matured was not different (P=0.18) from mean blood flow of 615 mL/min (SD=251 mL) obtained at first measurement (mean 19 days n=10) in fistulae that ultimately failed to mature. Mean blood flow of 894 mL/min (300 mL) at second measurement (mean 78 days, n=22) in fistulae that matured was significantly higher (P=0.006) than the mean flow of 485 mL/min (SD=150 mL) measured in (mean 52 days, n=8) fistulae that failed. This difference persisted (P=0.008) during the third measurement.

Four of 5 patients (80%) whose flows were less than 400 mL/min at first measurement failed to mature. Twenty-nine (81%) of 36 patients whose flows were over 400 mL/min at first measurement matured. Four patients with flows less than 400 mL/min at second measurement between 6 to 8 weeks failed to mature. Five patients who had flows over 600 mL/min at initial measurement between 2 to 4 weeks but had subsequent decrease in flows (to approximately 400 mL/min) at second measurement between 6 to 8 weeks failed to mature. Fistulae that had decreased flows initially (approximately 400 mL/min), but had increasing flows (500 to 600 mL/min) at second measurement, matured successfully.

Table 25-2. Brachial artery flows.

	N	Mature fistula mean mL/min (range, SD)	N	Fail fistula mean mL/min (range, SD)
US 1	26	795	10	615
(3 to 4 weeks)	(396-1220, 243)	(246-1000, 251)		
US 2	19	894*	7	485
(6 to 8 weeks)	(425-1710, 300)	(327-754, 150)		
US 3	7	762**	5	488
(11 to 13 weeks)	(712-1048, 200)	(394-555, 70)		

* *P* =0.006, ** *P* = 0.008

Discussion

A native vein fistula is the conduit of choice for long-term hemodialysis. It has increased hemodialysis access longevity and has fewer thrombotic episodes per year of access survival, compared with other vascular access modalities.[2] The prevalence of infection, bleeding, and pseudoaneurysm formation is less in native vein fistulae compared with PTFE or bioartificial conduits.[5] Use of native veins obviates the cost associated with artificial conduit material and makes native vein fistula cost effective. Despite these advantages, only 20% to 25% of ESRD population in the US have native vein fistula as conduit for long-term hemodialysis.[6] An initial failure rate of up to 30%,[7] patient body habitus, age, diabetes, previous needle sticks resulting in nonavailability of native veins, late referral for access creation, and lengthy postoperative periods for fistula maturation have been quoted as some of the reasons for not creating native vein fistulae.

In addition, the authors feel that a lack of objective methods to evaluate patients for native vein fistulae and evaluation of fistulae maturation are partly responsible for the present low rate of creation of native vein fistulae. Studies show that an increase in native vein fistula creation from 32% to 58% occurred with preoperative ultra sound vascular mapping.[8] We feel that use of duplex Doppler to assess fistula blood flow provides objective evidence of fistula maturation and further improve the fistula outcome.

Brachial artery flows in ESRD patients prior to access creation range from 6 to 78 mL/min (mean of 31 mL/min, unpublished data). After AV fistula creation, the flow ranges from 246 to 1710 mL/min. Our data showed that flows less than 400 mL/min early (2 to 4 weeks) after fistula creation, in the absence of anatomic problem, were predictive of fistula failure. Over 80% of patients with flows over 600 mL/min at first measurement, matured successfully. A few patients' fistulae (20% in this study) with flows above 600 mL/min at first measurement eventually failed. The patients had decreasing flow measurements at subsequent studies. Clinical findings and radiologic evaluation of these patients usually revealed evolving outflow vein stenosis. Only 1 fistula with flow less than 400 mL/min at initial estimation (at 15 days) matured. There was progressive increase in flow at subsequent measurements in this patient. No fistula with flows less than 400 mL/min at 2 months matured.

Longitudinal flow measurements in our patients also suggest that most flow changes occur between 1 and 2 months after fistula placement. The changes are predictive of fistula outcome. Our preliminary data challenges the concept of waiting indefinitely for native vein fistula maturation and the belief that fistulae take an extended time to mature. On the contrary, our data suggest that fistulae that fail to mature in 1 to 2 months have almost no chance of maturing thereafter. Our study suggests that it is never too late to place a native vein fistula in an ESRD patient regardless of the time of referral.

Conclusions

Brachial artery flow measurements with duplex Doppler scanning gave an accurate and reproducible method to assess blood flow in native vein radiocephalic fistulae. Serial measurement of blood flow 1 and 2 months following fistula creation were predictive of fistula maturation.

References

1. Feldman HI, Korbin S, Wasserstein A. Hemodialysis vascular access morbidity. J Am Soc Nephrol 1996; 7:523-35.
2. NFK-DOQI Vascular Access Work Group Members. NFK-DOQI clinical practive guidelines for vascular access. Am J Kidney Dis 1997; 30:S152-91.
3. Suchoki P, Conlon P, Knelson M, Harland RC, Schwab SJ. Silastic cuffed catheters for hemodialysis vascular access: Thrombolytic and mechanical correction of HD catheter malfunction. Am J Kidney Dis 1996; 28:379-86.
4. Atherikul K, Schwab SJ, Twardowski ZJ, et al. What is the role of permanent central vein access in hemodialysis patients? Sem Dial 1996; 9:92-403.
5. Hodges TC, Fillinger MF, Zwolak RM, et al. Longitudinal comparison of dialysis access methods: Risk factors for failure. J Vasc Surg 1997; 26:1009-19.
6. United States Renal Data System. USRDS 1995 Annual Data Report. Am J Kidney Dis 1995; 26:S1-186.
7. Palder SB, Kirkman RL, Whittlemore AD, et al. Vascular access for hemodialysis: Patency rates and results of revision. Ann Surg 1985; 202:235-39.
8. Robbin ML, Gallichio MH, Deierhoi CJ, et al. US vascular mapping before hemodialysis access placement. Radiology 2000; 217:83-88.

DISCUSSION

Panelist:
Surendra Shenoy, M.D., Ph.D.

Discussant: I am not sure why you looked to brachial artery flow. It is just simple to look at the fistula flow. We showed that if you looked at the flow the next day after you create a fistula, the next day you can determine with a fair degree of accuracy whether that fistula is going to work for dialysis or not. My research shows that those with low velocity, you can predict will never mature, and those with a reasonable velocity will. I think the cut off was about 0.4 meters per second. You can divide those groups. Now if you want to be absolutely certain whether they are going to mature or not, is actually to do another duplex. In about 2 to 3 weeks after your initial duplex, and that will separate the two quite adequately. So you do not have to wait very long at all. Then you can either revise that fistula or create another one. So you do not have to wait to long.

Dr. Shenoy: Well, I think probably this data again shows exactly the same thing except that we made the flow in the brachial artery. The reason for measuring the flow in the brachial artery is that it is much more reliable and you can easily reproduce it, as opposed to trying to measure the flows in the fistula. We felt in the immediate post-op phase, the fistula flow need not necessarily reflect the maturation, mainly because there are so many other added problems like edema and swelling, which can effect the fistula flows.

Discussant: How would you use this information to try to predict the next access that you use? In other words, if our Brescia fails, we go onto an elbow AV fistula or put in a loop graft. Do you think from this data that if the brachial artery flow had not increased, those won't work either? But, in fact, usually they do.

Dr. Shenoy: It is not really true when you extrapolate the data from radial artery to the brachial artery. I cannot prove this, but I think why the brachial artery flow does not go up is because it is not capable of dilating to increase the regional flow. It is like trying to suck water or blood through a straw, which is not capable of expanding or dilating.

Discussant: I enjoyed your study. I agree with you that brachial artery flow is the way to measure flow. I have some concerns with the conclusion that you are saying the fistula should not be made within 3 months of dialysis. We should try to make a fistula. Even if this fistula does not mature, we should try to plan for the management mainly in making a more proper fistula. But we should not wait until it is so late when at that time we may have to put the catheters. I think we have to take precaution measures in making our conclusion.

Dr. Shenoy: I think it is redundant to do a fistula and put the patient through 5 surgeries when he really does not need it and still you do not have a fistula when you really need it. That is the whole idea behind trying to optimize the timing of fistula creation.

Discussant: But it does not help you in the cases that the fistulas do not mature, then you are still stuck. If you started off at 3 months before you knew they were going to be on dialysis and it did not mature, then you do not have any access when they need dialysis. So I think what he is arguing for is a little buffer period in case that happens.

Discussant: Using the brachial artery flow, you would know at 2 months if this does not happen it is not going to happen. That might be a fistula that started with 400 at 2 months has gone to 600. That fistula still has a chance but there is a very small chance. Most of them declare themselves 1 way or other and you are done with it. You can plan the next access. You want the patient as close to dialysis to avoid a graft. The second thing is I firmly believe is that a fistula should be done at any cost, if you can do 1 and with the availability of good catheters. Catheters are pretty good. A month or 2 of catheter dialysis is not going to be a big difference in the long run of this patient if you can establish a fistula.

Discussant: You said something wrong. When the fistula fails to mature, in my experience, the mass majority of the stenoses are on the vein, rarely in the artery. So even a calcified artery can feed a good forearm fistula.

Dr. Shenoy: You are right. The data not shown is what we did with the fistulas that did not mature. We did try to improve in some of them. We did try to fix the existing problem. I agree with you 100% when fistulas do not get good flow there is a problem for inflow. Outflow problems are very easy to make out because you do a good clinical exam, and you do not feel a thrill or feel a pulse.

Discussant: I am a nephrologist and I can assure you that you cannot predict 3 months in advance when a patient is going to need dialysis. For that reason, I would urge you not to try to cut things that close. The problem is number 1, we do not know when the patient is going to need dialysis. We cannot take a calendar out and say on March the 21st we are going to start you on dialysis. It is something that you have to assess week by week, month by month. You may see a patient that you think is going to need dialysis very soon and then the patient may stabilize or improve. Dialysis is delayed much beyond from where you thought it would or the reverse may occur. The other thing is we all have experiences that we feel sure that the patient is going to need dialysis in the very immediate future and we have an access placed and it seems almost the access is therapeutic. The patient's renal function begins to improve and they may stabilize and you find out that a year later you still have not started them on dialysis. So I would urge you not to try to put in an access AV fistula 3 months before you think the patient is going to need dialysis, because you are frequently going to be wrong.

Discussant: There simply is nothing wrong with a patient having a fistula for a year that has never been used. We see patients like that all the time. There is no downside to it.

Discussant: I am a nephrologist and we have an extremely active pre-ESRD education program in Houston where the primary care physicians have been referring the patients early to us. It has taken us several years to develop that trend and train these guys, but it is very successful. I have been dealing with this now for 20 years with renal problems in dealing with pre-ESRDs since 1993. For the majority of diabetic and older patients, we find it takes longer for the fistulas to mature and so we are advocating early placement to AV fistulas. The benefit versus risk far out way the alternative where the patient shows up in the emergency room at 10 o'clock on Saturday night needing dialysis with no access at all. So I really am a strong advocate. Maybe I differ from some other people in this room. But I am a very strong advocate of early placement of AV fistulas.

26

ROLE OF FREQUENT BLOOD FLOW MEASUREMENTS IN PREDICTING HEMODIALYSIS GRAFT THROMBOSIS

Sunanda J. Ram, Ph.D., Carolyn G. Birk, B.G.S., Jack Work, M.D., and William D. Paulson, M.D.

Thrombosis of synthetic grafts is the major cause of morbidity in hemodialysis patients.[1] Thrombosis is usually caused by stenosis at the venous anastomosis or outflow vein of the graft. Because correction of stenosis may prevent thrombosis and prolong graft life, it has been proposed that grafts be monitored so that stenosis can be detected and corrected prior to thrombosis.[2] The dysfunction hypothesis provides the rationale for using graft blood flow (Qa) to predict thrombosis.[3] It states that progressive stenosis causes a decrease in Qa that reliably precedes and accurately predicts thrombosis.

Neyra et al. recently confirmed that a decrease in Qa indicates an increased risk of thrombosis.[4] These authors support the view that grafts should undergo monthly Qa monitoring with correction of stenosis if the decrease in Qa exceeds 15% or 20%. In order for such a monitoring program to be successful, however, Qa should have a high sensitivity and a low false positive rate (FPR) when predicting thrombosis. We have recently found that percent decrease in Qa has a sensitivity of only 74%, at an FPR of 25% during monthly monitoring.[5] Qa readings often fail to decrease prior to thrombosis, resulting in this poor predictive accuracy.

One possible explanation is that the decrease in Qa that precedes thrombosis is often too rapid and brief to be detected by monthly measurements. At a stenosis of 50% (which is reaching a level generally considered significant), the luminal cross-sectional area has already reduced by 75%. Thus, a small increase in stenosis could potentially lead to a rapid decrease in Qa with thrombosis occurring before the monthly Qa measurement. In addition, we have recently found that new grafts often develop progressive stenosis, which is followed by thrombosis, within weeks after placement.[6] This implies stenosis may progress more rapidly than is generally realized.

The foregoing suggests that Qa measurements taken at more frequent intervals may allow detection of a decrease in Qa before thrombosis occurs. In this study, we tested the hypothesis that biweekly Qa measurements provide a higher accuracy in predicting thrombosis than monthly measurements.

Materials and Methods

Patients. We prospectively studied 77 polytetrafluoroethylene (PTFE) grafts from 76 dialysis patients at the Dialysis Clinic, Inc. and Dialysis Center of Shreveport dialysis units in Shreveport, LA. Patients gave informed consent and underwent biweekly Qa measurements (at the beginning and middle of each month) from March 1998 through December 1999. Qa measurements were done by ultrasound dilution (Transonic Systems Inc, Ithaca, NY), as described previously.[5] Patients entered the study at different times and were followed until graft thrombosis or end of the study. Patients with thrombosed grafts were allowed to re-enter the study.

Monitoring protocols. We compared the accuracy of monthly and biweekly Qa measurements in predicting thrombosis. For predictive accuracy of monthly Qa (figure 26-1A), every other biweekly measurement was ignored so that a series of monthly measurements could be analyzed. For each graft, we randomly selected a measurement from the beginning or middle of a month to serve as the first monthly Qa (month -3, figure 26-1A). Months -3, -2, -1, and 0 indicate the timing of measurements for monthly Qa; month 0 was the last monthly measurement. For thrombosed grafts, knowledge of the timing of thrombosis allowed month 0 to be selected so that thrombosis occurred within the next month.

The biweekly Qa protocol (figures 26-1B-C) ensured that Qa was measured within 2 weeks of thrombosis. If thrombosis occurred in the first 2 weeks after month 0 (figure 26-1B), then biweekly Qa provided no advantage over monthly Qa, because the last Qa's for both were at month 0. On the other hand, if thrombosis occurred during the second 2 weeks after month 0 (figure 26-1C), then biweekly Qa had the advantage of an additional measurement after the last monthly Qa. Only grafts that thrombosed during the second 2 weeks after the monthly Qa had a potential to benefit from biweekly Qa. In theory, half of the grafts should thrombose in the first 2 weeks and half should thrombose in the second 2 weeks. For thrombosed grafts, we randomly selected month 0 so that the timing of thrombosis was equally distributed between the two 2 week periods (figure 26-1B-C).

Analysis. Data are reported as mean ± SE (standard error). Comparisons between means were made by paired *t*-test, significance was set at $P<0.05$. All grafts included in the study completed at least 4 monthly measurements so that the percent decrease in Qa over 3 months (ΔQa_{3mos}) could be computed (figure 26-1A). We have previously found that ΔQa_{3mos} is the most accurate of several Qa predictors of thrombosis.[5] ΔQa_{3mos} was computed from values at months 0 (Qa_0) and -3 (Qa_{-3}) by the following equation: $\Delta Qa_{3mos} = -100(Qa_0 - Qa_{-3})/Qa_{-3}$. The negative sign indicates that a decrease in Qa had a positive value.

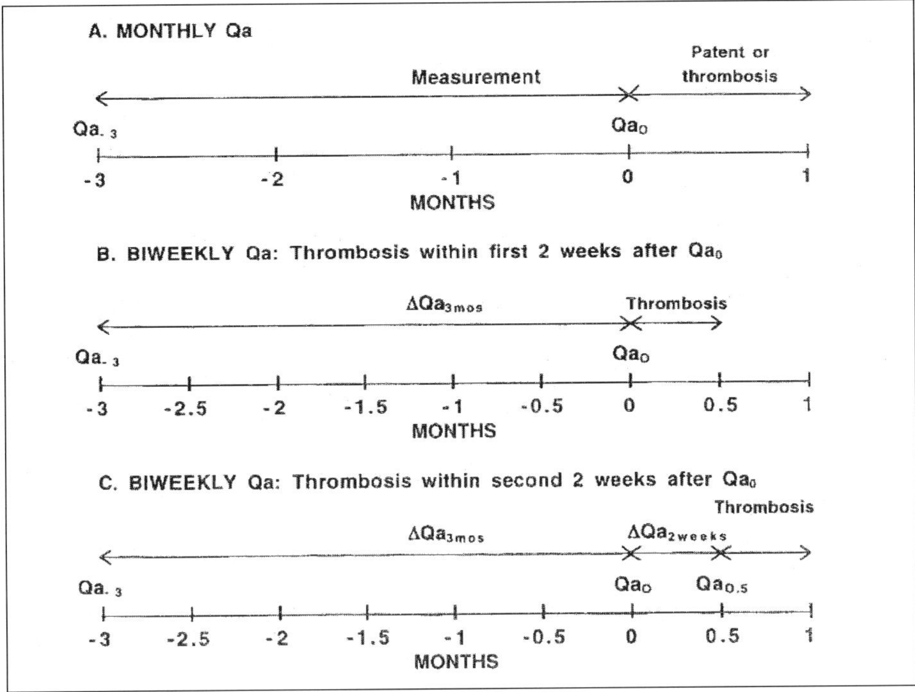

Figure 26-1. Study protocol. ΔQa_{3mos} and ΔQa_{2weeks} denote percent decrease in Qa over 3 months and 2 weeks, respectively.

For biweekly Qa, when thrombosis occurred in the first 2 weeks after month 0 (figure 26-1B), ΔQa_{3mos} was used to test predictive accuracy, since both monthly and biweekly Qa had the same last Qa. This also assured the highest possible predictive accuracy, because ΔQa_{3mos} was almost always larger than percent decrease over 2 weeks (ΔQa_{2weeks}). For grafts that thrombosed during the second 2 weeks after month 0 (figure 26-1C), we took advantage of the additional Qa measurement ($Qa_{0.5}$, at month 0.5) by using the ΔQa between months 0 and 0.5:

$$\Delta Qa_{2weeks} = -100(Qa_{0.5} - Qa_0)/Qa_0.$$

Predictive accuracy of ΔQa was tested by computing maximum-likelihood estimates of receiver operating characteristic (ROC) curves with ROCKIT 0.9B software for Apple Macintosh (Beta version) provided by Charles E. Metz.[7] ROC curves plot sensitivity versus false positive rate for predicting thrombosis at different threshold values of the predictor being tested. Figure 26-2 shows a hypothetical ROC curve. Sensitivity and false positive rate were defined as follows:

- *Sensitivity* (true positive rate): For thrombosed grafts, the proportion with $\Delta Qa \geq$ threshold value for predicting thrombosis.
- *False positive rate* (FPR = 1 – specificity): For nonthrombosed grafts, the proportion with $\Delta Qa \geq$ threshold value for predicting thrombosis.

The area under the ROC curve (AUC) is a measure of the overall predictive accuracy of a test. ROCKIT defines the curve and computes AUC ± SE. The Z statistic for paired data was used to compare AUCs;[7] significance was set at $P < 0.05$.

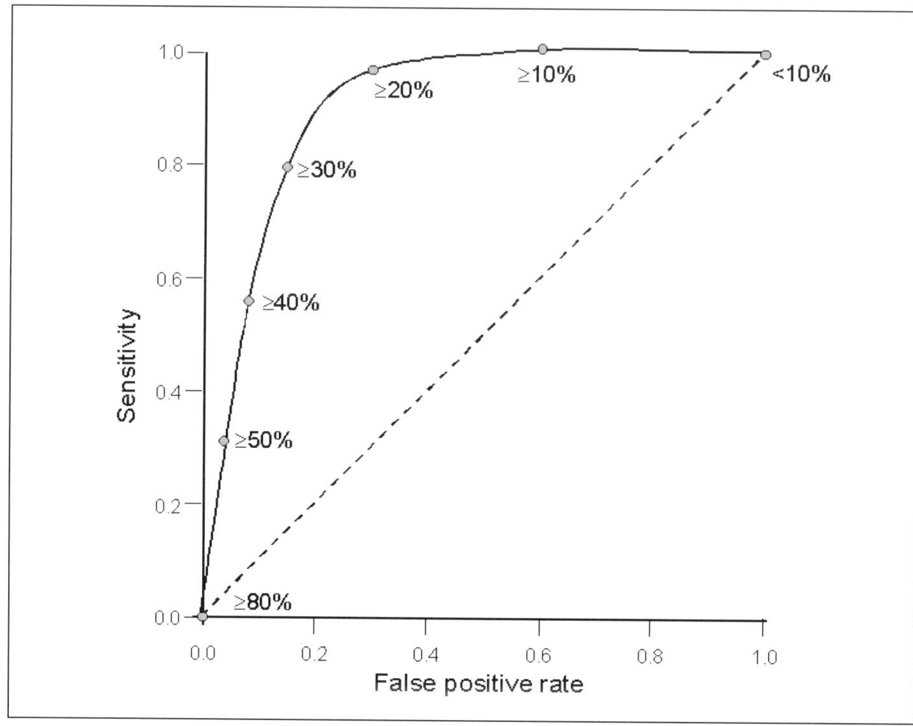

Figure 26-2. Example of hypothetical ROC curve that indicates high accuracy in predicting thrombosis. ΔQa values along curve are thresholds for predicting thrombosis. Values ≥ threshold predict thrombosis with indicated sensitivity and FPR. Threshold values decrease as the curve is traversed upward and to the right. Thus, the smaller the ΔQa used to predict thrombosis, the higher the sensitivity and FPR. A perfect predictor has AUC = 1.0. The solid curve has AUC = 0.90; it provides a high sensitivity at a low FPR. The dashed line at 45° indicates a predictor with no discriminative ability (AUC = 0.5; high sensitivity requires high FPR).

Results

Seventy-seven grafts from 76 patients were included in the study. Patient and graft characteristics are listed in table 26-1. All 76 patients were African American and 47% had diabetes mellitus. Thirty-three grafts (43%) thrombosed during the study. As previously reported[5], patient demographics and graft characteristics (location, configuration, graft age, and prior history of graft complications) did not differ between thrombosed and nonthrombosed grafts (comparison not shown).

Timing of thrombosis. Because the study tested whether biweekly Qa detects decreases in Qa that are missed by monthly Qa, we determined the timing of thrombosis after the last monthly measurement. Figure 26-3 shows that about half of all grafts that thrombosed (17 of 33) did so during the first 2 weeks following the last monthly Qa. Biweekly Qa would not have improved predictive accuracy in these

Table 26-1. Patient and graft characteristics.

Patient Information	No. (%)
African American	76 (100)
Male	28 (37)
Diabetes mellitus	36 (47)
Patient age at study entry (years)	56.3 ± 1.6*
Number of grafts	77
Location of grafts	
Forearm	27 (35)
Upperarm	42 (55)
Thigh	6 (8)
Chest	2 (3)
Graft configuration	
Loop	35 (45)
Straight	42 (55)
Graft age at study entry (days)	714.6 ± 82.1*

*Mean ± SE

grafts because monthly and biweekly Qa had the same last Qa before thrombosis (figures 26-1A, 26-1B). Biweekly Qa had an opportunity to improve predictive accuracy only in the grafts (16 of 33) that thrombosed during the second 2 weeks (figure 26-1C).

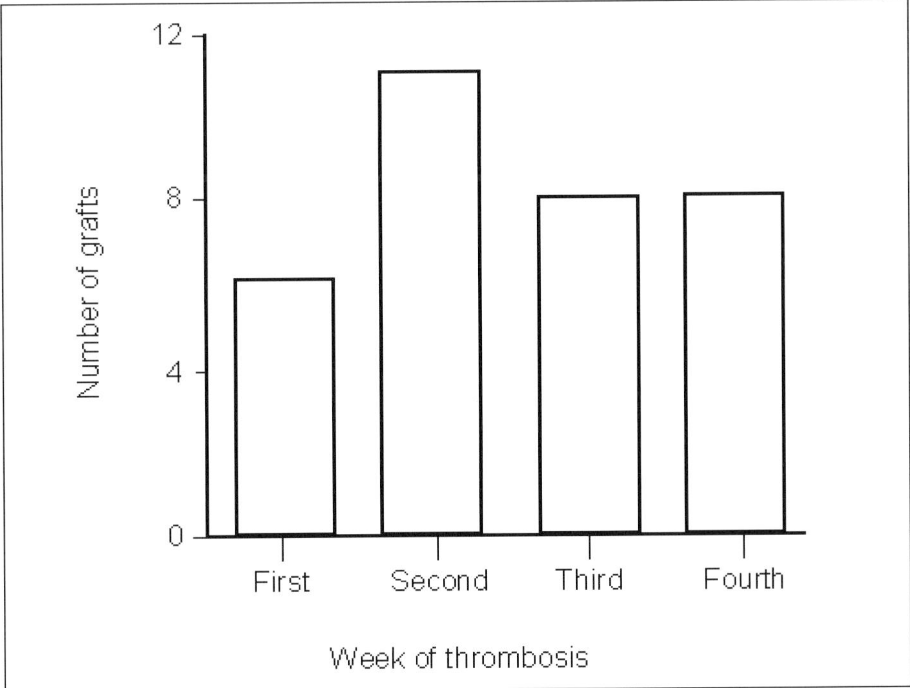

Figure 26-3. Timing of thrombosis after last monthly Qa measurement.

Percent decrease in Qa before thrombosis. We next studied the 16 grafts that thrombosed during the second 2 weeks to determine whether their percent decrease in Qa over 2 weeks (ΔQa_{2weeks}) was large compared with percent decrease over 3 months (ΔQa_{3mos}). The mean ΔQa_{3mos} was 16.3 ± 4.1%, while the mean ΔQa_{2weeks} was much smaller: 5.9 ± 4.7% (P=0.04). Thus, the last monthly measurements did not miss rapid decreases in Qa.

We examined the 16 grafts that thrombosed in the second 2 weeks in more detail by dividing them into 2 groups, depending on whether ΔQa_{3mos} was significant ($\Delta Qa_{3mos} \geq 20\%$). Seven grafts (44%) had $\Delta Qa_{3mos} \geq 20\%$, and their mean was 31.9 ± 3.2% (figure 26-4A). ΔQa_{2weeks} in these grafts was 14.3 ± 7.6%, indicating the additional ΔQa would augment ΔQa_{3mos} but not improve predictive accuracy because ΔQa_{3mos} was already large. Biweekly Qa had an opportunity to improve predictive accuracy in the remaining 9 thrombosed grafts that had $\Delta Qa_{3mos} < 20\%$ (ΔQa_{3mos} = 4.2 ± 3.0%). For these grafts, however, ΔQa_{2weeks} was only 0.73 ± 5.2% (figure 26-4B). This confirms that biweekly Qa did not detect a rapid decrease in Qa that was missed by monthly Qa.

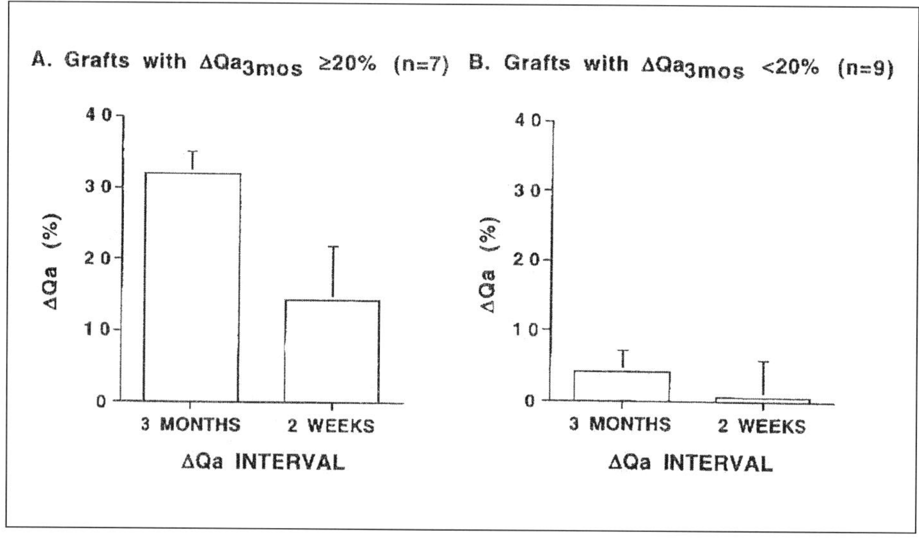

Figure 26-4. For 16 grafts that thrombosed during second 2 weeks after last monthly Qa measurement (figure 26-1C), comparison of percent decrease over 3 months (ΔQa_{3mos}) versus percent decrease over 2 weeks (ΔQa_{2weeks}).

Predictive accuracy of ΔQa. We used ROC curves to further show that biweekly Qa did not improve accuracy in predicting thrombosis (figure 26-5). The area under the curve (AUC) indicates the predictive accuracy of a test (see example, figure 26-2). The AUC for ΔQa_{3mos} was low (0.72 ± 0.07, figure 26-5). The curve indicates a sensitivity of 80% in predicting thrombosis requires a FPR of 50%. We next tested the benefit of substituting ΔQa_{2weeks} for ΔQa_{3mos} in the 16 grafts that thrombosed

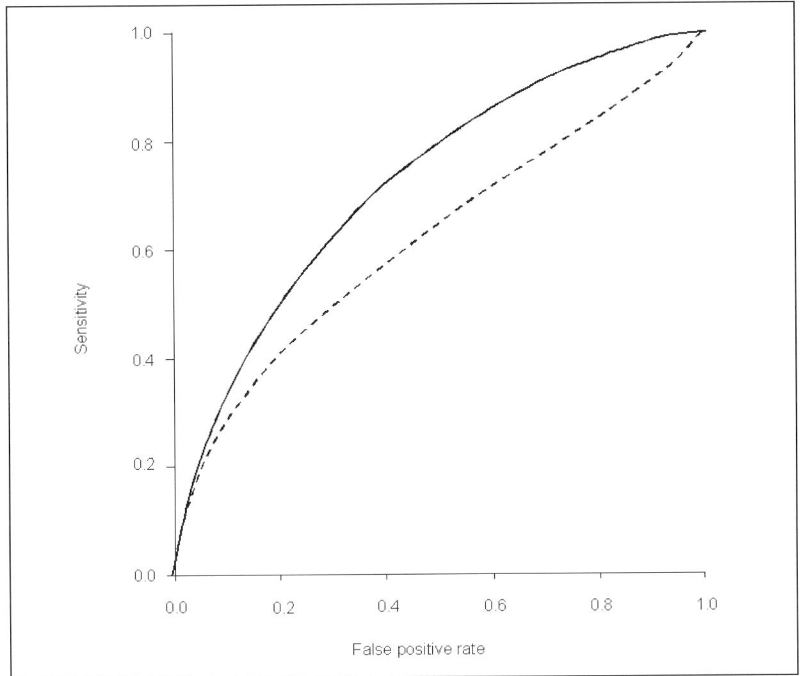

Figure 26-5. ROC curves show accuracy of percent decrease in Qa in predicting thrombosis. Solid curve shows predictive accuracy for ΔQa_{3mos}. Dashed curve shows predictive accuracy after substituting ΔQa_{2weeks} for ΔQa_{3mos} in grafts that thrombosed during second 2 weeks after last monthly Qa measurement (figure 26-1C).

Table 26-2. Distribution of ΔQa values for the 16 grafts that thrombosed during the second 2 weeks after the last monthly Qa.

	ΔQa			
	< 20%	20% to 39%	≥ 40%	Total
Net ΔQa over 3 months	9	6	1	16
Net ΔQa over 2 weeks	11	4	1	16

during the second 2 weeks after the last Qa measurement (see Analysis in Materials and Methods section). Table 26-2 shows that this reduced the number of grafts with $\Delta Qa \geq 20\%$ and yielded a lower AUC of 0.62 ± 0.09 ($P = 0.09$, figure 26-5). Thus, ΔQa_{2weeks} actually impaired predictive accuracy. We also found that using the largest decrease between $\Delta Qa2_{weeks}$ and ΔQa_{3mos} for these 16 grafts did not yield a significant improvement in AUC (0.75 ± 0.06).

Discussion

This study shows that biweekly Qa measurements do not improve accuracy in predicting graft thrombosis when compared with monthly Qa measurements. We found no evidence that biweekly Qa detects rapid decreases in Qa that are missed by monthly Qa. More than half of the grafts that thrombosed after the last monthly Qa measurement failed to show a decrease in Qa, regardless of whether the measurements were done monthly or biweekly.

One possible explanation for the failure of biweekly Qa to improve prediction of thrombosis is that biweekly measurements may not be frequent enough to capture the rapid decreases in Qa that might precede thrombosis. Thus, it is possible that a shorter interval between measurements might be more successful. Although this possibility deserves further investigation, it remains to be seen whether graft monitoring programs can carry out such frequent measurements, analyze data, identify grafts with decreases in Qa, and then schedule and correct stenosis before thrombosis occurs.

Another explanation for the failure of biweekly Qa to improve the prediction of thrombosis may be heterogeneity in mechanisms of thrombosis. It is possible that there are 2 populations of grafts: those that follow the dysfunction hypothesis by exhibiting a gradual decrease in Qa before thrombosis, and those that do not. Grafts that thrombose without warning may do so for a variety of reasons other than a rapid decrease in Qa, such as hypercoagulability (which may cause thrombosis with little or no stenosis), hypotension, and mechanical factors (such as sleeping on the graft arm). Hemodynamic variability strongly influences Qa and may impair the accuracy of Qa in predicting thrombosis.[5] For example, an increase in stenosis may be missed because a blood pressure increase has prevented the expected decrease in Qa.

In conclusion, Qa measurements at biweekly intervals failed to improve accuracy in predicting thrombosis when compared with monthly Qa measurements. Whether this was caused by decreases in Qa that were too rapid and brief to be detected with biweekly measurements, or other unidentified factors, is unknown. Failure of grafts to exhibit a gradual decrease in Qa as predicted by the dysfunction hypothesis significantly impairs the effectiveness of graft monitoring programs in preventing thrombosis.

References

1. Besarab A, Frinak S, Zasuwa G. Prospective evaluation of vascular access function: The nephrologist's perspective. Semin Dial (Suppl) 1996; 9:S21-29.
2. NKF-DOQI clinical practice guidelines for vascular access. National Kidney Foundation-Dialysis Outcomes Quality Initiative. Am J Kidney Dis 1997; 30(suppl 3) S150-91.
3. Paulson WD. Prediction of hemodialysis synthetic graft thrombosis: Can we identify factors that impair the validity of the dysfunction hypothesis? [editorial] Am J Kidney Dis 2000; 35:973-75.
4. Neyra NR, Ikizler TA, May RE, et al. Change in blood flow over time predicts vascular access thrombosis. Kidney Int 1998; 54:1714-19.
5. Paulson WD, Ram SJ, Birk CG, Zapczynski M, Martin SR, Work J. Accuracy of decrease in blood flow in predicting hemodialysis synthetic graft thrombosis. Am J Kidney Dis 2000; 35:1089-95.

6. Zaman F, Ram SJ, Dixit A, Work J, Paulson WD. Early hemodialysis graft thrombosis is associated with stenosis at venous anastomosis. J Am Soc Nephrol 1999; 10:223A.
7. Metz CE. Rockit 0.9B Software for Apple Macintosh (Beta Version). Chicago: University of Chicago Deptartment of Radiology; 1997.

DISCUSSION

Moderator:
Mitchell L. Henry, M.D.
Panelist:
Sunanada Ram, Ph.D.

Dr. Henry: If I understand your presentation, your arbitrary cut-off for whether flow decreased or did not decrease was a 20% change. If you plug that into your model with a 10% change or a 15% change how does that change all of your predictive abilities?

Dr. Ram: That is a very good question. Sensitivity has a false positive rate at a variety of thresholds and we can get values of sensitivity and false positive rate using a 10% threshold or a 15% threshold. When we reduce the threshold, we would increase the sensitivity; however, this would be at the cost of high false positive rate. We would be requesting intervention on a larger proportion of grafts.

Discussant: Not being a nephrologist, I guess I am not that familiar with some of these techniques. What is the day to day observer variability in single blood flow measurement? Dialysis patients come in with all states of hydration whether if they are dry or wet and then there are different people who are measuring and you did not say anything about that. I wonder how that might influence some of your observations?

Dr. Ram: There are large amounts of variation in day to day, or at least between the 2 weeks that we have used intervals in blood flow values. Also, blood flow is influenced a great deal by the patients' blood pressure and the blood volume. We have shown previously that we can correct the blood flow value by normalizing to the mean arterial pressure. However, when we do that we decrease the predictive accuracy of Qa in predicting thrombosis.

Discussant: If you look at the ones that clotted and did you compare the reasons for the clot with your progressive decrease in flow as oppose to those who did not have a decrease in flow or were clotted? Did you find that the operative findings were that there was stenosis in the ones without flow changes or was it things look good and it ran well for 6 months thereafter?

Dr. Ram: Well, you are correct. Thromboses can occur due to a variety of reasons. There are grafts with high blood flows that thrombose without showing us a decrease in blood flow before thrombosis. The important point here is that blood flow by itself can not be the sole predictor of thrombosis. The other criteria that would have to be taken into account so that we can increase predictive accuracy is a decrease before thrombosis. It goes without saying that about half the grafts do show us a decrease in blood flow before thrombosis, and blood flow is very valuable in predicting thrombosis in these grafts. We do need to find other criteria for predicting thrombosis in the other set of grafts that do not show predictive decreases.

Discussant: I just want to tell you about our experience at Vanderbilt in Nashville. When we started this program, we studied it on a monthly basis. We found out that on a monthly basis we were not seeing much difference because all the ones that were referred were referred early in the first and second months. Then we started seeing the trend getting better. So we jumped to 3 months and quarterly measurement did not show us any difference compared with the monthly measurement. We used also as a criteria the 25% that has been established in prior studies from Vanderbilt as far as a change for somebody who was at 1200 initially and then going down to 800. These patients were measured again before waiting for 3 months. There is a variation also within the same dialysis treatment in the first 2 hours versus the last 2 hours, to answer your question about the variation.

Dr. Ram: I think there are 2 issues here. Number 1 is the variation in blood flow within a given dialysis session. Now, we have shown earlier, when blood flow measurements are made throughout the 3 or 4 hours of dialysis, we find that there are relatively small changes in blood flow. The change in the patients' mean arterial pressure, however, are large so that it is difficult to standardize hemodynamic readability within the patient and determine that blood flow measurements be made early in dialysis or a given time in dialysis when there is hemodynamic stability. The other point regarding the use of Qa as a predictor of thrombosis. It is true that a decrease in Qa over time, such as 3 months, does increase the risk of thrombosis. However, risk alone is not enough. It is necessary to have a high sensitivity and a low false positive rate for a predictor to be clinically useful. The sensitivity and false positive rate that we have found in our study with monthly monitoring are about the same as was found with the Vanderbilt group, for example with Qa and delta Qa. It is just that our interpretation is slightly different. That interpretation is that half of the thrombosed grafts do not meet those criteria and this is what decreases the predictive accuracy of blood flow as the sole criteria for predicting thromboses.

Discussant: I think to answer the Vanderbilt people, the question isn't that access flow isn't useful. We all know if you set up an access flow base program that you can decrease thrombosis rates in your unit, to some extent. The problem is because of the variability week to week and month to month in flow, if you have a strict protocol, you have such a high false positive rate that you wind up doing a whole series of unnecessary tests because the whole premise of this is to pick up the stenosis that is repairable. I think we need to go back and rethink how much we should get into imaging, and even in the Vanderbilt group study, what predicts outcome is fixing stenoses.

27

PERCUTANEOUS FIBRIN SHEATH STRIPPING VERSUS TRANSCATHETER UROKINASE INFUSION FOR WELL-POSITIONED TUNNELED CENTRAL VENOUS DIALYSIS CATHETERS THAT MALFUNCTION: A PROSPECTIVE RANDOMIZED TRIAL

Richard J. Gray, M.D., Abraham Levitin, M.D., David Buck, M.D., Lisa C. Brown, R.N., Yvonne H. Sparling, M.S., Kathleen A. Jablonski, Ph.D., Amanuel Fessahaye, M.D., and Atul K.Gupta, M.D.

Funded through an unrestricted grant from Abbott Laboratories, North Chicago, IL. This paper was originally presented by Thomas Vesely, M.D., on behalf of Richard Gray, M.D.

The first-line therapy for dialysis catheters with suboptimal flow rates (less than 300 cc/min)[1] that are unresponsive to simple positional maneuvers or port reversal has usually been the instillation of a small quantity of urokinase in the dialysis unit for periods of up to 20 minutes.[2-4] This may be tried several times. Patients with catheters that fail a thrombolytic instillation are typically referred for a transcatheter venogram to confirm satisfactory catheter position and to be evaluated for the presence of a pericatheter fibrin sheath or thrombus.[1] Poorly positioned or kinked catheters are usually treated in a straightforward manner with standard interventional techniques.[4,5]

Pericatheter fibrin sheaths and thrombi have been treated with a variety of methods, such as percutaneous fibrin sheath stripping[4,6-9] and thrombolysis through the dialysis catheter[2,10-12], with return of catheter function for at least 1 dialysis session in most patients. Nevertheless, subsequent patencies after thrombolysis are unknown and the results following percutaneous fibrin sheath stripping have varied widely. These issues led us to conduct a prospective, randomized trial of a 4-hour urokinase infusion compared with percutaneous fibrin sheath stripping. We report here the results of this trial and review the pertinent literature.

Materials and Methods

Between April 30, 1996 and October 28, 1998, 57 patients with 57 poorly functioning dialysis catheters were enrolled into the study under the auspices of the hospital's institutional review board. There were 34 female and 23 male patients with a median age of 60 years (range 26 to 91 years). The study was explained to all patients, and a protocol consent form was signed. Each patient was enrolled only once, even if a new catheter was later inserted at the same or a new puncture site. During the course of the study, 54 other patients were excluded from enrollment for the following reasons: refusal to be stripped before (28 patients) or after (2 patients) randomization, refusal or inability to consent (17 patients), and contraindication to urokinase (7 patients). Risk factors for chronic renal failure included hypertension (23 patients), diabetes mellitus (18 patients), chronic glomerulonephritis (1 patient), systemic lupus erythematosus (1 patient), and multiple myeloma (1 patient). The cause of renal failure was uncertain in the other 15 patients. Ten patients had clinically apparent coronary artery disease, 7 had a history of coronary artery disease and congestive heart failure, and two had a history of congestive heart failure. There were 8 current smokers admitted into the study.

Forty-six catheters had been indwelling for a median 59 days (range 11 to 682 days) at the time of referral for catheter malfunction. Because the study took place at a tertiary referral center, exact indwell times were not known for the other 11 catheters. Vascular access surgeons or interventional radiologists had originally inserted the catheters. Most patients had failed 1 trial of Abbokinase® (Abbott Laboratories, North Chicago, IL) urokinase instillation in the dialysis clinic. Catheter types included the following: 45 PermCath® (Quinton Instrument Company, Bothel, WA), 7 Tesio® (Medcomp, Harleysville, PA), and 5 Hickman® (Bard Access Systems, Salt Lake City, UT) catheters inserted via the right internal jugular vein in 40 patients, right subclavian in 3, left internal jugular in 12, and the left subclavian vein in 2. All catheters had established baseline flow rates greater than or equal to 300 mL/minute[1] for at least 3 dialysis treatments after catheter insertion. Catheter malfunction was defined as a flow rate through 1 or both ports less than 250 cc/minute or a decrease through 1 or both ports greater than 50 mL/minute if the established baseline flow rate was greater than 300 cc/minute. Indications for treatment included blood flows less than 250 cc/minute through both ports (29 cases) and less than 250 cc/minute via the arterial (9 cases) or venous (1 case) port. Also, a flow rate decrease greater than 50 cc/minute below the established baseline flow through both ports (3 cases), a flow rate decrease greater than 50 cc/minute below the established baseline flow through the venous (3 cases) or arterial (1 case) port, and complete occlusion of the arterial (7 cases), venous (2 cases), or both (4 cases) ports were indications for treatment.

All catheters underwent transcatheter digital subtraction venography during very slow hand injections of 5 to 25 cc-iodinated contrast through each port consecutively. Tracking contrast either retrogradely along the catheter or flowing sluggishly away from the catheter tip was considered diagnostic of a pericatheter fibrin sheath. Filling defects were considered diagnostic of pericatheter thrombus. The venographic study was considered normal if contrast flowed immediately away from the catheter tip.

Using these criteria, 79% (45 of 57) transcatheter venograms were abnormal prior to treatment; 61% (35) revealed fibrin sheaths, 7% (4) fibrin sheath and thrombus, and 11% (6) had pericatheter thrombus. None showed large clots around the catheter. The studies were normal in 15.8% (9) and nondiagnostic (due respiratory motion) in 5.3% (3). Based on these contrast studies, the catheter tips were located in the right atrium of 22 patients, bridging the superior vena cava-right atrial junction in 24 patients, and in the superior vena cava above the right atrium in 11 patients. The superior vena cava was normal in 23 patients; it stenosed in 1 patient, and it could not be evaluated in 34 patients. A computer-generated randomization schedule was used to assign patients to the urokinase infusion or stripping group after the transcatheter venogram showed satisfactory catheter position and no mechanical problem such as a kink.

The median catheter indwell time at the time of treatment in the urokinase group (26 catheters) was 68 days (range 14 to 682 days) and in the stripping group (20 catheters), 35 days (range 11 to 306 days); the exact indwell times for the other 11 catheters were not known. The median test did not indicate a significant difference in the known pretreatment indwell times between the groups (P=0.388). The median test compares the proportions in each sample that are less than the combined median using a binomial test (ie, Fisher's exact test) that is sensitive to difference in location. It is the most powerful test for comparing skewed, asymmetrical distributions.

Urokinase infusion. A solution of 250,000 units urokinase dissolved in 250 cc 0.9 normal saline or 5% dextrose was administered at 30 cc/hour via both ports concurrently (60,000 units urokinase/hr total) over 4 hours and 10 minutes. The 4-hour infusion was chosen to facilitate treatment for outpatients. Urokinase was administered to 21 outpatients in either the Interventional Radiology Recovery Room or a 23-hour admission bed and to inpatients (8 patients), usually in their hospital beds. No other procedure medications were administered in this treatment group.

Percutaneous fibrin sheath stripping. Other investigators have described the technique in detail.[4,6-8] Briefly, all procedures were performed from a right (24 cases) or left (4 cases) common femoral access with a 25-mm (11 cases) or 35-mm (17 cases) Amplatz Nitinol snare (MicroVena, Vadnaise Heights, MN). The dialysis catheter was engaged with the snare, which was advanced over the catheter as far as possible, tightened, and pulled off the catheter tip. For Tesio catheters, the 2 catheters were stripped independently. The dialysis catheter hub was aseptically prepared and a guidewire was passed through the catheter to facilitate re-advancement of the snare over the dialysis catheter tip for additional stripping passes.[6] The number of stripping passes was determined at the operator's discretion, which resulted in wide variability in the number of passes performed. Four to 6 passes were made in 2 patients, 7 to 9 passes in 5 patients, 10 to 12 passes in 9 patients, and more than 12 passes in 9 patients. The number of passes was not recorded for 3 procedures. Versed® was administered to 23 patients; 19 of these patients also received fentanyl. One patient was pretreated with intravenous Cefoxitin®. This patient also received

Benadryl® due to a history of hives with iodinated contrast. Outpatients (n=25) were observed for 2 hours and 3 inpatients were transported to their rooms after hemostasis was achieved.

Follow-up. Post-treatment transcatheter contrast studies were performed at the operator's discretion, but the results were not used for patency determinations because clinical function was considered more important. Immediate clinical success was defined as at least 1 successful dialysis session with flow rates above the previously established baseline flow rate. Follow-up flow rates were obtained by the routine weekly review of dialysis clinic records. Primary patency was defined as a flow rate greater than the established baseline flow rate without additional intervention. Secondary patency was defined as a flow rate greater than the established higher baseline flow rate assisted by repeat treatment with the same treatment modality, either stripping or urokinase infusion. Study endpoints included restoration of catheter function by another treatment modality (eg, crossover to urokinase or stripping or catheter exchange), catheter removal for any reason (eg, catheter malfunction, permanent access available, or accidental catheter removal), or patient death. All analyses were performed with the Statistical Analysis Software System (STAT Version 7.0, SAS Institute, Cary, NC 1998). The nonparametric maximum likelihood estimator, Kaplan-Meier, was used to estimate survivor functions, and data was right censored. The difference between survivor functions was tested using the Wilcoxon statistic.

Results

Twenty-eight patients were treated with stripping and 29 patients with urokinase infusion according to the randomization schedule. Plots of the product-limit survival estimates are presented in figure 27-1.

Urokinase group. Thirteen (76%) of 17 transcatheter contrast studies following urokinase infusion were normal; 3 had fibrin sheaths and 1 had pericatheter clot. The other 12 patients were not evaluated angiographically after treatment because either the pretreatment study was normal (4 patients) or the operator chose against the procedure (8 patients).

The initial clinical success rate was 97% (n=28). The 15-, 30-, and 45-day primary patencies were 86% (n=21), 63% (n=13), and 48% (n=9), respectively. The median duration of additional satisfactory catheter function following infusion was 42 days (95% confidence interval for 22 to 364 days). As of this writing, 1 catheter is still being used without further treatment. Endpoints for primary patency included recurrent catheter malfunction treated by repeat urokinase infusion (3 patients), stripping (2 patients), or catheter exchange (5 patients). The other endpoints were catheter removals for recurrent malfunction (6 patients), matured permanent access (7 patients), or terminally ill patient (1 patient). One patient demanded the removal of the catheter and 3 patients died with functioning catheters. Because only 3 patients were retreated with urokinase when the catheter malfunctioned again (operator's discretion), the secondary patency curve would not be significantly different from the primary patency curve.

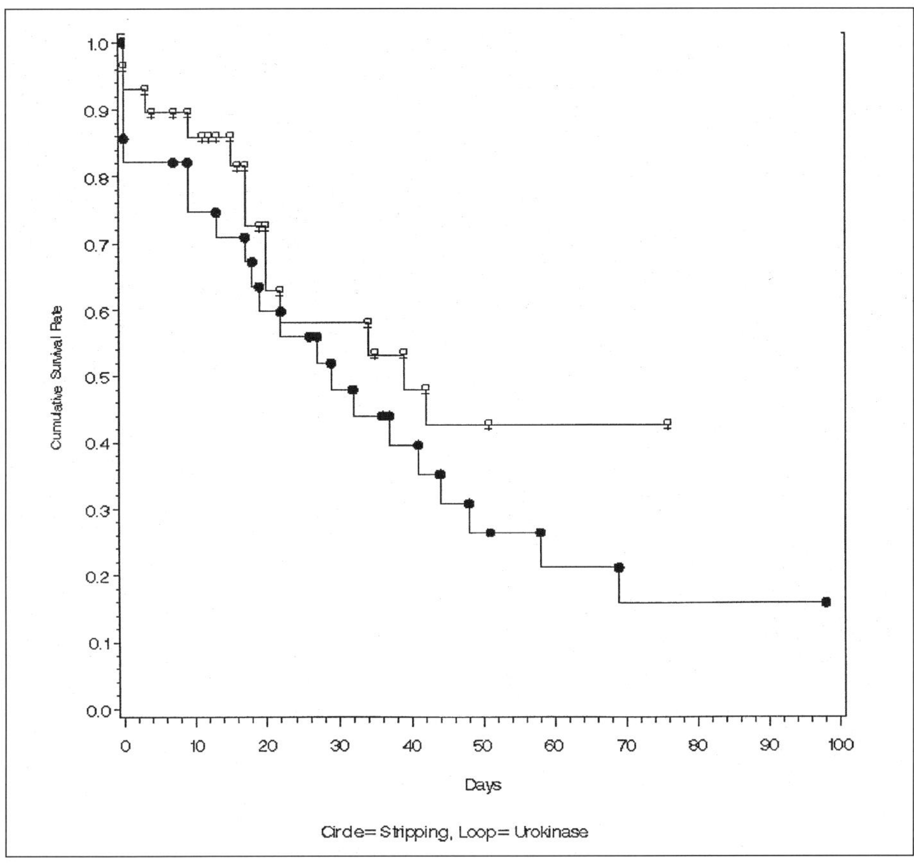

Figure 27-1. Urokinase and Stripping Survival Curves: Time to Primary Patency

Stripping group. Eighty-seven percent (20 of 23) of transcatheter contrast studies following stripping were normal; 1 had a fibrin sheath and 2 had pericatheter clots. The other 5 patients were not evaluated angiographically after treatment because of a normal pretreatment study (2 patients) or the operator chose against it (3 patients).

The initial clinical success rate was 89% (25 of 28). The 15-, 30-, and 45-day primary patencies were 75% (n=20), 52% (n=13), and 35% (n=8), respectively. The median duration of additional satisfactory catheter function following stripping was 32 days (with a 95% confidence interval for 18 to 48 days). As of this writing, 1 catheter is still being used without further treatment.

Endpoints of primary patency included restoration of catheter function by repeat stripping (3 patients), urokinase infusion (4 patients), or catheter exchange (6 patients). Other endpoints included catheter removal for recurrent malfunction (5 patients), or positive blood cultures (1 patient), permanent access (5 patients), transplant (2 patient), and accidental catheter removal (1 patient). Because only 3 patients were retreated by stripping when the catheter malfunctioned again (due to the operator's discretion), the secondary patency curve would not be significantly different from the primary patency curve.

Sample size calculation, interim and final statistical analysis. A sample size of 70 patients (35 in each group) was initially chosen based on an expected difference in immediate success rates between the treatment groups of 15%. The study had a type I error of 5%, and power of 80%. The initial clinical success and patency curves after 57 patients were enrolled were compared to the results obtained during an interim analysis after 44 patients were enrolled.[13] Because there were no notable differences or changes in the trends after the interim analysis and because the 95% confidence bands were broad, we concluded that enrollment of an additional 13 patients to reach the initial goal of 70 patients would not significantly change the final analysis. The study was therefore terminated after 57 patients were enrolled.

The Wilcoxon test indicated that the times to primary patency for the stripping and urokinase groups were not significantly different from each other (chi square=1.41, 1 degree of freedom, P =0.236).

Complications. There were 2 deaths in the urokinase group, 1 at 2 weeks and another at 1 month after the infusion. Both deaths were attributed to underlying disease and considered to be unrelated to the treatment. In the stripping group, 1 patient developed fever and positive blood cultures 5 weeks after treatment. Another patient presented with a symptomatic pericatheter innominate thrombosis necessitating catheter removal within days after the catheter had been unsuccessfully stripped.

Discussion

Central venous dialysis catheter malfunction is a serious problem necessitating removal of up to 28% of dialysis catheters because they do not function.[2,10,11,14-17] Catheters are removed for malfunction far more frequently than for symptomatic pericatheter thrombus and at a frequency similar to removal for infection (see table 27-1).[2,10,11,14-17] Dialysis catheter malfunction not requiring removal is extremely common, affecting 3% to 10% of all dialysis sessions,[2,16] and 87% of all catheters at some time prior to removal.[4] Until the removal of urokinase from the market by the Food and Drug Administration, simple urokinase instillation at the dialysis clinic restored immediate function to 74% to 81%[2,4] of dialysis catheters. Although this measure was performed blindly and its durability is unknown, it was sufficiently effective to be the appropriate first-line therapy1 because it was considered safe and

Table 27-1. Dialysis Catheter Removal.

Investigator	Catheters	Malfunction*	Infection	C.V. Thrombosis
McDowell[14]	172	5%	5%	0%
Cappello[15]	107	5%	5%	0%
Moss[2]	168	7%	8%	0%
Gibson[16]	94	9%	28%	1.6%
Schwartz[17]	118	17%	19%	0%
Lund[11]	222	28%	11%	1.2%
Trerotola[10]	250	19%	7%	0%
Duszak[18]	77	—	13%	0%

*Variable definitions

C.V. = central vein

inexpensive, and it expediently allowed dialysis to resume after a minimal delay during the same scheduled dialysis session.

Catheters that fail postural maneuvers, port reversal, and urokinase instillation can be malpositioned or kinked. Mechanical problems, however, are generally much less common than pericatheter fibrin sheath or clot formation[4,6,7,10] (see table 27-2) unless the catheter has been recently inserted. Malfunction in well-positioned catheters is typically due to the presence of a pericatheter fibrin sheath or a small amount of thrombus about the catheter tip.[4,6,7,10,18] Pericatheter fibrin sheath formation has been shown in a human autopsy study[19] to occur as early as 24 hours following placement and is thought to occur in 80% to 100% of central venous catheters within 2 to 7 days after insertion.[19-21] Fibrin sheaths propagate from the venous insertion site and from the tip toward the center of the catheter and can persist for weeks even after the catheter is removed.[19] When the pericatheter sheath and/or associated thrombus infringe on the functional endhole(s) of the catheter, decreased dialysis flow rates result.

Table 27-2. **Etiology of catheter malfunction.***

Investigator	No.	Episodes	Mechanical	Sheath/Clot
Crain[6]	24	44	4	40
Suhocki[4]	—	42	4	38
Rockall[7]	29	31	7	24
Trerotola[10]	63	63	23	40

* – most S/P failed urokinase instillation

No. – number of Catheters

Fibrin sheaths can be demonstrated with intravascular ultrasound[22] but are usually diagnosed on transcatheter venographic studies with[21] or without[4,6,8,9] pulling the catheter back prior to contrast injection. Since the sensitivity of transcatheter venography for the detection of fibrin sheaths is unknown, we included all malfunctioning, well-positioned catheters in this study, whether a fibrin sheath was detected on transcatheter venography or not. Regarding venographic technique, we believe that it is very important to inject contrast through the catheter slowly to avoid creating a hole in the fibrin sheath near the catheter tip. An iatrogenic fenestration from rapid contrast (or saline) injection can hinder angiographic diagnosis of the fibrin sheath because contrast can pass preferentially through the fenestration in the sheath, rather than retrogradely around the catheter. Furthermore, a subsequently administered transcatheter thrombolytic agent will also run through the iatrogenic fenestration instead of bathing the catheter from the tip proximally to the nearest naturally occurring fenestration. This will decrease the total surface area of the fibrin sheath exposed to the agent.

The results of studies reporting thrombolysis[2,10-12], including ours, are presented in table 27-3. The immediate success rates, defined as restoration of satisfactory function for at least 1 dialysis session, range from 55% to 97%. One investigator bolused a total of 250,000 units of concentrated urokinase into both ports and reported that this "nearly always"[12] worked for restoring immediate catheter function. Our study confirms the high rates of immediate functional restoration reported in prior studies. These treatments appear to be very safe; there were no bleeding complications

Table 27-3. **Thrombolytic infusion.**

Investigator	No.	Agent/Dose	Clinical Success	Additional Patency
Moss[2]	58	Streptokinase (12 hours)	97%	____
Uldall[12]	103	Urokinase (250,000 U bolus)	"nearly always"	____
Lund[11]	39	Urokinase (250,000 U/6 hrs)	79.5%	____
Trerotola[10]	11	Urokinase (250,000 U/6 hrs)	55%	31 days (mean)
Gray (current study)	29	Urokinase (250,000 U/4 hrs)	97%	48% at 45 days (primary)

attributed to the thrombolytic agent in any of these studies. Trerotola et al.[10] reported a 31 day mean period of additional function in their very small group of patients; otherwise, the durability of these treatments has not been previously studied. Our cumulative patencies after transcatheter thrombolytic infusion indicate that approximately half (48%) of treated catheters will maintain function for an additional 45 days after treatment. Although modest, this additional period of function will allow permanent access creation and maturation in many patients.

The investigators [4,6-9] in table 27-4 have reported the results of pericatheter fibrin sheath stripping. The initial success rates in these series, including ours, are generally high, and our overall complication rate was 6% (16 of 253). We found a modest durability, with 35% of catheters maintaining primary patency for 45 days. On the contrary, Brady et al.[9] and Crain et al.[6] reported 3 month primary patencies of 63% and 45%, respectively. Crain also used multiple strippings and optimistically reported that 81% of the treated catheters functioned satisfactorily for at least 1 year following the initial catheter insertion. Similarly, Suhocki et al.[4] emphasized that most treated catheters remained functional for the intended duration of use. Rockall et al.[7] were somewhat less optimistic, reporting a 61% (19 of 31) initial return of function. Their experience, however, illustrated the importance of evaluating for catheter malposition or kinks prior to percutaneous treatment. Contrary to the promising results of these 4 studies, Haskall et al.[8] experienced dismal patencies, with 92% (22 of 24) of catheters returning to the pre-treatment blood-liter process rate by the fifth post-stripping dialysis session. As a result, this group completely abandoned the stripping procedure.

Table 27-4. **Fibrin sheath stripping**

Investigator	No.	Clinical Success*	Additional Patency
Crain[6]	40	98%	45% at 3 months (primary)
Haskal[8]	24	92%	8% (2/24) at 2 weeks
Suhocki[4]	38	95%	3 months (mean)
Rockall[7]	31	61%	4.25 months (median)
Brady[9]	91	96%	51% at 3 months (primary)
Gray (current study)	28	89%	35% at 45 days (primary)

No. – number of catheters

* – at least one successful dialysis using variable criteria for success

Our results showed no statistically significant difference between a 4-hour urokinase infusion and fibrin sheath stripping for immediate restoration of catheter function and for maintenance of long-term patency. Although our results did not demonstrate a difference, a trend favoring urokinase is seen when looking at the Kaplan-Meier derived interval patencies, as well as the median time period of additional catheter function in both groups. Even if stripping and urokinase infusion have similar results, a thrombolytic infusion is our preferred therapy for several reasons. First, the patients prefer it. Our greatest difficulty enrolling an otherwise eligible patient for the study was patient refusal to undergo stripping after hearing about the lysis and stripping options. Second, transcatheter infusion is noninvasive, whereas stripping requires a venous puncture. Third, although stripping has been associated with potentially disastrous complications, transcatheter administration of thrombolytics has not.[2,10-12] One of the centers listed in table 27-4 reported an asymptomatic common femoral puncture site thrombus,[6] and another center[4] later published a case report of a septic pulmonary embolus caused by stripping.[23] Furthermore, 1 of our patients presented with a symptomatic pericatheter innominate vein thrombosis after an attempted stripping. For all of these reasons, thrombolysis is our preferred treatment compared with stripping.

After poor results for stripping had been demonstrated at their institution[8], Duszak et al.[18] began changing catheters through the same tract over a guidewire, while making an attempt to position the catheter tip beyond or outside the confines of the fibrin sheath. This was done either by repositioning the tip more centrally, or by manipulating a guidewire and the catheter tip through a fenestration in the fibrin sheath to a position outside of the sheath. They compared these catheter exchanges in a nonrandomized fashion with *de novo* catheter placement in the same patient population and found no significant differences in catheter patency or complication rates, including infections. Whether a catheter exchange or a thrombolytic infusion is preferable remains undetermined. As currently reimbursed by Medicare, a single catheter exchange is much less costly than an infusion. Catheter exchange over a guidewire spares the use of a vein[18] and usually allows a more expedient return to dialysis than an infusion. Nevertheless, the change requires an invasive procedure that can be complicated by prolonged pericatheter tract oozing.[18] Furthermore, patients would probably prefer a thrombolytic infusion because of its noninvasive nature.

In conclusion, our study demonstrated that urokinase infusion and stripping both allowed a reasonable period of additional function for well-positioned central dialysis catheters with poor flow rates. Unfortunately, there is little reported experience with other thrombolytic agents for catheter clearance. We are beginning a catheter clearance feasibility study to determine the effectiveness and safety of tissue plasminogen activator. Conceptually, tissue plasminogen activator administered in dose-equivalent infusions to urokinase should be similar in effectiveness and safety and may be faster than urokinase infusions. Although we did not detect a significant difference in outcome between urokinase and stripping, we prefer a thrombolytic infusion because it is noninvasive, preferred by patients, and safer. We reserve stripping for rare cases in which thrombolytic infusion fails or is contraindicated and catheter exchange or replacement cannot be performed.

Acknowledgements

The authors thank Mrs. Nancy Carnes for editorial assistance.

References

1. Schwab S, Besarab A, Beathard G, et al. NKF-DOQI clinical practice guidelines for vascular access. New York: National Kidney Foundation; 1997.
2. Moss AH, Vasilakis C, Holley JL, Foulks CJ, Pillai K, McDowell DE. Use of a silicone dual-lumen catheter with a dacron cuff as a long-term vascular access for hemodialysis patients. Am J Kidney Dis 1990; 26:211-15.
3. Schwab SJ, Buller GL, McCann RL, Bollinger RR, Stickel DL. Prospective evaluation of a dacron cuffed hemodialysis catheter for prolonged use. Am J Kidney Dis 1988; 11:166-69.
4. Suhocki PV, Conlon PJ Jr, Knelson MH, Harland R, Schwab SJ. Silastic cuffed catheters for hemodialysis vascular access: Thrombolytic and mechanical correction of malfunction. Am J Kidney Dis 1996; 28:379-86.
5. Egglin TKP, Rosenblatt M, Dickey KW, Houston JP, Pollak JS. Replacement of accidentally removed tunneled venous catheters through existing subcutaneous tracts. J Vasc Interv Radiol 1997; 8:197-202.
6. Crain MR, Mewissen MW, Ostrowski GJ, Paz-Fumagalli R, Beres RA, Wertz RA. Fibrin sleeve stripping for salvage of failing hemodialysis catheters: Technique and initial results. Radiology 1996; 198:41-44.
7. Rockall AG, Harris A, Wetton CW, Taube D, Gedroyc W, Al-Kutoubi MA. Stripping of failing haemodialysis catheters using the Amplatz gooseneck snare. Clin Radiol 1997; 52:616-20.
8. Haskal ZJ, Leen VH, Thomas-Hawkins C, Shlansky-Goldberg RD, Baum RA, Soulen MC. Transvenous removal of fibrin sheaths from tunneled hemodialysis catheters. J Vasc Interv Radiol 1996; 7:513-17.
9. Brady PS, Spence LD, Levitin A, Mickolich CT, Dolmatch BL. Efficacy of percutaneous fibrin sheath stripping in restoring patency of tunneled hemodialysis catheters. Am J Roentgenol 1999; 173:1023-27.
10. Trerotola SO, Johnson MS, Harris VJ, et al. Outcome of tunneled hemodialysis catheters placed via the right internal jugular vein by interventional radiologists. Radiology 1997; 203:489-95.
11. Lund GB, Trerotola SO, Scheel PF Jr, et al. Outcome of tunneled hemodialysis catheters placed by radiologists. Radiology 1996; 198:467-72.
12. Uldall R, Besley ME, Thomas A, Salter S, Nuezca LA, Vas M. Maintaining the patency of double-lumen silastic jugular catheters for haemodialysis. Int J Artif Organs 1993; 16:37-40.
13. Gray RJ, Fessahaye A, Gupta A, et al. Percutaneous fibrin sheath stripping versus Urokinase for malfunctioning central dialysis catheters [abstract]. J Vasc Interv Radiol 1998; 9:164.
14. McDowell DE, Moss AH, Vasilakis C, Bell R, Pillai L. Percutaneously placed dual-lumen silicone catheters for long-term hemodialysis. Am Surg 1993; 59:569-73.

15. Cappello M, DePauw L, Bastin G, et al. Central venous access for haemodialysis using the Hickman catheter. Nephrol Dial Transplant 1989; 4:988-92.
16. Gibson SP, Mosquera D. Five years experience with the Quinton Permcath for vascular access. Nephrol Dial Transplant 1991; 6:269-74.
17. Schwartz RD, Messana JM, Boyer CJ, et al. Successful use of cuffed central venous hemodialysis catheters inserted percutaneously. J Am Soc Nephrol 1994; 4:1719-25.
18. Duszak R Jr, Haskal ZJ, Thomas-Hawkins C, et al. Replacement of failing tunneled hemodialysis catheters through pre-existing subcutaneous tunnels: A comparison of catheter function and infection rates for de novo placements and over-the-wire exchanges. J Vasc Interv Radiol 1998; 9:321-27.
19. Hoshal VL Jr, Ause RG, Hoskins PA. Fibrin sleeve formation on indwelling subclavian central venous catheters. Arch Surg 1971; 102:353-358.
20. Ahmed N, Payne RF. Thrombosis after central venous cannulation. Med J Aust 1976; 1:217-20.
21. Brismar BO, Hardstedt C, Jacobson S. Diagnosis of thrombosis by catheter phlebography after prolonged central venous catheterization. Ann Surg 1981; 194:779-83.
22. Bolz K-D, Fjermeros G, Wideroe TE, Hatlinghus S. Catheter malfunction and thrombus formation on double-lumen hemodialysis catheters: An intravascular ultrasonographic study. Am J Kidney Dis 1995; 25:597-602.
23. Winn MP, McDermott VG, Schwab SJ, Conlon PJ. Dialysis catheter 'fibrin-sheath stripping': A cautionary tale! Nephrol Dial Transplant 1997; 12:1048-50.

DISCUSSION

Panelist:
Thomas M. Vesely, M.D.

Discussant: A philosophical question. Why would anyone want to do a procedure that involves a $600 snare or $500 worth of urokinase versus just exchanging the catheter, which would have a fraction of the cost?

Dr. Vesley: From a radiologist point of view, the next talk will be interesting. My point is that there are other methods that can be used to fix these sorts of things. The fibrinolytic infusion is probably cheaper, as the stripping procedure uses a $600 snare and exchanging the catheter, although the catheter is only a couple hundred bucks. I have to charge by my coding standards about the same. My stripping procedure costs more money. There is no question about that and you will also have to stick a femoral stick. So I personally do not do stripping. I am not a fan of stripping at all. I have rarely done it. I am a strong proponent of catheter exchange. But the reality is a catheter replacement is not nearly as cheap as it should be because of the fact that I get the bill for so much money for a really easy procedure and that happens to be the coding thing. I can change a catheter so fast and it is so easy to do but yet the bill for it is astounding. So when you actually talk about these procedures with expensive equipment and urokinase infusions, the costs are unfortunately similar. But I guess that is what we have to work on.

Discussant: I was just going to explain that same point. The cost of changing the catheter is far in excess of just the cost of the catheters because you have your radiology, your fluoroscopy charges, and particularly with these tunnel cuff catheters, they are small but of significant discomfort to the patient in removing this and putting a new 1 in. Another point, although we probably seldom think about it, in our institution we have unfortunately seen very significant morbidity and mortality even associated with just a simple catheter change. So it is not something to be taken likely or regarded as an inconsequential procedure. I think if you can clean them out with some urokinase that the patient is benefited.

Discussant: I would just reinforce the point that the catheter changes are not that benign particularly for the patient. In 2 years, when we come back hopefully we will be talking about how to salvage dialysis ports. They will not be quite as easy to change and we have used both catheter stripping as well as thrombolytic infusion recently salvaging ports.

Dr. Vesley: In my patient population, when a catheter is dysfunctional, we do a catheter angiogram to look for fibrin sheaths. But in my particular patient population, I rarely find the fibrin sheath. We usually use multi-side hole catheters and it is usually that the end hole is occluded and multiple side holes are occluded but just 1 or 2 side holes left open. That is our most common finding but we do not find fibrin sheaths that often. We bury our catheters into the right atrium, maybe that is what it is.

Discussant: I wonder if anybody has an experience with TPA, which is much cheaper?

Dr. Vesley: It is only cheaper if you get your pharmacist to divide the vile into the appropriate dose. It is the standard way to do it.

Discussant: I am somewhat concerned about people talking about mortality rates of catheter exchange. I have never heard of anyone dying from 1, but apparently that is occurring. I am also somewhat concerned about people talking about the patient discomfort from a catheter exchange in comparison to using a snare to stripping a sheath. That does not make a lot of sense to me.

Discussant: There is at least one case reported, and I believe it is a nephrology literature, of air embolism following catheter removal. It is not far fetched to believe that in a fellow's hands or a resident's hands who may be doing this you could get an air embolism following catheter exchange. It is possible but it is not probable.

Discussant: Somebody was asking about the experience with TPA as opposed to urokinase. I was a little surprised to be sitting here because in Canada we are no longer allowed to use urokinase.

Dr. Vesley: Oh no, we have not had urokinase available for over a year. So we are in the same boat.

Discussant: The only other experience I just wanted to share was contrary to what you say and not seeing very many sheaths. We see quite a lot of sheaths. One of the problems that we have with simple catheter exchange is especially if you are re-wiring to re-insert. Sometimes, and not uncommonly, you can put that new catheter exchange right back into the sheath that was existing and have a similar problem.

Dr. Vesley: That would be doing that technique inappropriately. You have to assume that that is what is happening. It is fairly easy to break up that sheath or re-route the new catheter outside that sheath. I am actually fascinated by the fact that people like yourself report a high incidence of fibrin sheath where as yet in my experience I hardly ever find it. Now you can fault me for saying I am a lousy radiologist and I am not looking for it correctly, but honestly we do but I do not know why I don't find them.

SECTION VII

28

OUTCOMES IN DIALYSIS VASCULAR ACCESS SURGERY: EFFECT OF HUMAN IMMUNODEFICIENCY VIRUS

Jeffrey A. Hertz, M.D., Henry C. Veldenz, M.D., F.A.C.S., James W. Dennis, M.D., and Keelee J. MacPhee, M.D.

Patients infected with human immunodeficiency virus (HIV) who subsequently develop acquired immune deficiency syndrome (AIDS) are living with their disease for longer periods of time.[1] As a result, complications of the disease are more prevalent. Included among the sequelae of the disease is HIV nephropathy, which progresses to renal failure in a significant portion of the HIV-positive population.[2] Decline in kidney function is 1 of many causes of end-stage renal disease (ESRD) that leads to the need for dialysis.

Despite continual progress in the creation of dialysis access, there is still significant morbidity associated with dialysis. Surgical placement of an indwelling venous catheter, an arteriovenous graft (AVG), an arteriovenous fistula (AVF), or a peritoneal dialysis catheter provides access for ESRD treatment. However, the patient who receives these access devises is at risk of developing serious complications (bleeding, graft infection, and peritonitis) as a result of their use. Access revisions are often needed because of malfunctions (such as thrombosis of AVGs) or infections, but these risks are not well characterized in the HIV-positive population. Despite an increasing experience with dialysis in HIV-positive patients, few data are available regarding the impact of HIV on dialysis complication and mortality. This study collected data on this population in terms of vascular access to better characterize this situation.

Materials and Methods

The medical records for all patients (N= 423) treated at a single dialysis center from July 1993 through January 1999 were reviewed. There were 101 patients lost to follow-up during the study period, due to transplantation or transfer to another dialysis facility. Dialysis records were reviewed for access procedures performed (AVG, AVF, peritoneal dialysis catheter, or indwelling vascular catheter), modes of dialysis, conversion rates between modes, access-related infections (graft infection, peritonitis, wound infection, or line infection), number of access revisions, and incidence of mortality. Infections that could not be attributed to dialysis access were not included in our analysis. Many patients experienced multiple modes of dialysis over the study period. Patients were grouped based on the mode of dialysis at the completion of the follow-up period, with either hemodialysis (HD) or peritoneal dialysis (PD) as the primary mode.

HIV status was determined by a positive Western blot, PCR-detected HIV levels, or CD4 T-cell suppression with clinical immunodeficiency. The HIV-negative group included all patients who were not tested or who did not meet the above criteria for HIV. Survival data were analyzed with Kaplan-Meier Analysis and log rank testing. Other outcomes were analyzed with either chi-square or Student *t*-test, with P<0.05 accepted as significant.

Results

There were a total of 423 patients in the study group. The HIV-positive and HIV-negative groups consisted of 36 and 387 patients, respectively. There were no significant differences in patient demographics between the 2 groups, except for patient age. The mean age for patients with HIV was 41 and for patients without HIV was 55. Overall survival for the HIV-positive and HIV-negative groups was 15.3 ± 2.2 months and 29.6 ± 1.1 months, respectively (P<0.001). Mortality was 79% for HIV-positive patients and 44% over the study period (P=0.001). These results are shown in table 28-1. Life-table analysis of patient survival for the 2 groups is summarized in figure 28-1.

While many patients experienced multiple modes of dialysis, patients were categorized according to the primary mode. Of the patients undergoing hemodialysis as the primary mode of dialysis, there were 24 HIV-positive and 295 HIV-negative patients. For those patients who were not lost to follow-up through either transplantation or facility transfer, mean survival times were 15.1 ± 2.4 months and 29.1 ± 1.1 months for the HIV-positive and HIV-negative groups, respectively (P<0.001). Similarly, there were 12 HIV-positive patients and 92 HIV-negative patients who experienced PD as their primary mode. Mean survival times for the 2 groups were 13.7 (2.8 months and 35.0 (2.3 months, for the HIV-positive and HIV-negative groups, respectively (P<0.001). These survival times are shown in tables 28-2 and 28-3.

Access mode (HD versus PD) conversion was similar between the 2 groups (18% for HIV-positive patients and 19% for HIV-negative patients, P not significant).

Table 28-1. Mortality data.

HIV Status	Mean Age (years)	Mortality (%)	Overall Survival (Months (SEM)
HIV-positive (n=36)	41	79	15.3 ± 2.2
HIV-negative (n=387)	55	44	29.6 ± 1.1
P Value	<0.001	<0.001	<0.001

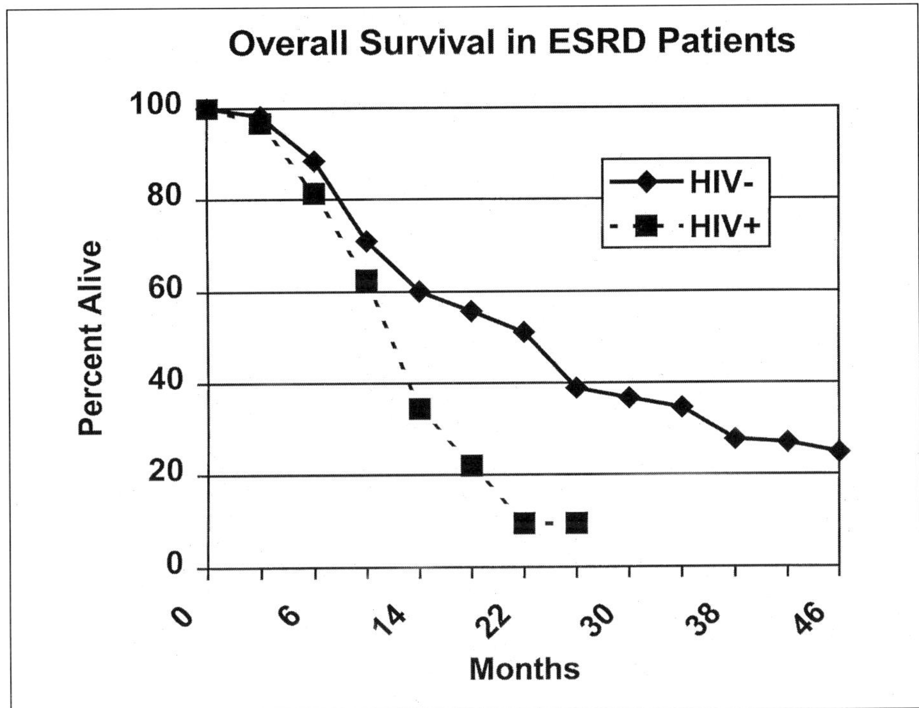

Figure 28-1: Life-Table Analysis.

Revision of access was also similar between the 2 groups (72% for HIV-positive patients and 64% for HIV-negative patients, P not significant). In addition, the use of either an AVG or autogenous fistula for HD in patients who were HIV-positive did not affect the rates of infection, mode conversion, or revision. This was also the case among patients without HIV infection.

Infectious complications were greater among patients with HIV infection at the end of follow-up. Eight (24%) of 33 patients with HIV developed infections, while 20 (7%) of 289 of patients without HIV had infectious complications (P<0.005). The organisms identified were similar between the 2 groups, primarily staphylococci (HD and PD infections) and gram-negative rods (PD infections). *Candida* peritonitis was also detected in PD patients in both groups. Opportunistic organisms did not account for any dialysis-related infectious complications. Dialysis access complications are summarized in table 28-4.

Table 28-2. **Hemodialysis as primary mode.**

Status	Survival (Months ± SEM)
HIV-positive	
(n=24)	15.1 ± 2.4
HIV-negative	
(n=295)	29.1 ± 1.3
P Value	<0.001

Table 28-3. **Peritoneal dialysis as primary mode.**

Status	Survival (Months ± SEM)
HIV-positive	
(n=12)	13.7 ± 2.8
HIV-negative	
(n=92)	35.0 ± 2.3
P Value	<0.001

Table 28-4. **Dialysis access complications.**

Status	Access Revisions (%)	Access Mode Conversions (%)	Infections (%)
HIV-positive	72	18	23
HIV-negative	64	19	7
P value	Not statistically significant	Not statistically significant	<0.005

Discussion

The prevalence of HIV infection in dialysis units has been estimated to be 1% to 2% in the early 1990s to as high as 12% to 23% in some series.[2-5] Understanding the problems associated with dialysis is especially important in this patient population, as they may be more likely to have problems tolerating dialysis-related difficulties, because of their immunosuppressed state. However, the morbidity and mortality in HIV-positive patients requiring dialysis, as compared with the non-HIV infected dialysis patients, is poorly understood.

HIV-positive patients tend to present to dialysis centers at a younger age than HIV-negative patients and their lifespan from the onset of dialysis is shorter than HIV-negative patients.[3-5] HIV-positive patients at our institution were younger than their HIV-negative counterparts by an average of 14 years. The survival of HIV-positive patients was also markedly less than in those patients who were HIV-negative, approximately 15 months versus 30 months. In addition to the many other causative factors that may contribute to their need for dialysis, these patients also suffer from HIV nephropathy, which by itself can result in renal failure.[6] Most patients who acquire HIV are in their 20s or 30s.[1] The onset of dialysis in HIV-positive patients would therefore occur approximately 10 to 15 years after infection with HIV.

It has previously been reported that the decreased survival time in HIV-positive patients is independent of the method of dialysis.[4] These results are confirmed by the current study. HIV-positive patients had similar survival times in both the HD and PD groups. The limited survival time after the onset of dialysis in HIV-positive patients suggested that the need for dialysis in this patient population is probably a contributing factor in their death. The shorter lifespan after the onset of dialysis for HIV-positive patients is likely due to infectious complications associated with their immunodeficiency. The method of dialysis, however, does not have an effect on patients' shorter survival time.

HIV status does not appear to have an effect on the success of dialysis. Hemodialysis and peritoneal dialysis were equally effective in the management of renal failure in HIV-positive patients. Revisions of AVGs, AVFs, or PD catheters were similar between the HIV-positive and HIV-negative patients. There were also no differences in the rates of conversion from AVFs to AVGs and conversion between HD and PD whether or not patients were infected with HIV.

Infectious complications have been previously investigated in HIV-positive patients undergoing minor surgical procedures.[7] It was noted that HIV-positive patients have an increased rate of surgical wound infection, so placement of AVGs, PD catheters, and performance of AVFs place HIV-positive patients at an immediate risk of infection. Also, HIV-positive patients are at further risk of infection due to the presence of prosthetic material, in the form of polytetrafluoroethylene (PTFE) grafts, PD catheters, or indwelling venous dialysis access catheters. Dialysis-related infection rates in patients with AIDS undergoing hemodialysis have been reported to be as high as 43% in1study, and intravenous drug use was a factor in those patients devleloping infections.[2,3,8] Another study found that 100% of the HIV-positive patients treated with PD developed peritonitis.[4] Our HIV-positive patient population had an overall infection rate of 23%, which was markedly greater than HIV-negative patients, who had an infection rate of 7%. Half of the infectious complications identified in our HIV-positive patients were in patients undergoing multiple modes of dialysis.

HIV-positive patients, because of their immunosuppressed state, are at risk for opportunistic infections. However, it has been shown in previous studies and the current study that the dialysis-related infectious complications seen in HIV-positive patients are with the same organisms found in HIV-negative patients receiving dialysis.[4,8,9] Staphylococci and gram-negative rods in HD and PD, respectively, were the most commonly observed organisms.

In conclusion, ESRD with HIV are younger and have a significantly increased access-related infection and mortality rate compared with patients without HIV, independent of dialysis access method. Further studies may elucidate the reasons for these differences. Hemodialysis and peritoneal dialysis are comparable methods of dialysis for HIV-positive patients. Currently, the use of an autogenous fistula is preferred in HIV-positive patients, as they are preferred with HIV-negative patients receiving hemodialysis. Further studies are needed to delineate the durability and potential benefits of PTFE over autogenous fistulae in hemodialysis access in HIV-positive patients.

References

1. Center for Disease Control and Prevention: National Center for HIV, STD and TB Prevention-Divisions of HIV/AIDS Prevention. HIV/AIDS Surveillance Report 1999; 11(1).
2. Curi MA, Pappas PJ, Silva MB Jr, et al. Hemodialysis access: Influence of the human immunodeficiency virus on patency and infection rates. J Vasc Surg 1999; 29:608-16.
3. Brock JS, Sussman M, Wamsley M, et al. The influence of human immunodeficiency virus infection and intravenous drug abuse on complications of hemodialysis access surgery. J Vasc Surg 1992; 16:904-12.
4. Kimmel PL, Umana WO, Simmens SJ, et al. Continuous ambulatory peritoneal dialysis and survival of HIV infected patients with end-stage renal disease. Kidney Int 1993; 44:373-78.
5. Perinbasekar S, Brod-Miller C, Pal S, Mattana J. Predictors of survival in HIV-infected patients on hemodialysis. Am J Nephrol 1996; 16:280-86.
6. Murthy BVR, Pereira BJG. A 1990s perspective of hepatitis C, human immunodeficiency virus, and tuberculosis infections in dialysis patients. Semin Nephrol 1997; 17:46-63.
7. Emparan C, Iturburu IM, Portugal V, et al. Infective complications after minor operations in patients infected with HIV: Role of CD4 lymphocytes in prognosis. Eur J Surg 1995; 161:21-23.
8. Nannery WM, Stoldt HS, Fares LG II. Hemodialysis access operations performed upon patients with human immunodeficiency virus. Surg Gynecol Obstet 1991; 173:387-90.
9. Tebben JA, Rigsby MO, Selwyn PA, et al. Outcome of HIV infected patients in continuous ambulatory peritoneal dialysis. Kidney Int 1993; 44:191-98.

DISCUSSION

Panelists:
Henry C. Veldenz, M.D.
Jeffrey A. Hertz, M.D.

Discussant: Did you correlate the patients who did have infection with absolute CD4 counts?

Dr. Hertz: No, we did not. We did not have the data on everybody, and the infections and timing with their most recent CD4 counts were difficult to determine.

Discussant: What percent of these HIV patients had a graft versus a venous catheter?

Dr. Hertz: Several of the patients had combined modes, and either had grafts and ultimately had peritoneal dialysis, or ultimately had catheters, or vice versa. It was difficult to determine which patients had only 1 mode versus multiple modes and to really categorize their infections just based on that. Patients with multiple modes overall did have more infectious complications.

Discussant: Just out of curiosity, were there any needles stick exposures during the multiple operations the patients had?

Dr. Hertz: None that were reported, no. That certainly is a consideration in terms of choosing which method you are going to offer your patients.

29

THE ADVANTAGES OF FEMORAL CATHETERS FOR HEMODIALYSIS

Peter Dejanov, M.D., Angel Oncevski, M.D., and Vesna Gerasimovska, M.D.

In hemodialysis units, the use of central venous catheters has been increasing because of the relative ease of their use. Catheters do not need to mature, and there is no need for surgery or a puncture. Also, these units feature good blood flow and are easily inserted into patients at bedside.

The catheters are used in emergency situations, such as acute renal failure or episodes of hyperkalemia, and in cases of acute access complication. They can also be used while clinicians are waiting for an arteriovenous fistula (AVF) to become functional. In addition, these units are used for permanent access when patients have exhausted all subcutaneous blood access sites and are not candidates for peritoneal dialysis, or when patients have a short life expectancy due to cancer, advanced age, or other factors.

Different materials are available for central venous catheters. They can be stiff or soft, and with single or dual lumen. In addition, central venous catheters can be inserted surgically or percutaneously, as cuffed or uncuffed catheters. Several sites, such as femoral, subclavian, or jugular veins, may be used for insertion. Femoral vein catheterization in hemodialysis is not considered a desirable option for either temporary or long-term vascular access.

Modern femoral catheters are made of materials that are more flexible and biocompatible than earlier catheters, so they cause less trauma and are less prone to the problems of infection and thrombosis than in the past. Such devices can remain in place for a long time, and offer excellent safety without immobilization or even hospitalization of the patients, thus decreasing treatment costs. The success of catheter placement relies on an educated staff that is able to control infections through rigorous maintenance of the catheters.

Material and Methods

Different types of catheters have been used during a 25-year period of cannulation in the Department of Nephrology Vascular Access Unit of Skopje, Macedonia. During the past few years, we have mostly used the Gam-Cath catheter.

During the past 25 years, 4964 cannulations were performed in our unit. Of these, 4411 were femoral cannulations (4312 temporary access catheters and 99 tunneled catheters). Tunneled catheters were able to provide permanent access in 2 situations, by way of 1 straight modification (from the puncture site in the inguinal region to the knee) and 1 loop modification (from the puncture site in the inguinal region to the abdominal wall).

The distribution of femoral, subclavian, and jugular cannulations is presented in table 29-1. The Seldinger technique was used in all cannulation procedures, and maintenance of the catheters was performed after each hemodialysis session.

Table 29-1. Distribution of catheters over a 25-year period.

Catheter type	Temporary	Permanent	Total (%)
Femoral	4312	99	4411 (88.86)
Subclavian	287	123	410 (8.26)
Jugular	95	48	143 (2.88)
Total (%)	4694 (94.56)	270 (5.44)	4964 (100)

Results

The complication rates of femoral/subclavian cannulation procedures for the period from 1985 to 1992 are shown in table 29-2. The complication rates over a period of 10 years are presented in table 29-3. Table 29-4 shows the presence of bacteria from routinely analyzed catheter tips in surgeries on 102 patients with 105 cannulations (84 femoral, 21 subclavian), from 1996 to 1997. Duration of catheters placed for femoral and subclavian catheterizations between January 1997 and June 1998 for 200 patients with 228 cannulations (188 femoral and 40 subclavian) is shown in table 29-5. Table 29-6 shows the outcomes for femoral or subclavian cannulation sugeries performed from January 1997 to June 1998, on 200 patients with 228 cannulations. Table 29-7 presents the outcomes for femoral catheters performed on 97 patients from January 1998 to December 1998. Detailed characteristics for proved catheter-related bacteriaemia (CRB) are presented on table 29-8. Table 29-9 shows the results of efforts to increase femoral cannulations on an outpatient basis.

Table 29-2. **Complication rates for femoral and subclavian cannulations between 1985 and 1992.**

Femoral cannulation n=1621	Number	%	Subclavian cannulation n=210	Number	%
Catheter related bacteremia	80	4.93	Catheter related bacteremia	4	1.9
Thrombosis	10	0.61	Thrombosis	3	1.42
Arterial puncture	16	0.98	Arterial puncture	4	1.90
Lethal outcome	3	0.18	Lethal outcome	3	1.42
Retro peritoneal hematoma	4	0.24	Pneumothorax	2	0.95
			Hemathorax	1	0.47
			Inappropriate position	10	4.76
Total	113	6.97	Total	27	12.9

Table 29-3. **Complication rates for femoral and subclavian cannulations between 1985 and 1995.**

Complication type	No. of femoral catheters (%)	No. of subclavian catheters (%)	P value
Arterial puncture	19 (0.89)	37 (1.86)	Not significant
Insufficient flow	173 (8.15)	37 (9.84)	Not significant
Local infection	106 (4.99)	18 (4.78	Not significant
Sepsis	21 (0.99)	10 (2.65)	0.007
Catheter clot	12 (0.56)	6 (1.59)	0.03
Malposition	N/A	13 (3.45)	0.00
Lethal outcome	3 (0.14)	3 (0.79)	0.01
Retroperitoneal hematoma	5 (0.23)	N/A	N/A
Pneumothorax	3 (0.79)	N/A	N/A
Hemathorax	2 (0.53)	N/A	N/A
Total with complication	339 (15.98)	99 (26.32)	N/A
Total without complication	1782 (84.02)	277 (73.68)	0.04
Total catheters	2121	376	N/A

N/A is not available.

Table 29-4. Distribution of bacterial infections from routinely analyzed catheter tips for 102 patients with 105 cannulations (84 femoral, 21 subclavian) between 1996 and 1997.

Infection-causing bacterium	Percentage of infected femoral tips (n=84)	Percentage of infected subclavian tips (n=21)
Staphylococcus coagulase negative	58.0	56.4
Staphylococcus aureus	18.1	20.1
Enterococcus	16.1	20.5
Escherichia coli	4.6	1.4
Streptococcus viridans	1.6	0
Pseudomonas aeruginosa	1.6	1.6

Table 29-5. Duration of catheters for 200 patients with 228 cannulations (188 femoral and 40 subclavian) between January 1997 and June 1998.

Duration of femoral catheters 6 to 124 days		Duration of subclavian catheters 6 to 83 days	
Days	% of total	Days	% of total
1 to 7	16	1 to 7	7.0
8 to 14	25.4	8 to 14	16.3
15 to 30	44.3	15 to 30	50.6
31 to 60	12.3	31 to 60	24.1
Greater than 60	2.0	Greater than 60	2.0

Table 29-6. Femoral and subclavian outcomes for 20 patients with 228 cannulations performed between January 1997 and June 1998.

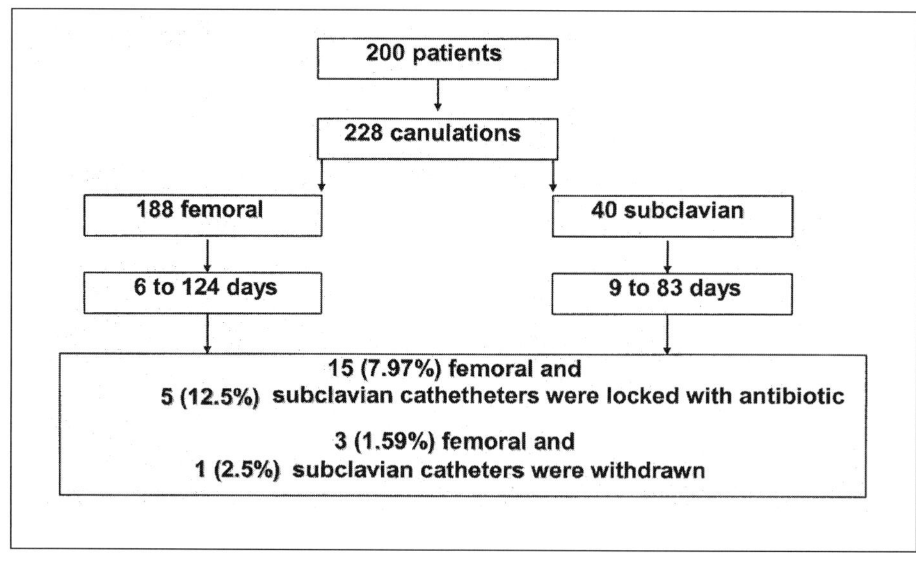

Table 29-7. Outcomes of 97 patients with femoral catheters between January 1998 and December 1998.

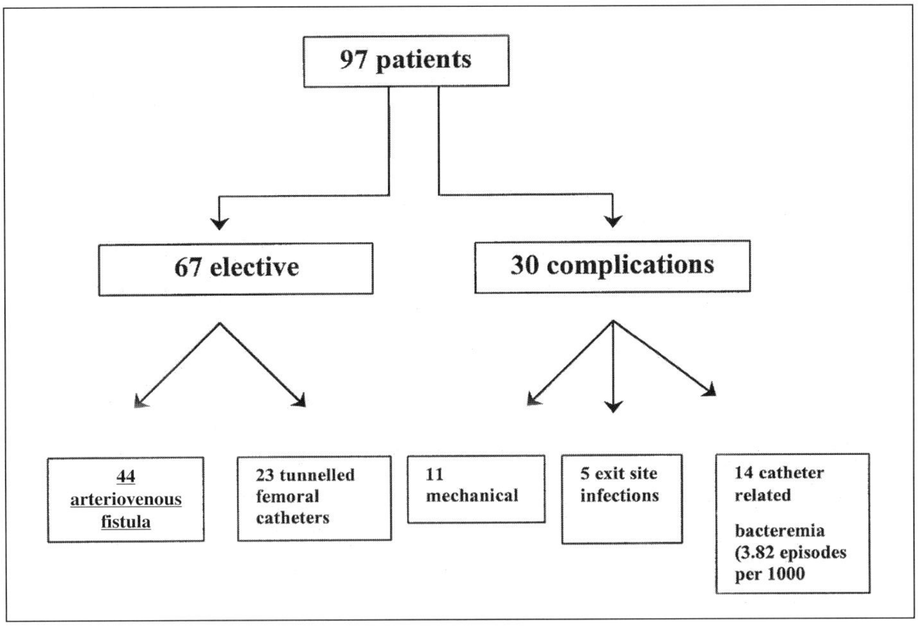

97 patients

67 elective

30 complications

44 arteriovenous fistula

23 tunnelled femoral catheters

11 mechanical

5 exit site infections

14 catheter related bacteremia (3.82 episodes per 1000

Table 29-8. Characteristics of patients with proved chronic renal bacteremia (DM=Diabetes mellitus; ON=Obstructive nephropathy; BNL=Bilateral nephrolithiasis; CRF=Chronic renal failure).

Age	Sex	Diagnosis	Days	Microorganisms isolated
37	M	DM	37	S aureus (tip+blood culture+swab)
54	M	DM	45	S aureus (tip+blood culture+swab)
59	M	ON	24	S aureus (tip+blood culture)
65	M	DM	29	S aureus (tip+swab); K aerogenosa
67	M	ON	25	Enterococcus (tip+swab);
				Acinobacter (swab+blood culture)
71	M	ON	41	Enterococcus (tip+blood culture)
32	F	BNL	13	Streptococcus viridans (tip+blood culture)
66	M	CRF	16	S aureus (tip); Enterococcus (tip)
19	F	SLE	32	Methicillin-resistant S aureus (tip+blood culture+swab)
66	F	DM	16	Enterococcus (tip+blood culture+swab)
55	M	CRF	45	S aureus (tip+blood culture+swab)
42	F	DM	84	Staphlococcus coagulase negative (tip+swab)
52	M	DM	40	Pseudomonas aeroginosa (tip+blood culture)
34	F	SLE	36	Streptococcus viridans (tip+blood culture)

Table 29-9. Proportion of cannulations performed on an outpatient basis.

Year	Total femoral cannulations	Femoral cannulation on an outpatient basis	
1998	308	84	27%
1999	337	131	43%

Discussion

In contrast with articles in the literature and the DOQI guidelines for vascular access, which recommend nonfemoral cannulation routes, our vascular access unit has used all available methods of cannulation access over the past 25 years. Our unit used femoral accesses 25 years ago, then switched to using subclavian and jugular accesses soon after that, and we now use femoral accesses again.

Over an 8-year period, subclavian catheters had a higher rate of thrombosis, arterial puncture, lethal outcome, and total complication. The femoral catheter group's only comparative drawback was its higher rate of infection. In an attempt to reduce the infection rate in the femoral catheter group, we started rigorous maintenance of every catheter after each hemodialysis session. In addition, our unit implemented a rigorous staff education program and used UV lighting in every room for dialysis and dressing of the patients. Also, over the past 7 years, we positioned locked antibiotics into the lumen of the catheters.[1-3] Catheter-related infections have been controlled over this period of time.

Antibiotics (usually cephalosporins) featured not only antimicrobial effects, but also antithrombotic[4-7] and coumarin-like effects[8] that helped reduce the rate of stenosis end thrombosis. Cephalosporins, like other beta-lactam antibiotics, have the ability to cause bleeding and other disturbances of hemostasis. When locked into the catheter lumen, however, the antibiotics were not only safer, but they also achieved a favorable concentration against large numbers of bacteria. This technique could help to prevent occurrence of stenosis or thrombosis of the femoral, subclavian, and jugular veins. Cephalosporins were also used due to their possible immuno-stimulating effects.

We did not use prophylactic antibiotics. Instead, we waited for clinical signs of catheter-related infection to occur. First, we flushed antibiotics into the circulation through arterial and venous lines. Next, we flushed half the antibiotics into circulation, locking the other half into the catheter lines, so that the antibiotics remained in place for half an hour before being pushed with saline and locked with heparin.

The next phase was to lock the antibiotics after hemodialysis sessions to keep the antibiotic in the lumen of catheters between hemodialysis sessions without heparin.

Finally, we flushed half of the total antibiotic into circulation and locked the other half into the lumen of the catheter, forcing it into circulation. The catheter was heparinized between hemodialysis sessions. If the catheter did not work after 3 hemodialysis sessions, it was removed.

Some figures changed over the 10-year period of data analyzation are shown in table 29-3. Over a period of 2 years, our unit used subclavian catheters, in an attempt to reduce hospitalization stays for patients with either AVF problems (eg, thrombosis or stenosis with inappropriate blood flow) or short life expectancies due to cancer or advanced age. This phase increased the number of subclavian cannulations from 210 to 376. We still believed during that time that subclavian catheters could be more convenient for patients. After analyzing an 8-year period of cannulations, from 1985 to 1992, however, we noticed that thrombosis rates, arterial puncture rates, lethal outcome rates, and total complication rates were higher for the subclavian catheter group. After this, femoral catherization became the preferred method.

We observed the presence of bacteria from routinely analyzed catheter tips (table 29-4) even though we did not find any differences in the presence of bacteria in the 2 groups. We also found that the duration of placement for femoral or subclavian catheters was similar and that the use of locked antibiotic in subclavian catheters was more frequent than in femoral catheters (table 29-5). Subclavian catheters were removed more frequently than femoral catheters (table 29-5). All of these observations supported the use of femoral, rather than subclavian, catheters.

When we analyzed the group of 97 femoral catheters, we obtained quite acceptable results for the infection rate (14 patients with CRB or 3.82 episodes per 1000 catheter days). This is especially true because 6 patients were diabetic and 2 had systemic lupus erythematosus (SLE) and were at an increased risk for infection.

In summary, our results showed the following benefits of femoral catheterization:

- The rate of early complications was less than the rate of early complications for the subclavian catheter group.
- The rate of late complications (thrombosis, stenosis, or infection) was either lower or equal to that of the subclavian catheter group.
- Femoral catheter infections occurred less frequently than subclavian or jugular catheter infections.
- Maintenance of femoral catheters was easily performed.
- Femoral catheters were cannulated on an outpatient basis.
- Straight and loop versions (according to the position of the abdominal wall) of femoral catheters were used for long-term dialysis.

Based on our results, we now prefer femoral catheters for both temporary and permanent access. We perform femoral cannulation procedures on an outpatient basis, and achieved a femoral cannulation rate of 39% for last year. We reduced the number of subclavian cannulation procedures (n=5 during the last year) and used jugular catheters for permanent use only.

References

1. Dejanov P, Oncevski A, Gerasimovska V. Locking of hemodialysis catheters with proper antibiotics in catheter related infections. Paper persented at: Angloaccess for Hemodialysis, Second International Multidisciplinary Symposium 1999.
2. Dejanov P, Oncevski A, Polenakovik P, Dejanov I. Use of proper group of antibiotics in catheter related infections. XXV Congress European Society of Artificial Organs; Bologna, Italy, November 11-13, 1998. Int J Artif Organs 1998; 21:636 [abstract].

3. Dejanov P, Oncevski A, Polenakovik M, Sikole A. Antithrombotic effects of antibiotics in catheter infection. XXIV Congress European Society of Artificial Organs; Budapest, Hungary, October 16-18, 1997.
4. Nakano T, Terawaki A, Arita, H. Influence of beta-lactam antibiotics on platelets. II. In vitro effects of some beta-lactam antibiotics on the biochemical responses of rat platelets. J Pharmacobiodyn 1987; 10:408-20.
5. Cazzola M, Matera MG, Santangelo G, et al. Effects of some cephalosporins and teicoplanin on platelet aggregation. Int J Clin Pharmacol Res 1993; 13:69-73.
6. Sattler FR, Weitekamp MR, Sayegh A, Ballard JO. Impaired hemostasis caused by beta-lactam antibiotics. Am J Surg 1988; 155:30-39.
7. Shearer MJ, Bechtold H, Andrassy K, et al. Mechanism of cephalosporin-induced hypoprothrombinemia: Relation to cephalosporin side chain, vitamin K metabolism, and vitamin K status. J Clin Pharmacol 1988; 28:88-95.
8. Bechtold H, Lorenz J, Weilemann LS, et al. Possible coumarin-like mechanism of action for cephalosporins. Klin Wochenschr 1984; 62:885-86.

30

ORGANIZING VASCULAR ACCESS MANAGEMENT: THE NURSING ROLE

Kerri A. Welch, R.N., C.N.N.

The dialysis community is extremely interested in giving quality vascular access care, especially since the National Kidney Foundation's release of the Dialysis Outcomes Quality Initiative (DOQI) Guidelines.[1] The task of managing hemodialysis access can be overwhelming. There are many people and places involved, and information is exchanged through numerous caregivers. The key to managing this overwhelming responsibility is organization. RenalCare Associates saw the need to funnel all of this information through 1 source and developed the Vascular Access Coordinator position.

RenalCare Associates, located in Peoria, IL, oversees more than 600 hemodialysis patients in central Illinois. These patients are treated in 8 different outpatient facilities and served by 3 hospitals, with some patients traveling more than 60 miles to get to Peoria. This practice consists of 9 nephrologists and 1 transplant/vascular surgeon. There are also 2 other surgical practices and 2 radiology groups serving these patients.

Components of an Organization Managing Vascular Access

There are 4 key components to organizing and managing vascular access: 1) a vascular access team (VAT), 2) a medical director, 3) a vascular access coordinator (VAC), and 4) a vascular access database (VAD). The idea behind the VAT was to develop a group of caregivers interested in giving quality access care. Initially, the

VAT members consisted of the nephrologist medical director, a surgeon from each of the 3 groups, an interventional radiologist, and a dialysis nurse. The vascular access coordinator, (VAC) who uses a VAD, joined the team shortly thereafter.

All members recognize a need to funnel information through 1 source. It is also imperative that the data be tracked in an organized fashion. The nephrologist serves as the team leader and oversees the care of the patient. The surgeons and radiologists confer and exchange relevant information relating to procedures, techniques, and complications. The dialysis nurse and VAC share the patient's perspective and broach issues relating to the day-to-day management of access care. The team meets quarterly to discuss quality improvement and to review the data. Physicians are provided with individual and program-wide data giving valuable information on performance relating to such areas as incidence of fistula placement (figure 30-1), thrombosis rate, and procedure patency rates. All of the reports are directly related to DOQI guidelines and are generated from the InnoVAD™ database (Innovative Vascular Access Database, Lakewood, CO). Viewing the data as a team sparks informative and valuable discussions enabling quality issues to be addressed.

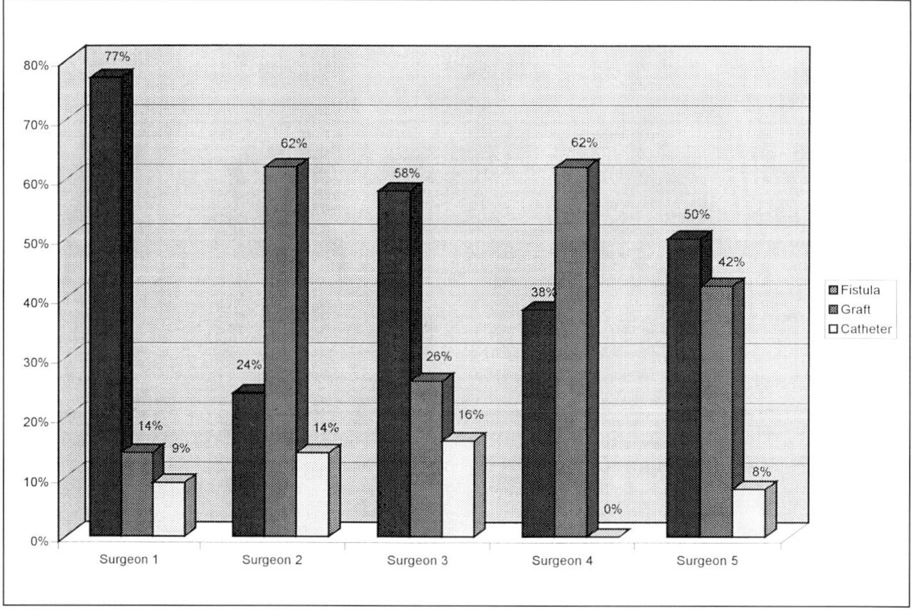

Figure 30-1. Access incidence by surgeon.

The medical director leading the VAT has an important role. At RenalCare Associates, the medical director is one of the partners, with a specialty in vascular access. The medical director is very involved with the daily concerns of the VAC; the 2 also meet weekly to review and treat complicated access problems. The Medical Director and VAC develop treatment protocols, patient and staff education, and database improvements. The medical director also serves as a liaison between VAT members.

The VAC's role is to centralize all information about vascular access. Prior to hiring a VAC, there had been no structured algorithm to handle vascular access complications and no way to track data from various sources. Outcomes such as the thrombosis rate, for example, were estimated. Information on a patient's graft clotting would have been managed as shown in figure 30-2. When the clot was noted, the dialysis RN would page the nephrologist on call and await a response. (Note that the on-call physician may not be the patient's primary physician.) Meanwhile, the nurse would have moved the patient to the waiting room and managed other dialysis patients, concurrently handling problems ranging from staffing issues to mechanical failures with the dialysis machines or the water system.

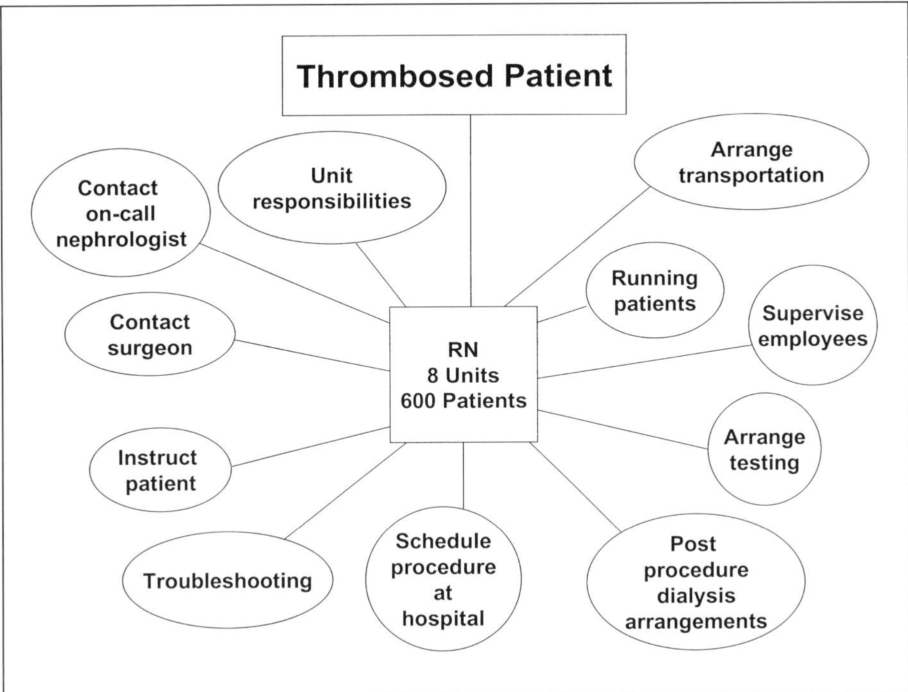

Figure 30-2. Information management regarding thrombosed graft.

If the nephrologist who subsequently returned the nurse's call asked for a history regarding the vascular access, the nurse would have offered only the information on the hard chart in her file, which may or may not have been complete, especially since it may take 2 weeks or longer to receive radiology and surgery reports. The nurse would have been able to offer information on other interventions only by reading through the physicians' and nurses' notes, which would have taken a considerable amount of time.

Thus, the physician was sometimes forced to make a decision on limited information. Further, if patients required radiology or surgery, it would have been the nurse's responsibility to arrange patient transportation and to make arrangements for the patient to dialyze at a later time. Despite the fact that 2 large outpatient units were located within a short distance of the hospitals, patients were most commonly dialyzed in the acute setting due to nurse time constraints in locating an outpatient chair. Obviously, this practice was inefficient and costly.

Results and Discussion

Under the new algorithm (figure 30-3), the dialysis nurse makes 1 phone call to the VAC to say that the access is clotted and to determine whether or not the unit has an open chair to dialyze the patient within the next 24 hours. At this point, the VAC organizes everything that needs to occur. The VAC notifies the surgeon and primary physician about the problem and offers a full access history. The VAC acts as the liaison between the 2 physicians and facilitates referrals to radiology or surgery departments. The VAC schedules the procedure and faxes vital information, including the access history, medications, allergies, and demographics. If a chair at the patient's home unit is not available or time does not allow the patient to return to his or her home unit, the VAC will make dialysis arrangements where it is most suitable geographically. The VAC also communicates relevant information to the dialysis unit. Making patient transport arrangements is the only task delegated to dialysis unit personnel.

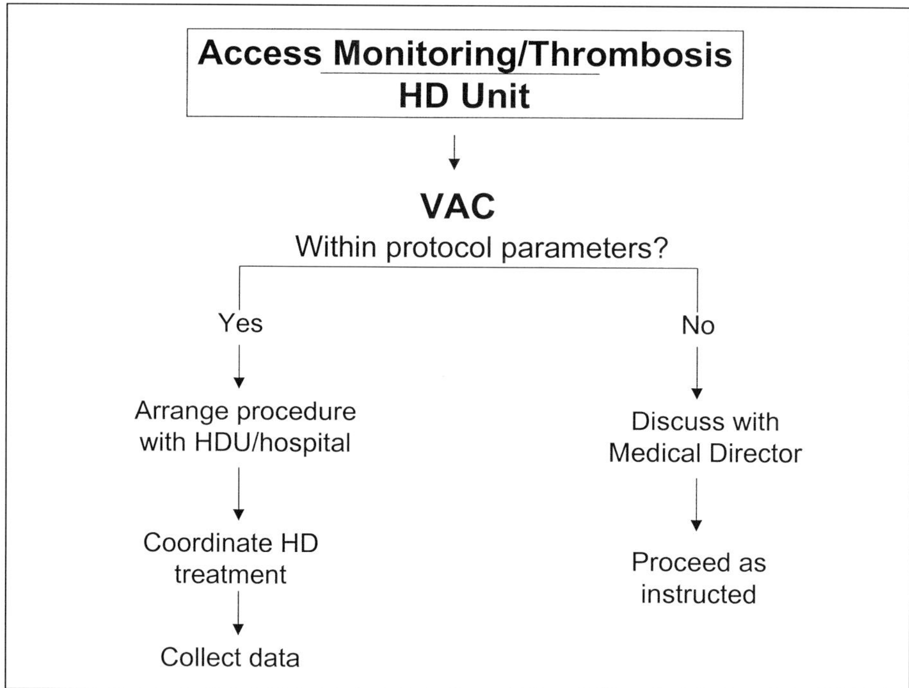

Figure 30-3. Algorithm to address clotted grafts.

Prior to hiring a VAC, only 40% of access procedures were done on an outpatient basis in RenalCare Associates' program but currently 72% are conducted on an outpatient basis (figure 30-4). After 1 year, the program-wide thrombosis rate was 1.5%. The VAC and medical director initiated a screening program using the Transonic® ultrasound dilution method. Patients are screened every other month. One technician at each unit is trained to perform the recirculation and access flow testing. A center-specific protocol was created by the medical director, allowing the

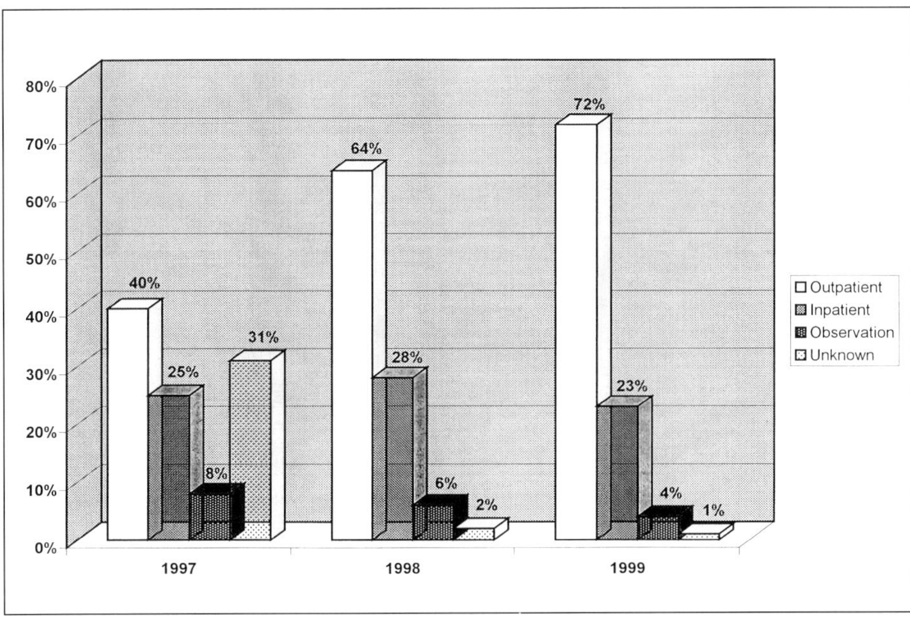

Figure 30-4. Admission status by year.

VAC to order procedures. The VAC reviews flows, labs, pressures, and any clinical complications occurring before deciding whether to order a shuntogram. Since initiating the screening program, the institution's thrombosis rate has decreased to 1.1%, and rates within 3 units have decreased to less than 0.5%.

Within the past year, the vascular access group has also begun tracking the history of pre-dialysis patients with newly created accesses. Often, these patients had been left unaccounted. Ideally, fistulas would be placed several months before dialysis is needed and the patient would return for an office visit with the surgeon 2 weeks after fistula placement. In a collaborative effort between the VAC and surgeon's office nurse, patients are now called 1 week post-fistula placement. The patient is encouraged to follow up in the office, but, if an office visit is not possible, the nurse will explain over the phone about hygienic care of the access, signs and symptoms of infection, feeling for the buzz, and the importance of exercising the fistula. Squeeze balls are mailed to patients who need them. Each patient is called every 2 to 3 weeks to see how he or she is progressing.

Thus, having a database to track interventions is an essential component to the success of organized vascular access management. At RenalCare Associates, patient information is entered into InnoVAD™ when dialysis is initiated. With clerical assistance, the VAC enters a patient's demographics and history of all interventions relevant to vascular access. Through the VAT, an intervention log was created for the surgeons and radiologists to complete after the procedure (figure 30-5) and fax to the VAC. InnoVAD™ allows the user to generate both clinical reports and outcome analyses for comparison with DOQI guidelines. Such reports are a vital part of our Continuous Quality Improvement (CQI) program. As part of this program, the VAC reports to the CQI Committee quarterly. Program wide, unit specific, and physician-specific reports are generated that are shared with dialysis staff and access

Date ____/____/____

Patient name________________

Admission status
❑ inpatient ❑ outpatient
❑ observation

Reason for Procedure
❑ Thrombosis
❑ Abnormal shuntogram
❑ First access intervention
❑ Inadequate flow
❑ Infection
❑ Hemorrhage
❑ Recirculating
❑ Other________________

Intervention Physician
(please enter physicians name)

____
Primary procedure

____
Secondary procedure

Primary and Secondary procedure
(Please write **1** for primary procedure and **2** for secondary procedures)
____ Angioplasty open
____ Angioplasty percutaneous
____ Angioplasty with stent
____ Banding
____ Catheter stripping
____ Catheter removal
____ Fistula revision
____ Graft removal
____ Graft revision
____ Incision and drain
____ Ligation
____ Shuntogram
____ Thrombolysis pharmacological
__________dosage UK
__________dosage Heparin
____ Thrombolysis mechanical
____ Thrombolysis, pharmaco-mechanical
____ Thrombectomy, surgical
____ Other________________

Angioplasty Results

Before:_______ % stenosis

After: <30% or >30% stenosis
(circle one)

Shuntogram results
❑ Arterial anastomosis stenosis
❑ Central venous stenosis
❑ Outflow vein stenosis
❑ Venous anastomosis stenosis
❑ Intragraft Stenosis
❑ Other ________________

Intervention Access

Location : ❑ Right ❑ Left

Site :
❑ Forearm ❑ Femoral
❑ Upper leg ❑ Subclavian
❑ Upper arm ❑ Internal jugular

❑ Other ________________

Anesthesia: ____ Loc ____ Gen ____ Block

EBL: ____________ ml

New Access Placed ?
(If yes, complete the following information)

Location: ❑ Right ❑ Left

Site:
❑ Forearm ❑ Femoral
❑ Upper leg ❑ Subclavian
❑ Upper arm ❑ Internal jugular

❑ Other ________________

Type:
❑ Fistula
❑ Gore ringed gortex

❑ Other ________________

Medcomp catheter :
❑ Permcath SL 17cm
❑ Permcath SL 28cm
❑ Temp cath SL 12cm
❑ Temp cath SL 15cm
❑ Temp cath SL 20cm
❑ Tesio cath MBR 37cm art 40cm ven

❑ Other ________________

Notes/Drawings/Future Plans:

Figure 30-5. Intervention log – operative note.

team members. Certificates of achievement have been given to those units achieving DOQI recommended standards, such as a thrombosis rate of 0.5%. Some friendly competition between the units increases morale and facilitates discussion about potential improvements. Since distribution of the unit-specific reports, nurses and technicians are more aware of potential problems that might be communicated to the VAC earlier, thereby allowing interventions and avoiding complications.

InnoVAD™ also creates a patient-specific access history report that is invaluable to caregivers involved in vascular access management. The report shows all interventions on the patient's current access and includes a list of all previous accesses. The access history follows the patient during every intervention, including office visits, radiology or surgical procedures. The VAC and Medical Director find this report extremely useful when reviewing complicated access cases. Further, the report provides a valuable intervention time line and a chart that maps access flow readings reported via the Transonic®. After each intervention, the access history report is faxed to the patient's home unit and added to his or her chart.

Conclusion

Care of vascular access may be organized efficiently by using the following 4 components: a vascular access team, a medical director, a vascular access coordinator, and a specialty database, such as InnoVAD™. The result is improved care of vascular access and better DOQI outcomes. Better communications between the many caregivers involved leads to improved approaches to quality care. While we have seen many advantages and improvements since changing the way we manage vascular access, there continue to be challenges. Over the last 2 years, we have recognized that having a freestanding vascular access center and an interventional nephrologist would be valuable assets to our access management program. With continued commitment to the organized management of vascular access care, we hope to further improve the quality of care given to hemodialysis patients.

Reference

1. Schwab S, Besarab A, Beathard G, et al. NKF-DOQI clinical practice guidelines for vascular access. New York: National Kidney Foundation; 1997.

31

VASCULAR ACCESS IN THE ELDERLY

M.K. Lazarides, M.D., D.N. Staramos, M.D., C. Maltezos, M.D., and V.D. Tzilalis, M.D.

The recently published National Kidney Foundation Dialysis Outcome Quality Initiative (NKF-DOQI) clinical practice guidelines stated that the first choice of access in patients requiring chronic hemodialysis is the wrist radial-cephalic arteriovenous (AV) fistula.[1] Our clinical impression over the years, however, was that autologous AV fistulae, especially distal wrist fistulae, had an inferior patency rate in elderly patients. The purpose of this article was to compare the patency of autologous and graft bridging (prosthetic) AV fistulae in patients greater than 70 years of age in a nonrandomized study and to review the literature on this controversial subject.

Patients and Methods

The study sample included all new access procedures performed in elderly (defined here as older than 70 years of age) patients who presented with end-stage renal disease (ESRD) between January 1990 and December 1998. A total of 154 consecutive procedures were performed in 131 patients. Patients greater than 75 years of age constituted 60% (n=79) of the 131 in the studied population. Forty-two (32%) of the 131 were older than 80 years of age. An interim analysis of part of these data has been previously published.[2] The mean age of the patients was 76.3 years (range 70 to 89 years) and 82 of them were men. Seventy-four autologous AV fistulae and 80 prosthetic AV fistulae were performed with PTFE grafts in various configurations (table 31-1). Temporary or permanent accesses with intravenous catheters and corrections of previous access procedures were excluded. Our policy was to offer autologous fistulae to all suitable patients needing hemodialysis. The use of prosthetic grafts was for patients who were overweight or who had no autologous option available. Clinical evaluation, including tourniquet application and

Table 31-1. Configurations of the 154 access procedures performed during a 9-year period in patients older than 70 years of age.

Number of autologous AV fistulae		Number of prosthetic AV fistulae	
Radiocephalic AV fistulae at wrist	44	Brachioaxillary straight PTFE AV grafts	74
Brachiocephalic AV fistulae at elbow	23	Forearm "loop" PTFE AV grafts	3
Basilic transpositions	7	Femorofemoral "loop" PTFE AV grafts	3
TOTAL	74	TOTAL	80

vein percussion, was used as preoperative assessment; however, in the last 3 years, an intraoperative maneuver was employed to reveal any stenotic lesions in the proximal vein.[3] All procedures were done under local anesthesia, and a single dose of vancomycin plus a 2-day course of an intravenous cephalosporin was given in the prosthetic AV fistulae group.

Cumulative patency of the access procedures and the survival of patients were assessed using life-table analysis and presented as Kaplan-Meier curves. Access failure was defined not only as thrombosis but as any problem that required surgical intervention or a new access creation (eg, inadequate maturation, infection necessitating graft removal, false aneurysm correction, and revisions due to limb-threatening steal). Censored endpoints were death, loss of follow-up, end of hemodialysis due to either transplantation or renal function improvement, and access patency to the end of the study period. Patencies were compared using the Gehan's Wilcoxon test. Data management and statistical analysis were performed using the statistical software package STATISTICA (StatSoft Inc, Tulsa, OK).

Results

The primary cumulative patency of the autologous procedures (n=74) was 70%, 58%, and 52% at 1, 2, and 3 years, respectively. The corresponding primary cumulative patency of the prosthetic AV grafts (n=80) was 71%, 61%, and 47%, which was not a statistically significant difference (P=0.8, figure 31-1). The secondary cumulative patency of the autologous procedures was equal to the primary patency because no revisions were performed. The previous policy was due to the very low success rate after correction procedures for failed native fistulae. We favored the creation of proximal new autologous access or conversion to a synthetic one in all cases. This handling has been suggested by others previously.[4]

The secondary patency of the prosthetic AV grafts was 82%, 71%, and 65% in 1, 2, and 3 years respectively, and the difference compared with the patency of autol-

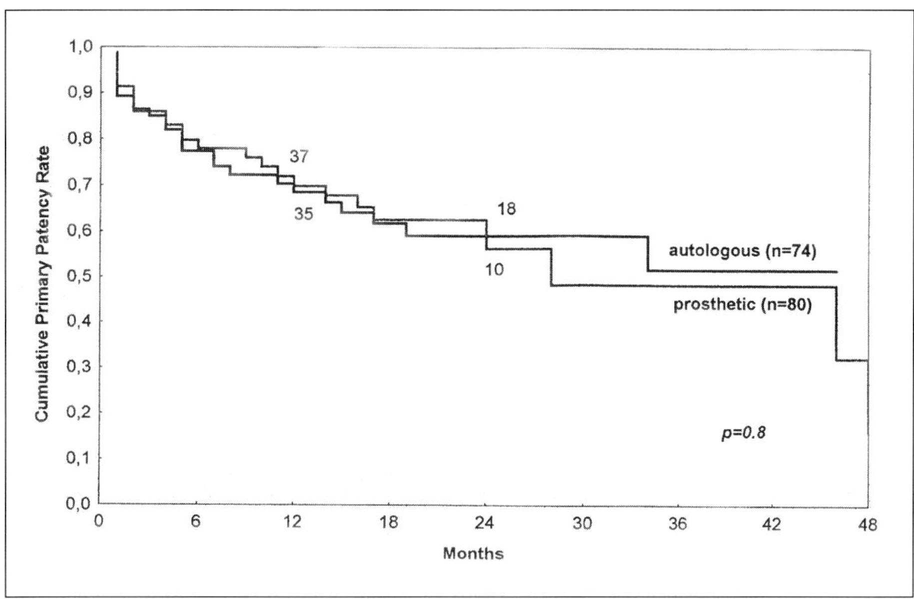

Figure 31-1. Primary cumulative patency rate of autologous versus prosthetic AV fistulae in ERSD patients (70 years of age).

ogous fistulae was statistically significant (P=0.04, figure 31-2). In the prosthetic group, a total of 17 reoperations were performed in 16 patients, including 3 thrombectomies, 6 thrombectomies with a jump graft at the venous anastomosis, 4 correction operations for limb-threatening steal, 2 removals of infected grafts, and 2 false aneurysm corrections. There were 0.18 surgical revisions for the prosthetic AV

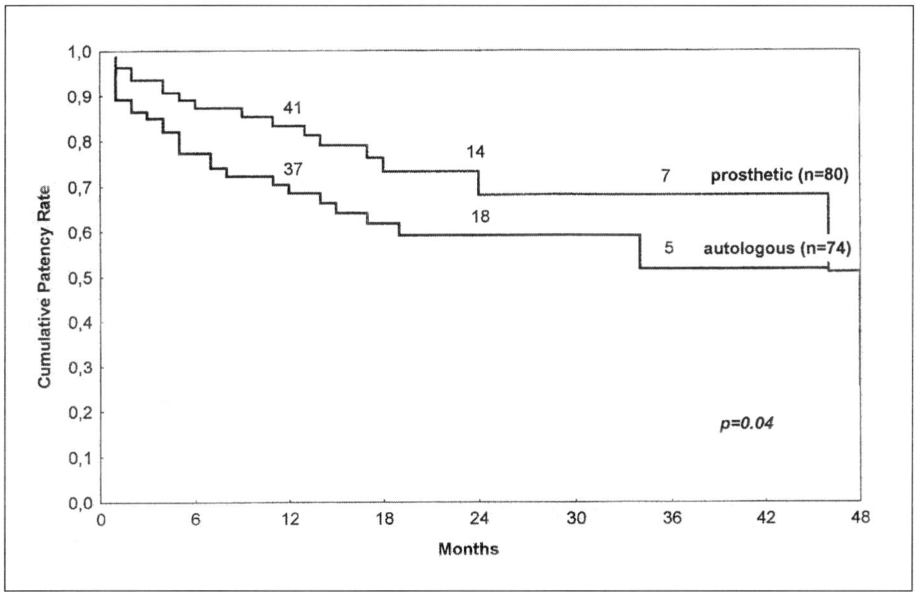

Figure 31-2. Secondary cumulative patency rate of autologous versus prosthetic AV fistulae in ERSD patients (70 years of age).

fistulae per graft per year. The primary access failure specifically for the upper arm AV grafts (n=74) was 4% (limb-threatening steal not included if corrected).

Patients with prosthetic AV fistulae as the initial procedure necessitated an average of 1.5 operations (either new or corrections) in order to maintain a functional access during the study period. Patients with native AV fistulae at initial access required 1.7 operations.

The yearly mortality rate of patients in this series was quite high, with 84 patients dying during the study period; however, no deaths were immediately related to angioaccess creation. The cumulative patient survival rate at 3 years was 25% (figure 31-3). The cumulative survival rates at 3 years for those patients older than 75 years of age (n=79) and for those older than 77 years (n=53) were 20% and 13%, respectively. Concurrently, the computed cumulative survival rate for ESRD patients between 65 and 69 years of age (n=78) was 48%.

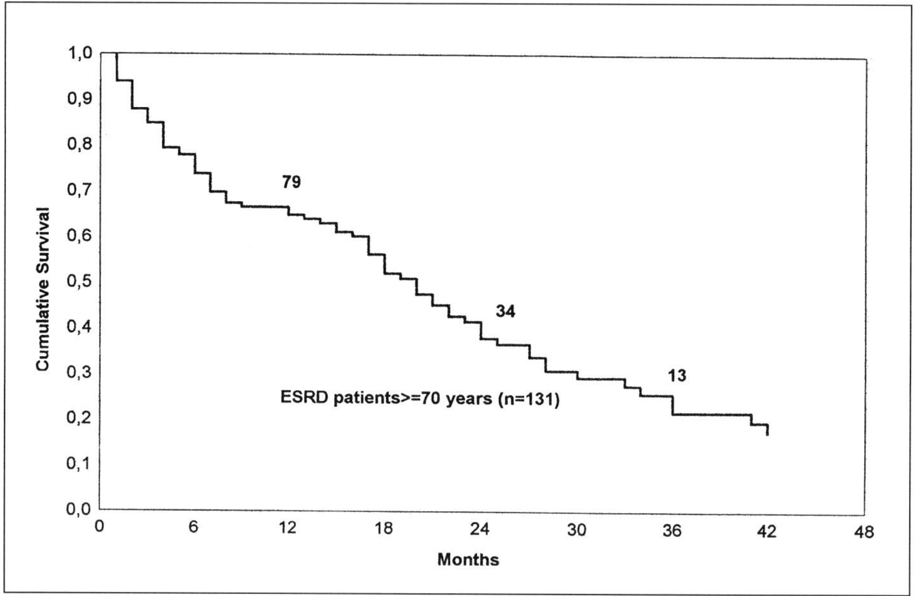

Figure 31-3. Survival rate of all ERSD patients (70 years of age in a 9-year period).

Discussion

Recently published NKF-DOQI guidelines on vascular access stated that the first-choice access in patients requiring chronic hemodialysis is the wrist radial-cephalic AV fistula.1 Because autologous AV fistulae are superior to grafts, DOQI guidelines recommend an aggressive strategy to increase the number of native fistulae, with AV bridge grafts reserved for patients whose vein anatomy does not permit the construction of an autologous AV fistula. Once a forearm fistula has matured and has been used for dialysis, it rarely clots, with most patients enjoying function for many years. Controversy exists, however, regarding the optimal access for elderly ESRD patients. Fifteen years ago, Hinsdale et al. reported that autologous fistulae construction was less feasible in elderly patients and that proximal access sites may be preferred in this particular subgroup.[5]

Since then, the argument persists for the initial construction of proximal accesses instead of forearm fistulae in patients older than 65 years of age.[6,7] Miller et al. introduced the term fistula adequacy, which defined patency and maturation with a flow of at least 350 mL/min on at least 6 dialysis sessions per month. The same study suggested that forearm fistulae matured adequately in only 12% of patients aged 65 years or older, while upper arm fistulae were adequate in 54% of the same population.[6] The authors suggested that it might be reasonable to construct the initial fistula in the upper arm rather than the forearm in this particular subgroup of elderly patients.

Additionally, Woods et al. established that the risk of failure for fistulae, but not grafts, varies significantly with the age of the patient.[7] Prischi et al. also stated that the relative risk for AV fistula failure in 70-year-old patients was 6 times higher than in patients 30 years old.[8] These findings agree with similar data presented from a survey in the area of Athens, which showed a significant association between age and autologous access failure, but not prosthetic AV grafts.[9] Didlake et al. also found that the patency rates of prosthetic AV grafts was equivalent in groups older and younger than 65 years of age.[10] In many other clinical series, autologous distal fistulae were not associated with inferior patency in elderly patients. In a recent large series of snuffbox AV fistulae, patients older than 70 years showed no less fistula longevity than other patients.[11] Golledge et al., in a prospective study of 107 primary radiocephalic fistulae, found that there was no evidence that older patients had a poorer patency. In fact, Golledge's group reported that older patients had a more favorable outcome.[12] Additionally, Gomez-Campdera and colleagues reported that native AV fistulae could be successfully created in more than 70% of cases in a series of 125 ESRD patients over 65 years of age.[13] Sands and Miranda also suggested that the number of fistulae that can be created in elderly patients is higher than most authors acknowledge.[14]

Obviously, previous studies are contradictory. The main problem with native AV fistulae in the elderly is the inferior reported patency rates compared with those reported for younger patients.[15] Only 1 article, however, reported comparative patencies of native and bridge graft AV fistulae in the elderly in a life table format.[7] In this article, a slight advantage for native AV fistulae over grafts was noticed in patients older than 65 years of age (1 year patency, 57% versus 49% for synthetic grafts). Our results demonstrated that the secondary patency of the prosthetic grafts was superior to that of autologous AV fistulae in patients older than 70 years of age, at a statistically significant level. A possible explanation may be the inferior quality of the veins in the elderly.[16]

The disagreement of the 2 studies may be explained by the subjective cut-off age used to define the elderly population (65 versus 70 years), the inclusion in the former study of various prosthetic AV graft configurations, and the report of only primary patencies, when secondary patency is more advantageous in prosthetics. Both studies were nonrandomized with obvious selection bias, as graft fistulae were created only when creation of autologous ones was not feasible. A superior patency for AV grafts should be expected in a randomized trial in which patients with optimal veins would be allocated to the prosthetic group.

No randomized trials compare the various access types in the elderly, so the decision regarding the optimal initial procedure in this subgroup of patients is complex. In our view, the application of the general DOQI guidelines in the elderly, regarding the first choice access procedure, is based on weak evidence. This problem was further complicated by the significant discrepancies regarding survival of the various ESRD age groups. In our department the 3-year mortality of the 65 to 69 years age group (not included in the study) was half than that of the older than 70 years age group.

The increased interest in elderly ESRD patients is due to a tremendous demographic change within the ESRD population in the past 20 years. It is interesting that elderly patients, who were excluded from dialysis in the early years, are now the fastest-growing segment of the total dialysis population. In the early 1960s, patients who were older than 45 years of age were excluded from consideration for dialysis treatment in Seattle. During the 1980s in the United Kingdom, the elderly were denied access to renal replacement therapy.

Broader acceptance criteria allowed patients of any age to enter dialysis therapy and produced a dramatic increase in their number. In America in 1972, less than 20% of ESRD patients were older than 65 years of age. In 1996, nearly 1 in 2 (47%) were 65 or older. It has been estimated that persons over 65 years of age comprise more than 60% of the total number of ESRD patients at present.[17] The European Renal Association Registry has reported a similar trend. In 1977, only 9% of the patients starting renal replacement therapy were older than 65 years of age, while by 1992 this proportion had increased to nearly 37%. Also in Canada in 1989, 35% of ESRD patients were older than 65 years, compared with 25% in 1981.[17] Not surprisingly, mortality is higher among elderly dialysis patients. Held et al. reported a 5 year survival rate of 10% for Americans between 75 to 84 years[18], while the Canadian study reported a 3-year survival probability of 36% for ESRD nondiabetics who were 65 years old or greater.[19] The 2- and 5-year survival rates computed from recent data for 70-year-old ESRD patients were 47% and 15%, while rates for those 75 years of age were 35% and 10%, respectively.[20] The present study revealed similar findings, with a 3-year cumulative survival rate of 25% for ESRD patients greater than 70 years of age and only 13% for those older than 77 years of age.

In elderly patients there is a lessened need for conservation of access sites as a result of the limited life expectancy. This explains the almost exclusive use of proximal straight brachio-axillary arm AV grafts in our study. Using mainly this prosthetic configuration, we achieved an optimum revision rate of 0.18 per graft/year, as it is well known that upper arm proximal accesses have superior patency rates.[9,21,22] Hodges et al. reported a revision rate of 0.5 per access/year to maintain secondary prosthetic graft patency, using forearm loop grafts in 82% of cases.[4] Johnson reported revision rates of 0.4 for native and 1.08 for prosthetic accesses per patient-year.[23]

The primary access failure specifically for the upper arm AV grafts was 4% within the suggested DOQI guidelines (5% for upper arm grafts).[1] On the basis of this report we have no enthusiasm to perform distal native AV fistulae in patients over 70 years of age and we prefer the construction of proximal arm AV grafts. We do, however, perform autologous fistulae, mainly proximal ones, in selected patients of this age with favorable anatomy, as these accesses have equal or superior patency compared with the prosthetic ones.[9] Following this plan, we have never had a patient with all possible access sites exhausted, and in only 3 patients were we forced to create, as tertiary angioaccess, a femorofemoral loop AV graft. Despite the extended use of proximal prosthetic accesses in our study, the incidence of limb threatening steal necessitating revision was only 5% (4 cases), which was within the reported limits in the literature.[24] The incidence of infection was only 2.5% (2 out of 80 prosthetic grafts), far less than the 10% limit set by DOQI.[1]

Several considerations must be considered when choosing access for elderly patients, including: (1) immediate need of dialysis, (2) expected survival of the proposed access, (3) expected survival of the patient, (4) vascular anatomy, (5) patients preferences, and (6) experience of the surgeon.[13] In our view, the ideal initial access in the elderly should be the one with the shortest maturation time, longest medium-term patency, and lowest revision rate. In this specific subgroup of patients, parameters such as long-term patency and conservation of proximal access sites are of minimal importance because of the patient's limited life expectancy.

The superior medium patency in the prosthetic group in our study, along with an extremely low revision rate, indicate that the use of the proximal AV arm grafts may be used as alternative initial access procedures in elderly ESRD patients. An additional advantage of the prosthetic grafts was the shorter maturation time (1 to 3 weeks) associated with grafts compared with autologous AV fistulae (greater than 6 weeks),[25] especially because maturation time in elderly ESRD patients may be up to twice as long as the time required for younger patients.[26]

Access failure and the necessity of access creation or revision result in significant strain on the personal and emotional life of the patient. In the present study, patients with autologous AV fistulae as the initial procedure needed more operations in order to maintain a functional access during the study period than those having prosthetic grafts (average 1.7 versus 1.5). Our results justify the design of a randomized study comparing the 2 access types, namely, the autologous and the proximal prosthetic upper arm AV fistulae, in ESRD patients older than 70 years of age. In such a study, parameters related to quality of life, such as the total number of procedures needed to maintain a functional access and maturation time, should also be considered.

References

1. NKF-DOQI clinical practice guidelines for vascular access. National Kidney Foundation-Dialysis Outcomes Quality Initiative. Am J Kidney Dis 1997; 30(suppl 3) S150-91.
2. Staramos DN, Lazarides MK, Tzilalis VD, Ekonomou CS, Simopoulos CE, Dayantas JN. Patency of autologous and prosthetic arteriovenous fistulae in elderly patients. Eur J Surg 2000; 166:777-81.
3. Lazarides MK, Staramos DN, Tzilalis VD, Simopoulos KE, Dayantas JN. Evoked thrill: A simple intraoperative maneuver predicts early patency of AV fistulas. J Vasc Surg 1998; 27:750-52.
4. Hodges TC, Fillinger MF, Zwolak RM, Walsh DB, Bech F, Cronenwett JL. Longitudinal comparison of dialysis access methods: Risk factors for failure. J Vasc Surg 1997; 26:1009-19.

5. Hinsdale JG, Lipkowitz GS, Hoover EL. Vascular access for hemodialysis in the elderly: Results and perspectives in a geriatric population. Dial Transplant 1985; 14:560-65.
6. Miller PE, Tolwani A, Lusky CP, et al. Predictors of adequacy of arteriovenous fistulas in hemodialysis patients. Kidney Int 1999; 56:275-80.
7. Woods JD, Turenne MN, Strawderman RL, et al. Vascular access survival among incident hemodialysis patients in US. Am J Kidney Dis 1997; 30:50-57.
8. Prischi FC, Kirchgatterre A, Brandstatter E, Wallner M, et al. Parameters of prognostic relevance to the patency of vascular access in hemodialysis patients. J Am Soc Nephrol 1995; 6:1613-18.
9. Lazarides MK, Iatrou CE, Karanikas ID, et al. Factors affecting the lifespan of autologous and synthetic access routes for haemodialysis. Eur J Surg 1996; 162:297-301.
10. Didlake R, Raju S, Rhodes RS, Bower J. Dialysis access in patients older than 65 years. In: Vascular access for hemodialysis-II. Sommer BG, Henry ML, eds. Chicago: W.L. Gore & Associates and Precept Press 1991:166-72.
11. Wolowczyk L, Williams AJ, Donovan KL, Gibbons CP. The snuffbox arteriovenous fistula for vascular access. Eur J Vasc Endovasc Surg 2000; 19:70-76.
12. Golledge J, Smith CJ, Emery J, Farrington K, Thompson HH. Outcome of primary radiocephalic fistula for haemodialysis. Br J Surg 1999; 86:211-16.
13. Gomez Campdera FJ, Polo JR, Sanabia J, Tejedor A. First choice vascular access in patients over 65 years of age starting dialysis. Nephron 1996; 73:342-43.
14. Sands J, Miranda CL. Increasing numbers of AV fistulas for hemodialysis access. Clin Nephrol 1997; 48:114-17.
15. Leapman SB, Boyle M, Pescovitz MD, Milgrom ML, Jindal RM, Filo RS. The arteriovenous fistula for hemodialysis access: Gold standard or archaic relic? Am Surg 1996; 62:652-57.
16. Shina MJ, Neumayer MN, Healy DA, Atnip RG, Thiele BL. Influence of age on venous physiologic parameters. J Vasc Surg 1993; 18:749-52.
17. Grapsa I, Oreopoulos DG. Practical ethical issues of dialysis in the elderly. Semin Nephrol 1996; 16:339-52.
18. Held PJ, Brunner F, Odaka M, et al. Five year survival for end stage renal disease patients in the United States, Europe and Japan 1982 to 1987. Am J Kidney Dis 1990; 15:451-57.
19. Churchill DN, Taylor DW, Cook RJ, et al. Canadian hemodialysis morbidity study. Am J Kidney Dis 1992; 19:214-34.
20. Latos DL. Chronic dialysis in patients over age 65. J Am Soc Nephrol 1996; 7:637-46.
21. Culp K, Flanigan M, Taylor L, Rothstein M. Vascular access thrombosis in new hemodialysis patients. Am J Kidney Dis 1995; 26:341-46.
22. Bittner HB, Weaver JP. Brachioaxillary interposition graft as a successful tertiary vascular access procedure for hemodialysis. Am J Surg 1994; 167:615-17.
23. Johnson CP, Zhu YR, Matt C, Pelz C, Roza AM, Adams MB. Prognostic value of intraoperative blood flow measurements in vascular access surgery. Surgery 1998; 124:729-38.

24. Lazarides MK, Staramos DN, Panagopoulos GN, Tzilalis VD, Eleftheriou GJ, Dayantas JN. Indications for surgical treatment of angioaccess-induced arterial steal. J Am Coll Surg 1998; 187:422-26.
25. Besarab A, Frinak S, Zasuwa G. Prospective evaluation of vascular access function: the nephrologigst's perspective. Semin Dial 1996; 9(Suppl1):21-29.
26. Haish CE. Vascular access in the high-risk patient. In: Henry ML, Ed. Vascular access for hemodialysis-VI. Chicago: W.L. Gore & Associates and Precept Press 1999; 315-26.

32

CPT AND ICD-9 CODING FOR DIALYSIS ACCESS: A PRACTICAL GUIDE

Ingemar J.A. Davidson, M.D., Ph.D., F.A.C.S., Diana J. Adams, R.H.I.A., and Carolyn E. Munschauer, B.A.

Using the Current Procedural Terminology (CPT) and the International Classification of Diseases, 9th Revision, Clinical Modification (ICD-9-CM) manuals properly for vascular access coding is challenging because of the complexity of clinical diagnoses and procedures in dialysis patients. This complexity is often intensified by the level of urgency of most medical decisions and surgeries. Proper coding requires sound surgical judgement and proper documenting of the sequence of often staged access procedures.

The CPT is a statistical coding system used for reimbursement purposes. Insurance companies and Medicare are not required to use the CPT system. Thus, insurance companies, Medicare, and other third party payers have their own guidelines that often differ from the CPT. The use of the ICD-9 coding system, however, is required by Medicare because of a federal mandate in the late 1980s.[1] The lack of clear coding rules has led to a confusing second set of guidelines developed by coding experts who attempt to interpret the rules for Medicare and third party payers. Coding training seminars have become an industry preying on doctors threatened by audits and fines for not following rulings that they did not realize existed. The current situation has created unnecessary tension between the medical community and payers, which is also hurting patients and the public in terms of treatment delays and increased cost. Measures to improve clarity and understanding are badly needed and could benefit society as a whole.

Nonintentional, erroneous coding is commonplace. Only proper coding will result in appropriate reimbursement. Undercoding will always guarantee underreimbursement. Improper overcharging will result in one of the following: delays, overpayment, or, most likely, no payment at all from insurance companies.

Interpreting the coding systems can be challenging. For example, the coding systems have inconsistent definitions of the term "global surgical package." In the 2000 CPT, the global surgical package definition is not clearly delineated in the text and is described through several different venues of "reporting more than one procedure/service," "add-on codes," "separate procedures," and "starred procedures or items." It is standard when reporting postoperative follow-up visits for documentation purposes to use CPT 99024 for the global surgical package code. Such visits typically include suture removal, evaluation of the outcome of surgery, and a check for complications.[2] Note that initial pre-operative services are not included in this package guideline through Medicare; however, some third-party payers, through their own global package definition, may bundle visits prior to the procedure. Verification of insurance policies per the provider contract is required when filing claims for these services. Each insurance payer also has defined global time periods. For example, Medicare has a 0 day global period for endoscopy, 10 days for minor (usually office) procedures, and 90 days for major surgeries (table 32-1). Again, verification of insurance contract policies to determine their defined global period is mandatory when filing claims for these services.

Table 32-1. Medicare 90-day major global package summary.

Included in the global package definition are the following:
1. All normal preoperative visits beginning with the day prior to a major surgery.
2. Intraoperative services as a necessary part of the surgical procedure.
3. All medical or surgical services required of the operating surgeon due to complications that do not require additional trips to the operating room.
4. Services such as: dressing changes; wound incision care; removal of packings, drains, sutures, staples, lines, or wires; irrigation; removal of urinary catheters, IV lines, nasogastric tubes, rectal tubes; changes and removal of tracheostomy tubes.
5. Postoperative visits for 90 days for all settings related to recovery from surgery.
6. Same day visit is not paid separate from the procedure.
7. Postoperative pain management by the operating surgeon.
8. Supplies, except for the surgical tray for specified procedures in an office setting.

Therefore, the most common vascular access case scenarios outlined below reflect the complexity that goes into surgical judgment, preoperative medical morbidity, urgency, patient referral pattern, and facility[3], and may not always be reimbursed by insurance companies. The outcome standards outlined in this chapter reflect or exceed the National Kidney Foundation Dialysis Outcomes Quality Initiative (NKF-DOQI) guidelines.

Tables 32-2 and 32-3 show commonly used CPT codes for procedures and surgical management, as well as modifiers. Table 32-4 lists the most commonly used ICD-9 codes associated with vascular access surgical cases. They are used to support the degree of complexity and the use of modifiers. Table 32-5 shows the most

Table 32-2. Common CPT Codes in vascular access surgery.

Category	Procedure	CPT code	Comment
Primary AVF	Create	36821	
	Declot, no revision	36831	Balloon
	Declot, with revision	36833	Balloon
	Revise only	36832	No thrombectomy
	Interposition	36834	For aneurysm-separate procedure
	Ligate/Band	37607	
	Angioplasty	35460	Modifier
PTFE	Create	36830: If 2 separate dialysis grafts are addressed, use modifier 59.	
	Declot no revise	36831: If 2 separate dialysis grafts are addressed, use modifier 59.	Balloon
	Declot with revision	36833: If 2 separate dialysis grafts are addressed, use modifier 59.	Balloon
	Revise only	36832	No thrombectomy
	Interposition	36834	For aneurysm-separate procedure
	Ligate/Band	37607	
	Angioplasty	36005 diagnosis, 37201 lytic	
	Remove (infection)	35903	
Tenckhoff	Insert	49420 temperature, with 99025 if NP 49421* permanent	
	Manipulate	49400 inject contrast/air	
	Remove	49422 permanent E/M temp	
Catheters	Cuff, independent lumens	36533 first, 36533 second	Modifier 51 exempt
	Cuff, independent lumens, manipulate	36534	Requires fluoro
	Cuff, independent lumens, out	36535	
	Permcath, in	36491 cut down, 36489 percutaneous	
	Permcath manipulate	36493	Requires fluoro
	Permcath, out	E/M	
	Percutaneous, in	36489	
	Percutaneous, out	E/M	
	Declot Catheter	36550	
Angiography	Thrombolysis	37201	
Transcatheter	Retrieval FB (percutaneous)	37203	Not covered by Medicare-Not approved for AV shunt
	Stent placement (percutaneous)	37205 for 1 vessel 37206 for additional	Not covered by Medicare-Not approved for AV shunt
	Stent place, open	37207 for 1 vessel 37208 for additional	
Vascular injection	AV shunt	36145	Includes catheter placement or needle
Vascular lab studies	AV acx study	93990-26	Inflow, body-hard copy
	Veins (compression)	93971-26 unilateral 93970 bilateral	

Table 32-3. Common modifiers used in vascular access surgery.

Physician billing modifiers	
Modifier	**Description**
22	Unusual procedural service (time is not a factor)
24	Unrelated E and M service by same physician during post op period (ICD-9 code is different)
25	Significant, separate E and M by same MD same day as procedure or other service (ICD-9 code does not have to be different, but documentation must support a separate visit)
26	Professional component (separate from technical component) utilized with radiology codes when that service is performed by the surgeon following guideline of separate report of the service performed
50	Bilateral procedure at same operative session when CPT code does not have bilateral description.-LT(left) and/or -RT (right) may be more appropriate pending supporting documentation
52	Reduced services-elimination or reduction of service at MD discretion.
53	D/C procedure after starting. (documentation must state why procedure was canceled)
54	Surgical care only 1 MD does procedure, another provides pre- and postoperational management
55	Post-operation management only 1 MD does procedure, another pre- and postoperational management
56	Pre-op management only 1 MD does procedure, another pre- and postoperational management
57	Decision for surgery- E and M service resulting in decision to perform surgery (may be utilized in association with the global package concept)
58	Staged/related procedure same physician in postoperational period-prospective, extensive (may be utilized when the procedure requires stages to be performed before completion)
59	Distinct procedure service (eg, refers to different sites or operative sessions, according to NCCI guidelines)
62	Two surgeons-primary surgeons performing distinct parts of total procedure-2 operative reports are required that demonstrate what each surgeon did
76	Repeat procedure by same physician-same procedure twice or more by same MD
77	Repeat procedure by another physician-same procedure twice or more by different MDs
78	Return to operating room for related procedure during post-operation period (ICD-9 code must reflect complication)
79	Return to operating room for unrelated procedure during post-operation period-if same day as original, use 76
80	Assistant surgeon
82	Assistant surgeon when no qualified resident is available
Ambulatory surgery (ASC) facility only modifiers-not for inpatient or physician use	
These modifiers are to be used by the facility when billing for services performed in a free standing ambulatory surgery center. They are not to be used by the surgeon.	
Modifier	**Description**
50	Bilateral procedure at same operative session
52	Reduced services-elimination or reduction of service at MD discretion
59	Distinct procedural service-independent from other service same day
73	D/C procedure prior to administration of anesthesia NOT elective cancellation
74	D/C procedure after administration of anesthesia, and/or after starting procedure
76	Repeat procedure by the same physician the same procedure twice or more by the same MD
77	Repeat procedure by another physician same procedure twice or more by different MDs

Table 32-4. Common ICD-9 codes in vascular access surgery.

ICD-9 code	Explanation
042	HIV-also list manifestations, ie, 585
585	Chronic renal failure-including nausea, edema, and anuria
276.6	Fluid overload
276.7	Hyperkalemia
250.01	Diabetes, I, controlled
250.03	Diabetes, I, uncontrolled
250.00	Diabetes, II, controlled
250.02	Diabetes, II, uncontrolled
403.01	Hypertension with ESRD, malignant-use 585
403.11	Hypertension with ESRD, benign-use 585
403.91	Hypertension with ESRD, unspecified-use 585
278.00	Obesity, unspecified
278.01	Obesity, morbid
278.1	Obesity with fat pad (localized)
451.89	Central venous thrombosis, including IJ, EJ, SCV
451.82	Venous thrombosis, UE superficial, including antecubital, cephalic, basilic
451.83	Venous thrombosis, UE deep, including brachial, radial, ulnar
459.2	Edema D/T venous compression
787.01	Nausea with vomiting
787.02	Nausea only
787.03	Vomiting only
996	Complications associated with certain special procedures (ie, internal anastomoses, patch grafts)
996.1	Mechanical complications of vascular devices, implant, graft-not embolus or athero sclerosis
996.62	Infection and inflammatory reaction secondary to internal catheter, graft, shunt
996.73	Other complications (NOS) renal dialysis devices, imp-embol, fibrosis, hemorrhage, pain, stenosis, thrombosis

commonly used V and E codes. Table 32-6 depicts a decision-driven algorithm for common vascular access procedures.

The authors realize that coding may vary because of differences in opinions, practice styles between individual surgeons, and geographical locations. This article serves as a guide or example of 1 approach. Also, because of the changing practices with outpatient access centers where radiology and surgery procedures are performed in 1 setting, proper CPT coding related to vascular access becomes even more crucial, not just for reimbursement, but also for statistical and patient management purposes.

Scenario No. 1. Elective outpatient. This case represents patients with known renal disease and a serum creatinine level of 4 to 5 mg/dL (glomerular filtration rate [GFR] 20 to 25 mL/min) in a diabetic, or less than 7 mg/dL (GFR 15 to 20 mL/min) in a renal failure patient with no other morbidity. The access is placed

Table 32-5. V and E codes for vascular access.

These ICD-9 codes are for secondary diagnoses only. Many V codes describe the patient's status but not necessarily the medical necessity of the procedure. E codes refer to external causes and are never primary or principal codes when coding or billing for services rendered. Medical necessity must be proven and documented and most often will be classified to categories of "malfunction of an internal device" or "complications of ESRD."

ICD-9 code	Explanation
V09	Infection with drug resistant microorganisms: Use fourth and fifth digits to identify resistance
V12.51	Patient with history of venous thrombosis, may impact current care
V42.0	Renal transplant status
V42.83	Pancreatic transplant status
V44.6	Artificial opening status, nephrostomy, ureterostomy, or urethrostomy
V45.1	Renal Dialysis status-presence of dialysis shunt
V45.73	Acquired absence of kidney
V49.6	Upper limb amputation status-use fourth digit to identify level
V49.61	Thumb
V49.62	Other finger(s)
V49.63	Hand
V49.64	Wrist
V49.65	Below elbow
V49.66	Above elbow
V49.67	Shoulder
V49.7	Lower limb amputation status-use fourth digit to identify level
V49.71	Great toe
V49.72	Other toe(s)
V49.73	Foot
V49.74	Ankle
V49.75	BKA
V49.76	AKA
V49.77	Hip
V56.1	Fitting and adjustment of dialysis extracorporeal catheter, including removal, replacement, or cleaning
V56.2	Fitting and adjustment of peritoneal dialysis catheter, including removal, replacement, or cleaning
V58.3	Attention to surgical dressings and sutures, including change and removal
V58.61	Long-term use of anticoagulants, still in use
V67.0	Follow-up examination: surveillance of patient after surgery is completed
E870.2	Accidental cut, perfusion, and/or hemorrhage during dialysis or perfusion
E871.2	FB left in during dialysis or perfusion
E872.2	Failure of sterile precautions during dialysis or perfusion
E874.2	Mechanical failure of instrument or apparatus during dialysis or perfusion
E878.2	Operation with anastomosis, bypass or graft, natural or artificial, cause abnormal reaction or late complication, without problems at the time of procedure
E879.1	Kidney dialysis as cause of abnormal reaction or late complication, without problems at the time of procedure

Table 32-6. Suggested algorithm for various vascular access settings.

Office visit
99203-99205 new patient
99213 - 99215 established patient
Code level depends on history, physical exam

Surgical consult for access –inpatient
99252 - 99255
Code level depends on history, physical exam and medical decision making

Duplex doppler exam
93990 - Access
93971 - Venous unilateral
93970 - Venous bilateral

#6
#7
#4

Admit to hospital (preoperation) for comorbidity not suitable hospital stay
If observation or 23 hour - no bill, part of global package if surgery is performed
If inpatient –99222 first day, 99232 each additional day– requires modifiers

#1
#2
#5

Access surgical procedures: creation/insertion
36821 - Primary AV fistula (seperate procedure)
36830 - PTFE
49421 - peritoneal catheter
Dual lumen catheters: 36491 - cut down; 36533 - cuffed; 36489 femoral (percusion) line (with 99025 if first visit)

Access surgical procedures: declot/ revise
36831 - Declotting (balloon)
36833 - Declotting with revision
36834 - Resection of aneurysm

#3

Admit postoperation for complication or insufficient recovery
If observation or 23 hour-no surgery bill, part of global package
If medical complication, admission

#4

Discharge - if no surgical procedure performed
99217 - if observation or 23 hour
99238 (< 30 min); 99239 (>30 min) if inpatient with no time specified

#2 #3 #6
#4 #5 538 #7
#5 #1

Postoperative visits/no charge visits

before anticipated need for dialysis to allow for healing and maturing. The office visit includes pertinent history and physical examination elements. Often, patients have little knowledge or understanding of options and benefits, which results in extended time for discussions. In a young patient not previously hospitalized or exposed to IV infusions, a primary AV fistula is a more likely possibility in this scenario.

Scenario No. 1. Elective outpatient

Procedure	Suggested CPT/ICD-9 code
Office visit	99203-99205†
Operative procedure:	
Primary AV fistula	36821-separate procedure. Per CCI bundled into 35860, 36825, and 36834
PTFE	36830
Peritoneal catheter	49421*‡
Moncrief peritoneal catheter	49421*-58 insertion‡ 49999 externalization (with operation note)
Postoperative visits	99024§
Examples of ICD-9 coding: For a more complete list of ICD-9 codes, see table 32-4	Chronic renal failure secondary to diabetes or hypertension: 585

† Code level depends on the nature of the presenting problem and how the history, physical exam, and medical decision making are documented. The decision on an evaluation and management (E and M) level is not time dependent-it is based on the number and complexity of systems reviewed. Consult the E and M guidelines in the CPT manual for detailed description.

‡ Third-party payers may also have specific guidelines concerning starred procedures. Medicare does not recognize the starred procedure concept. Thus, starred procedures may be bundled into the more comprehensive procedure through the insurance company's surgical package.

§ Statistical code only for postoperative visits related to the procedure with no charge attached. Subsequent visits related to the procedure have already been reimbursed through the global package concept and are tracked through the statistical code of 99024 only. All access categories will have postoperative visits coded 99024.

Scenario No. 2. Elective inpatient. This patient is similar to scenario No. 1. This patient, however, has a higher medical risk, because of morbidity that requires a hospital stay. Examples include advanced age, heart disease, social or mental factors, amputations or other physical disability.

Scenario No. 2. Elective inpatient

Procedure	Suggested CPT/ICD-9 code
Office visit	99203-99205†
Admit to hospital	Observation or 23 hours: 99218-99220†
(Days or weeks later)	If inpatient without time specified 99221-99223† first visit 99221-99233 each add day† Once surgery is done, visits are bundled into a global package
Operative procedure:	
Primary AV fistula	36821
PTFE	36830
Peritoneal catheter	49421*‡
Moncrief peritoneal catheter	49421*-58 insertion‡ 49999 externalization (with operation note)

Scenario No. 2. Elective inpatient. *(continued)*

Procedure	Suggested CPT/ICD-9 code
Discharge, if no surgery is performed.	If observation: 99217 (48 hour observation
Once surgery is done, discharge is bundled into a global package	status only). If inpatient without time specified: 99238 (<30 minutes), 99239 (>30 minutes)
Postoperative visits	99024‡
Examples of ICD-9 Coding: For a more complete list of	Chronic renal failure secondary to diabetes or hypertension: 585
ICD-9 codes, see table 32-4	Morbidities requiring hospital admission for usual outpatient procedure§ BKA V49.75; AKA V49.76

† Code level depends on the nature of the presenting problem and how the history, physical exam and medical decision making are documented. The decision on E and M level is not time dependent-it is based on the number and complexity of systems reviewed. Consult the E and M guidelines in the CPT manual for detailed description.

‡ Third-party payers may also have specific guidelines concerning starred procedures. Medicare does not recognize the starred procedure concept. Thus, starred procedures may be bundled into the more comprehensive procedure through the insurance company's surgical package.

§ Diagnoses represent secondary ICD-9 codes, and are for billing purposes only in developing the severity of illness profiles and databases. These are important in identifying those patients who may run a higher risk due to these secondary conditions.

Scenario No. 3. Outpatient becoming inpatient after surgery. This scenario is very similar to scenario No. 2. The procedure is planned as an outpatient procedure. For unforeseen reasons, such as insufficient recovery after surgery, vomiting, medical problems, chest pain, or EKG changes, the patient often requires hospital admission for 24 hours.

Scenario No. 3. Outpatient becoming inpatient after surgery.

Procedure	Suggested CPT/ICD-9 code
Office visit	99203-99205†
Operative procedure:	
Primary AV fistula	36821
PTFE	36830
Peritoneal catheter	49421*‡
Moncrief peritoneal catheter	49421*-58 insertion‡ 49999 externalization (with operation note)
Dual-lumen catheter	36489* percutaneous‡ 36491* cut down‡ 36533*, 36533* independent lumen‡
Admit same day after surgery	Involves the bundling of the patient into the surgical global package and may not be billed separately. Admission usually occurs because of a complication that may be related to the surgery. If admission is medical, ie, patient requires dialysis for hyperkalemia, medicine service will admit and consult.

Scenario No. 3. Outpatient becoming inpatient after surgery. *(continued)*

Procedure	Suggested CPT/ICD-9 code
Discharge, if no surgery is performed.	If observation occurs, 99217
Once surgery is done, discharge is bundled into global package.	If inpatient without time specified 99238 (< 30 minutes), 99239 (>30 minutes)
Postoperative visits	99024§
Examples of ICD-9 Coding:	Chronic renal failure secondary to diabetes
For a more complete list of	or hypertension: 585
ICD-9 codes, see table 32-4	Second category for reason for admit: EKG change (postoperational arrhythmia): 997.1 Nausea and vomiting: 787.01 Insufficient anesthesia recovery: 995.2

† Code level depends on the nature of the presenting problem and how the history, physical exam and medical decision making are documented. The decision on E and M level is not time dependent-it is based on the number and complexity of systems reviewed. Consult the E and M guidelines in the CPT manual for detailed description.

‡ Third-party payers may also have specific guidelines concerning starred procedures. Medicare does not recognize the starred procedure concept. Thus, starred procedures may be bundled into the more comprehensive procedure through the insurance company's surgical package.

§ Statistical postoperative code only with a no charge value attached. Subsequent visits related to the procedure have already been reimbursed through the global package concept and are tracked with the statistical code of 99024 only.

Scenario No. 4. Inpatient staged procedures. Scenario No. 4 represents an inpatient on medical service for such conditions as ESRD, congestive heart failure, fluid overload, type 2 diabetes, hyperkalemia, ketoacidosis, shortness of breath, or HIV. The patient is usually known to have ESRD with rapidly worsening uremic symptoms. Variations of case scenario No. 4 represent perhaps the most common of all scenarios. The staged procedures (type and timing) depend on the patient's condition and the clinician's medical judgment, facility sophistication, patient comorbidity, and social factors. It is the author's experience that stabilizing a patient with a dual lumen catheter for 2 to 4 weeks as an outpatient can improve the outcome of a permanent access. For example, a forearm that is bruised from intravenous (IV) accesses and blood draws can improve over time, increasing the likelihood of a primary AV fistula or successful PTFE placement.

Scenario No. 4. Inpatient staged procedures.

Procedure	Suggested CPT/ICD-9 code
Surgical consult for access	99251-99255† If initial consult leads to decision for surgery the same day, use modifier-57 with consult code
Operative option No. 1: Patient too sick for operation	
1a. Placement of femoral line (emergent dialysis), or	36489*‡
1b. Percutaneous dual lumen central line (not recommended) Patient to option No. 2 or 3 when stable	36489*‡

Scenario No. 4. Inpatient staged procedures. *(continued)*

Procedure	Suggested CPT/ICD-9 code
Operative option No. 2: patient stable for operation	
2a. Dual lumen cuffed catheter (R internal jugular preferable) Patient to option 4 when stable	36491* cut down, 36533, 36533* independent‡ lumens
Operative option No. 3: patient stable for operation	36491* cut down, 36533, 36533* independent lumens‡
3a. Placement of Dual lumen cuffed	
catheter, and Primary AV fistula,	36821
or PTFE,	36830
or PD catheter,	49421*‡
or Moncrief peritoneal catheter	49421*-58 insertion‡
	49999 externalization (with operation note)
Operative option No. 4 **4a.** Elective placement of primary AV fistula or PTFE or PD or Moncrief peritoneal catheter	Repeat scenario No. 1, or No. 2, or No.3
Examples of ICD-9 Coding: For a more complete list of ICD-9 codes, see table 32-4. The medical service, the admitting service, codes for diagnosis. The surgeon should also do this, especially for the catheter placement for emergent dialysis, and to substantiate staged surgical procedures, patient transfer to the surgical service, or multiple operative procedures during the admission.	Chronic renal failure secondary to diabetes or hypertension: 585 Shortness of breath: 786.09 Fluid overload: 276.6 Uremia: 586 Bacteremia (unspecified): 790.7 Sepsis (generalized): 038.9

† Code level depends on the nature of the presenting problem and how the history, physical exam, and medical decision making are documented. The decision on E and M level is not time dependent-it is based on the number and complexity of systems reviewed. Consult the E and M guidelines in the CPT manual for a detailed description.

‡ Third-party payers may also have specific guidelines concerning starred procedures. Medicare does not recognize the starred procedure concept. Thus, starred procedures may be bundled into the more comprehensive procedure through the insurance company's surgical package.

Scenario No. 5. Infected dual lumen catheter. This is a fairly common scenario with some clinical urgency involved. The decision algorithm will vary depending on a patient's status. Prompt removal of an infected catheter and an I and D of an infected PTFE graft are often warranted. Temporary femoral line for 24 to 48 hours will bridge the patient to a cuffed dual lumen catheter 48 to 72 hours later under antibiotic coverage, when the patient is afebrile, and clinically improved with lower white cell count. If possible, primary AV fistulae should be placed at this time, but placement of PTFE grafts or PD catheters should wait 7 to 10 days. The patient may then be discharged and reverted to scenario No. 1, 2, 3, or 4 (operative option 4).

Scenario No. 5. Infected dual lumen catheter.

Procedure	Suggested CPT/ICD-9 code
5a. Admit for fever or rule out sepsis	If admitted to surgery, 99221-99223 first visit 99231- 99233 each additional day until surgical procedure is performed†
5b. Surgical consult for sepsis	If admitted to medical service, 99253-99255† If initial consult leads to decision for surgery the same day, use modifier-57 with consult code
5c. Removal of dual lumen catheter	36535 when surgical procedure is required for removal. Operation report must be submitted with code
5d. Femoral line placement	36489*‡
5e. New access placement	Dual lumen catheter 36489* percutaneous, 36491* cut down,‡ 36533, 36533* independent lumens‡ possible primary AVF 36821
5f. Discharge only if surgery not performed. Otherwise, bundled into global package	99238 or 99239
5g. Revert to scenario No. 1, 2, 3, or 4 (operative option 4) while on antibiotics for permanent access placement.	Now repeating scenario No. 1, 2 , 3, or 4 (option 4)
Examples of ICD-9 coding: For a more complete list of ICD-9 codes, see table 32-4	Chronic renal failure secondary to diabetes or hypertension: 585 Fever: 780.6
The medical and admitting service codes for diagnosis. The surgeon should also substantiate staged surgical procedures or patient transfers to the surgical service	Catheter sepsis: 996.62 Generalized sepsis: 038.9 Renal dialysis status: V45.1

† Code level depends on the nature of the presenting problem and how the history, physical exam and medical decision making are documented. The decision on an E and M level is not time dependent-it is based on the number and complexity of systems reviewed. Consult the E and M guidelines in the CPT manual for a more detailed description.

‡ Third-party payers may also have specific guidelines concerning starred procedures. Medicare does not recognize the starred procedure concept. Thus, starred procedures may be bundled into the more comprehensive procedure through the insurance company's surgical package.

Scenario No. 6. Clotted AV access. Scenario No. 6 represents perhaps 50% of all access procedures and is characterized by the unpredictable causes, as well as outcomes, of access failure. Many patients are treated with both radiology and surgery. Ideally, surgeons and radiologists work cooperatively and interdependently, performing the procedures that benefit the patient the most. Vascular surgicenters unite these 2 specialist groups together. At these centers, which are being established nationwide, patients may be referred to either surgery or radiology if either department fails an attempted intervention or if problems arise during a procedure.

Scenario No. 6. Clotted AV access.

Procedure	Suggested CPT/ICD-9 code
Office visit (referred from dialysis, nephrology, radiology, or self-referred)	Established point 99212-99215† New point 99202-99205†
Duplex Doppler exam	93990 (access), 93971 (venous unilateral), 93970 (venous, bilateral) are codeable separately if performed in the office setting with appropriate modifiers meeting insurance requirements.
6b. Operative procedure, same day or next outpatient	
6b1. Declotting only (balloon), or	36831-separate procedure
6b2. Declotting plus revision	36833
6b3. Failed declotting plus dual lumen catheter Discharge to home, revert to scenario No. 4, Operative option No. 4.	36831/36833; 36489* percutaneous, 36491* cut down, 36533, 36533* independent lumens‡
6b4. Failed declotting plus dual lumen catheter plus new PTFE or other permanent access	36831/36833; 36489* percutaneous, 36491* cut down, 36533, 36533* independent lumens‡ 36830 (PTFE)
6c. Refer to radiology. Radiology: declot (mechanical), Declot (chemical, ie, TPA), angioplasty	36821 (Primary) Office visit, Doppler codes only
6c1. Successful: discharge to home	Radiology D/C
6c2. Failed-dual lumen catheter placed-radiology	Radiology codes
6c3. Failed-dual lumen catheter placed-surgery	Surgery codes: 36489* percutaneous, 36491* cut down, 36533, 36533* independent lumens‡
6c4. Failed, revert to scenario No. 4, option No. 4	
Examples of ICD-9 coding: For a more complete list of ICD-9 codes, see table 32-4	Chronic renal failure: 585 Renal dialysis status: V45.1 Complications of renal dialysis device: 996.73 Accidental cut during dialysis: E870.2 Operation with anastomosis as cause of abnormal reaction or later complication, without mention of problem at time of procedure: E878.2 (ie, intimal hyperplasia) Kidney dialysis as a cause of abnormal reaction or later complication, without mention of problem at the time of procedure: E879.1, ie, dialysis induced metabolic hyperkalemia, hypovolemia

† Code level depends on the nature of the presenting problem and how the history, physical exam, and medical decision making are documented. The decision on E and M level is not time dependent-it is based on the number and complexity of systems reviewed. Consult the E and M guidelines in the CPT manual for detailed description.

‡ Third-party payers may also have specific guidelines concerning starred procedures. Medicare does not recognize the starred procedure concept. Thus, starred procedures may be bundled into the more comprehensive procedure through the insurance company's surgical package.

Scenario No. 7. Miscellaneous vascular access problems.

Procedure	Suggested CPT/ICD-9 code
Office visit	Established point 99212-99215† New point 99202-99205†
Duplex Doppler exam	93990 (access), 93971 (venous unilateral), 93970 (venous, bilateral) are codeable separately if performed in the office setting with appropriate modifiers per insurance requirements.
Fistulogram	36145 (on table)
7b. Outpatient OR procedure Revision of vascular access	36832 separate procedure
Primary AV fistulae	
Stenosis	
7b1. Reanastomosis	36832 (revision)
7b2. Patch angioplasty	36832 (revision)
7b3. Interposition graft	36832 (revision); 36834 (aneurysm)
7b4. Resection of aneurysm	36834 separate procedure if performed alone,
fistula-arterial steal	otherwise bundled
7b5. Ligation/banding	37607
7c. PTFE graft problems	
Infection	
7c1. I and D	10140 separate procedure, use modifiers 78 or 79 to identify cause
7c2. Bypass graft	36832 (revision)
7c3. Removal	35903
Pseudoaneurysm	
7c4. Resection	36832
7c5. Ligation	37607
Examples of ICD-9 coding: For a more complete list of ICD-9 codes, see table 32-4	Examples of ICD-9 coding: Chronic renal failure: 585 Renal dialysis status: V45.1 Code problem as exists: 996 Complications peculiar to specified procedures (ie, internal anastomoses, patch grafts) 996.1 Mechanical complications of vascular devices, implant, graft-not embolus or atherosclerosis 996.62 Infection and inflammatory reaction secondary to internal catheter, graft, shunt

Scenario No. 7. Miscellaneous vascular access problems. *(continued)*

Procedure	Suggested CPT/ICD-9 code
	996.73 Other complications (NOS) of renal dialysis device, implanting embolus, fibrosis, hemorrhage, pain, stenosis, thrombosis
	E870.2 Accidental cut, or hemorrhage during dialysis or perfusion
	E871.2 Foreign body left in during dialysis or perfusion
	E872.2 Failure of sterile precautions during dialysis or perfusion
	E874.2 Mechanical failure of instrument or apparatus during dialysis/perfusion
	E878.2 Operation with anastomosis, bypass or graft, natural/artificial, as cause of abnormal reaction or later complication, without mention of problem at procedure, ie intimal hyperplasia
	E879.1 Kidney dialysis as cause of abnormal reaction or later complication, without mention of problem at time of procedure, ie stenosis from needle punctures

† Code level depends on the nature of the presenting problem and how the history, physical exam, and medical decision making are documented. The decision on E and M level is not time dependent-it is based on the number and complexity of systems reviewed. Consult the E and M guidelines in the CPT manual for detailed description.

Scenario No. 8. Failed thrombectomy with return to operating room. Failed declotting (rethrombosis) for no obvious technical reason is commonplace. National statistics indicate that 50% of grafts fail within 3 to 6 months after declotting, with rates similar for both radiology and surgery departments. Repeat procedures with appropriate coding are billable and must be reimbursed. No bill should be issued only if no attempt was made to correct a technical problem, as indicated below.

Scenario No. 8. Failed thrombectomy with return to operating room.

Procedure	Suggested CPT/ICD-9 code
Office visit	99212-99215†
Duplex Doppler exam	93990 (access), 93971 (venous unilateral), 93970 (venous, bilateral) are coded separately if performed in the office setting with appropriate modifiers meeting insurance requirements.
Operative procedure: same or next day outpatient	
8b1. Declotting (Balloon)	36831
Fistulogram	36145 (on table)
8b2. Declotting plus revision	36833
Fistulogram	36145 (on table)

(continued)

Scenario No. 8. Failed thrombectomy with return to operating room. *(continued)*

Procedure	Suggested CPT/ICD-9 code
8b3. Failed declotting without revision and return to the operating room on the same day	
a) If fistulogram done in first procedure with out evidence of lesion and second exploration=hyperplasia or vascular anomaly	36833 separate procedure
b) If fistulogram done in first procedure without evidence of lesion and second exploration=no hyperplasia or vascular anomaly	36833
c) If fistulogram done in procedure has evidence of lesion and no revision attempted	no bill
d) If second exploration reveals technical problem	no bill
8b4. Failed declotting with revision and return to OR same day	
a) If second exploration reveals hyperplasia or vascular anomaly	
b) If second exploration reveals no hyperplasia or vascular anomaly	36833
c) If second exploration reveals technical problem	36833 no bill
8b5. Failed declotting plus dual lumen catheter. Discharge home, revert to scenario No. 4, option No.4	Bill declot as appropriate from above, add 36489* percutaneous, 36491* cut down, 36533, 36533*‡ independent lumens.
8b6. Failed declotting plus dual lumen catheter plus new PTFE or other permanent access.	Add 36830 (PTFE); 36821 (Primary AVF) to 8b5
Examples of ICD-9 coding: For a more complete list of ICD-9 codes, see table 32-4. Documentation of the differences in the outcome of the first procedure in this scenario may determine level of reimbursement for the second procedure, if any. All of these outcomes assume that a fistulogram was performed as part of the thrombectomy, and that appropriate action was taken based on these results, ie,	Chronic renal failure: 585 Renal dialysis status: V45.1 Code problem as exists: 996 Complications peculiar to specified procedures (ie, internal anastomoses, patch grafts) 996.1 Mechanical complications of vascular devices, implant, graft-not embolus or athero sclerosis 996.73 Other complications (NOS) of renal dialy sis device or implant, including embolus, fibrosis hemorrhage, pain, stenosis, thrombosis

Scenario No. 8. Failed thrombectomy with return to operating room. *(continued)*

Procedure	Suggested CPT/ICD-9 code
revision of the access. Failure of a thrombectomy and/or revision in the immediate postoperative period can be the result of many factors. The "no bill" designation is used here to reflect possible factors that could reasonably have been addressed during the initial procedure, ie failure to correct a stenosis as demonstrated by fistulogram.	E870.2 Accidental cut, or hemorrhage during dialysis or perfusion E878.2 Operation with anastomosis, bypass or graft, natural/artificial, as cause of abnormal reaction or later complication, without mention of problem at procedure E879.1 Kidney dialysis as cause of abnormal reaction or later complication, without mention of problem at time of procedure
	458.2 Postoperative hypotension (iatrogenic)

† Code level depends on the nature of the presenting problem and how the history, physical exam, and medical decision making are documented. The decision on E and M level is not time dependent-it is based on the number and complexity of systems reviewed. Consult the E and M guidelines in the CPT manual for detailed description.

‡ Third-party payers may also have specific guidelines concerning starred procedures. Medicare does not recognize the starred procedure concept. Thus, starred procedures may be bundled into the more comprehensive procedure through the insurance company's surgical package.

References

1. The International Classification of Diseases, 9th Revision, Clinical Modification 2000. Salt Lake City, UT: Medicode Publications; 1999.
2. Physicians Current Procedural Terminology 2000. Chicago: American Medical Association; 1999.
3. H.R. 2650. Sponsor: Rep. Stark FP (introduced 07/29/99). The Medicare Physician Self-Referral Improvement Act (HR 2650 IH).

DISCUSSION

Moderator:
Mitchell L. Henry, M.D.
Panelists:
Kerri A. Welch, R.N., C.N.N.
Miltos K. Lazarides, M.D.
Ingemar J.A. Davidson, M.D., Ph.D., F.A.C.S.

Discussant: I have a question regarding the vascular access team. I think that getting the medical director team, the surgeons, and the nurses together should not be as difficult, just given the level of frustration that we all have with access but the thing might be the database. I was wondering if you could tell us a little bit more about the database, whether it is commercially available, whether it is in development now, whether if it works on the internet, how it integrates with say Microsoft programs, and just anything you can tell us about it in about a couple of minutes?

Ms. Welch: It is available and in your syllabus there is a web site and you can download some of the reports from that. It is built on a Microsoft access platform, and it is wonderful.

Discussant: Question for Dr. Davidson. We have had a series of denials from Medicare recently denying payment for vascular surgery consultation for an inpatient encounter, if what was done was placement of the cuffed catheter. In other words, like a Tesio catheter. If we do that, they deny the consultations saying that the degree of the procedure was minor and a consultation is not in order. We have appealed it by saying, I am asked to see this patient in consultation to make a decision about the plan for dialysis access, not just for acute access, but also for the future access for permanent access. It is all documented and laid out. The decision-making is all documented, but they deny that. Have you encountered that or do you have any comment about that?

Dr. Davidson: Yes, I have encountered stuff like that and you did the right thing. Complain and fight it. I think we all need to fight this and I think we need to evaluate these patients initially and do it right and as long as you document, you are right. If you saw the patient, you did the work, you didn't write much or anything then you do not have a case. But if you document and follow these kind of steps that Medicare has outlined. You can print these 97 and 95 guidelines and you can make your own forms and templates and just follow them. Then the audits will love you and I think you will win that kind of case. Just do not give up. I think if you are persistent they will profile you and respect you and they try not to get back to you if you are persistent. That is my impression.

Discussant: I have a question for Dr. Lazarides or any surgeon in the room. You went over the issue in elderly patients in terms of their life expectancy rate and then looking at what type of access should you put in first, either distal or proximal, and the issue of having something that will require minimal intervention over the long run. My question is, is there ever a role or any information or data out there that shows that a thigh graft would be the access of choice in older folks who have very small BMIs or who do not have a long life expectancy in terms of reducing their overall expected or future interventions for their access maintenance?

Dr. Lazarides: As the primary access, I would say no. I am not suggesting that. I told you that I used 3 thigh grafts for the access in cases where the upper limbs were exhausted. However, as far as I know, thigh grafts have significant morbidity and my personal impression is to avoid such kind of grafts in initial procedures.

Discussant: This is for Dr. Davidson. I bet other people have encountered an access graft that has been worked on many times, and it is thrombosed. You declot the graft, and you revise the graft, and then the graft does not run well, or thromboses on the table. You shoot a venogram on the table and you have a graft that you feel is unsalvageable you abandon the graft and maybe put in catheters or do a new access. Now you have done several procedures here. You have done a declot, revision, and it doesn't work. You have done a venogram and make your decision based on that. In my experience based on that they will not pay for the declot revision that did not work. They will not pay for the venogram. You spend several hours and you are paid for a catheter.

Dr. Davidson: Number 1, I think you did the right thing. You helped the patient. You spent a lot of time. The modifier you should list the most expensive first, and then you get paid 50% for the second one and maybe 50% for a few more and I think if you documented that you should get paid, fight it.

Discussant: It may be different in Texas but...

Dr. Davidson: I heard that yesterday and some things are just not being paid for. Still, in my case, I will still do what is right for the patient, and I think we need to be guided by that, and I think that is at least my ethical view on all this. We cannot be run by and make decisions to operate or do medical interventions based on codes. We need to be doctors and decide what needs to be done. Sometimes we get hurt because there are no codes, or we are not being paid. I would still do what is right, because in the long run you get rewarded in some fashion.

Discussant: Another question for Dr. Lazarides. It is very surprising in your population that you place more than 50% of grafts. It sounds like all the conventional American surgical papers and no Americans surgeons claim that today in this meeting. You are the only 1. There is only 1 conclusion, that you need to work better with the radiologist for preoperative mapping and second for revision of your failing on thrombosing fistulas.

Dr. Lazarides: Thank you. I would like to mention that my percentage of synthetic grafts is within the DOQI limits. In this difficult subgroup of patients, I have 50% autologous accesses. However, I have to admit that you are not an average radiologist. The results of your colleagues are far worse. I don't know if the patients in Greece must be happier, but I am not referring these patients to the local radiologist.

Dr. Henry: Ms. Welch, there are a couple of questions here for you. One is, who pays for the extra personnel, which I assume is you, as well as somebody that would manipulate the database and spit the numbers out for your CQI issues?

Ms. Welch: I am employed by the nephrology group.

Dr. Henry: The other question here, and it really is not a question, it is really a statement. It says no one ever seems to address the care that occurs in some dialysis units with sterility, failure to rotate sites, appropriate compression of grafts, failure to identify problems early on, etc. Having obviously a great deal of experience in that area, do you want to comment on that? I would say those are things we take for granted. We have spoken a lot about this at these meetings over the last years. All those issues are very important in nursing roles, and technician roles that can play a part in success or failure that as well.

Ms. Welch: I totally agree. We see that there is a definite need for education in our units. We especially push for fistulas and that is what we want. Most of the people, the techs, are used to cannulating grafts, so that is part of my job, also, to educate the staff and it is definitely in the forefront of our minds.

Discussant: I just have a little comment in terms of the number of dialysis grafts that have been placed in the United States. At least half of the patients that I see as a referral have already been on hemodialysis for more than 6 years. Most of them have had their fistulas and most of them have failed and now I am putting in prosthetic grafts. It is not that I do not want to put in grafts. It is just that these patients are getting older and the age adjusted mortality rate is dropping so they are living longer. We are having to provide more angio access after their fistulas have failed. So I think this is 1 of the reasons why we are seeing more grafts being placed today.

Discussant: Ms. Welch, I enjoyed your talk a great deal. The question I had for you is what would you consider to be the minimum dialysis population for which a vascular access coordinator would be cost effective?

Ms. Welch: As a full-time person like myself, I would say around 300 patients.

Dr. Henry: That is a good question. That is a good estimate. I do not know what the answer is. If you really did a careful cost analysis I think those positions pay for themselves very readily in the long run. Unfortunately, it is not the physician practices that necessarily see those cost savings. It may be the carriers, it may be the hospitals, and it may be other people that are involved and not the people who are actually paying the salaries of those individuals.

Ms. Welch: I think that is part of the problem where it is hard to get an access coordinator hired. I definitely do not generate revenue. But like you said in the long run, I think that we have saved a lot of money over the last few years.

Discussant: As one who pays Kerri's salary I can tell you it is not cost effective in the short run. But Mitch, your point is exactly right. We think in the long run, it very much will be cost effective. We will hope to be able to have data to follow that and see that. We have seen missed dialysis treatments in the outpatient units fail, and that is revenue to the dialysis unit. Now as physicians we have an interest in our dialysis units, so we benefit from that, but that is not always the case. Again, we see a shift in patterns of procedures and changes, but as nephrologists, in the short run that does not benefit us in any way. But it is clearly benefiting our patients to organize the care in the way it has happened. As payment systems change and particularly if vascular access is capitated as HCFA was talking, then we think that it is going to be very cost effective.

Dr. Henry: We are based in an academic center. Our offices are physically in the hospital and medical center complex but we have a person who does very similar things as Kerri does. We actually cost share her salary between the surgeons and nephrologists and the hospital. So there is a cost sharing within it and again a lot of the benefits are not necessarily cost savings but the patients really enjoy having a single person that they can talk to that can help things go much more smoothly.

Discussant: I wanted to follow up on that. I think this is the key issue here. What we are talking about it cost shifting and who is going to pay for it up front and the analogy is anticoagulation clinics. We know that, for example, an anticoagulation clinic will reduce the number of thrombotic and bleeding episodes a patient has so the system will save money if you have got these kind of systems built in. But who is going to pay for running the clinic and who is going to pay for the coordination. It costs the nephrology group, I am sure it costs them money to build this ideal system. When the patient clots and then they go to the hospital, you know it does not cost the dialysis clinic anything for that patient to be hospitalized quite frankly, but the cost for managing that remains in the system. It has just been shifted from 1 place to another and maybe that is the advantage of having a capitated system.

Discussant: I am an access coordinator from Akron, Ohio and I am hired by the dialysis units. They examined, prior to me coming on to the position, a year's worth of mistreatments. It has saved well over a couple hundred thousand dollars in mistreatments after I was hired on. So that is one of the ways they justify paying my salary.

Dr. Levine: As far as the access coordinator, I think it gets down to what your goal is. Speaking as an interventional nephrologist and speaking of somebody who has overseen the access monitoring for 400 to 450 hemodialysis patients, there is so much data being generated. With our goal being to prevent thrombosis, I just do not have the time because I am in the interventional suite doing the procedures and so there is no question we needed to have an access coordinator. In the end you have to think if what you are trying to do for your patients and if you are trying to do what is best, I think you have no choice if you have a large dialysis population.

Discussant: I would like to congratulate Dr. Lazarides on the outcomes in his older patients. In Sweden, we create 80% AV fistulas. But, we think that grafts have better results in all the patients over 75 years old because radiologists cannot help here. These patients that do not have proper vessels and they have 3, 4, or 5 operations and finally they are getting grafts. Very often we recommend a graft from the beginning in this patient who has no proper vessels.

Discussant: I support the coordinator concept. I was at Parkland before I left academics and vascular access was a mess. We did 350 to 400 per year and it was perceived as a surgical problem. Then, when I showed the data, the department hired a coordinator who was a retired dialysis nurse who kept everyone straight and in order. The cancellation rate of surgical cases for access was higher before she came on and cleaned up everything. The problems are not mainly surgical, they are patient teaching information. The access coordinator saves hundreds and thousands of dollars for Parkland per year.

Index

W-Z